Multicultural Approaches to Health and Wellness in America

Multicultural Approaches to Health and Wellness in America

Volume 1: Key Issues and Medical Systems

Regan A. R. Gurung, Editor

Foreword by Michael Winkelman

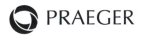 PRAEGER

AN IMPRINT OF ABC-CLIO, LLC

Santa Barbara, California • Denver, Colorado • Oxford, England

Library of Congress Cataloging-in-Publication Data

Multicultural approaches to health and wellness in America / Regan A.R. Gurung, editor ; foreword by Michael Winkelman.
   pages cm
  ISBN 978-1-4408-0349-9 (pbk. : alk. paper) — ISBN 978-1-4408-0350-5 (ebook)
1. Health attitudes—United States—Cross-cultural studies. 2. Health behavior—United States—Cross-cultural studies. 3. Transcultural medical care—United States. I. Gurung, Regan A. R.
  RA776.9.M85 2014
  362.1—dc23   2013031733

ISBN: 978-1-4408-0349-9
EISBN: 978-1-4408-0350-5

18 17 16 15   2 3 4 5

This book is also available on the World Wide Web as an eBook.
Visit www.abc-clio.com for details.

Praeger
An Imprint of ABC-CLIO, LLC

ABC-CLIO, LLC
130 Cremona Drive, P.O. Box 1911
Santa Barbara, California 93116-1911

This book is printed on acid-free paper ∞
Manufactured in the United States of America

To my father, Douglas Narendra Raj Gurung,
for inspiring me to always consider the extraordinary
and think beyond the bounds of the normally accepted.

Contents

Foreword

The world has experienced increasing cultural pluralism in recent years, a diversity of cultures within societies that makes personal, social and institutional relations more complex and challenging. Diversity is produced not only by the many immigrant cultures and their healing traditions, but also by health care preferences shaped by a number of cosmopolitan medical traditions. These include millennia-old traditions such as Ayurvedic medicine, Chinese medicine, and Tibetan medicine as well as more recent practices such as Homeopathy and Naturopathic Medicine. These are further complemented by many formerly local traditions such as shamanism, curanderismo, Islamic medicine, and others, such as herbalism, which have become internationalized.

These diverse health care resources that are part of the client's cultural background, worldview, care preferences, and expectations further complicate professional obligations and personal needs to address the roles of culture in client relationships. Cultural differences can play a significant role in thwarting the effectiveness and quality of client interactions, making appropriate responses to cultural differences a professional responsibility and institutional need.

The reality of cultural pluralism means that helping professionals need to develop intercultural relations skills and adapt culture-specific approaches that are sensitive to client background. These culturally appropriate responses are generally labeled as cultural sensitivity, but just what are these intercultural skills and cultural competencies? Development of appropriate and effective responses to address these differences involves varying degrees of ability to respond to cultural differences at personal, interpersonal, and organizational levels. The commitment to cultural sensitivity requires the rejection of simplistic platitudes of equal treatment and approaches which are "color blind," and the development of sensitivity to the particular situations of each individual derived from the impact of the client's culture and broader social relations (such as discrimination) on their lives.

Developing culturally competent professional services begins with self-assessments of one's personal knowledge, beliefs, and behaviors, as well as intercultural attitudes, skills, and experiences. Competence in intercultural relations begins in cultural self-awareness, skills in intercultural relations, and knowledge about cultural groups served. Cultural self-awareness includes recognition of one's own cultural influences on values, beliefs, and judgments, as well as the influences derived from the professional's work culture. Awareness of the effects of these personal and professional influences on client relations is necessary for developing a culturally sensitive approach. Without a personal cultural self-awareness, biases will be unconsciously imposed on clients and their ability to respond undermined. For this reason and others, personal values assessments are a basic aspect of developing cross-cultural awareness and sensitivity. Such assessments (Winkelman 2005) provide a basis for not only personal awareness, but also greater tolerance and perspectives that facilitate avoidance of conflicts and their resolution.

Cross-cultural perspectives and skills necessary to meet the professional obligations begin with making personal assessments and adjustments and developing a personal commitment to engage in processes of personal transformation. These personal commitments then need to be followed by developing a foundation for culturally sensitive and competent approaches through acquiring a range of cultural understandings and knowledge of many aspects of intercultural dynamics. The ability to effectively deal with the challenges presented by intercultural dynamics involves skills and perspective that can expand our ability to effectively overcome the barriers and conflicts presented by cultural differences.

An important perspective for initiating cross-cultural development begins with the realization that we are not normally and naturally disposed to sensitive responsiveness to cultural differences. Rather, what is natural is an ethnocentric view in which our own personal and cultural assumptions are viewed as normal. Our own developmental environments create our perception of what is normal. This context is not merely a physical, but system that is fundamentally cultural.

It is knowledge of that cultural context that is key to both personal developments of cross-cultural competencies as well as sensitivity to the cultural formation of clients, which is essential to appropriate responses to them. Cultural perspectives are focused on cultural strengths approach that views cultural differences not in terms of pathology and deviance but rather as resources. Such perspectives require an understanding of the client's cultural system and the strengths that are found in its community organizations and practices, particularly those related to its natural support systems. The various health care systems covered here in *Multicultural Approaches to Health and Wellness* exemplifies the core natural support systems of a culture.

Religious and spiritual healing systems are probably more core to natural support systems than any other aspect of culture (Winkelman 2009). These cultural systems of health—ethnomedicines—are central aspects of the cultural environment wherein lie the client's conceptual frameworks, as well as the natural resources that can be utilized for interventions. These areas of culture provide the key to the strengths approach which emphasizes a social empowerment derived from strengthening their ability to solve their problems using the social networks of their own social group and the cultural resources of their society.

Effective health care is not merely reducing social barriers to access but also facilitating the use of resources within their cultural system. This focus upon strengths and empowerment must, by necessity, consider cultural resources and traditions that give people meaning and organization to their lives. These are principally found within religious and spiritual traditions and their inevitable intersection with the indigenous cultural healing traditions. This cultural focus strengthens people's sense of community, a necessary component of healthy psychological functioning. Strengths perspectives enhance the integration of individuals within their communities, a significant aspect of the emotional life of individuals and an important aspect of overall wellbeing. This connection of individual and community is an inherently empowering process.

Understanding these connections of individuals with their communities and the cross-cutting ties within cultures are enhanced by psychocultural and cultural systems perspectives (Winkelman 2001, 2005, 2009). Systems perspectives help in overcoming the "blaming the victim" approach inherent in psychoanalytic and deviance approaches, instead locating the problem in the interdependent relations between the individual and numerous cultural and social influences. Cultural systems perspectives help identify the myriad influences and cultural resources, enabling the development of more appropriate intervention strategies based in the numerous subsystems of cultures and their broader social networks and opportunities. The notion of systems perspectives is implicit in many views of cultural competence that emphasize the importance of personal, interpersonal and organizational levels of competence:

• Personal, including cultural self-awareness and cross-cultural adaptation skills;

- Interpersonal, particularly clinical skills and intercultural relations abilities; and
- Knowledge of cultural systems and organizational culture and their impacts on behavior.

What is necessary to manage effectively cultural differences is not merely awareness of other cultures but rather more sophisticated skills. Mere awareness of other cultures needs to be supplemented with knowledge of cultural patterns of behavior and how to effectively adapt to them with intercultural skills. An awareness of the significance of cultural differences must be supplemented with a more nuanced approach based in modifications in our behavior that makes us sensitive to the normative social expectations of others. Some may think that they "treat everybody the same," but closer examination would reveal that such people do not in the same way treat their siblings, girl- and boyfriends, parents, teachers, police, strangers, and the homeless. Even culturally encapsulated people make varied adjustments in their behavior depending on the specifics of the person with whom they are interacting—"different strokes for different folks." But how should we deal with differences?

Cultural capacity levels range from destructiveness (ethnocentrism) to incapacity and blindness, through various degrees of cultural sensitivity adaptation. Cultural sensitivity begins with the appropriate use of knowledge about people's cultural background, combined with the ability to respond to intercultural processes with a range of intercultural skills appropriate to effectively manage cultural differences. Cultural sensitivity provides a more nuanced response than mere awareness of cultural differences while competence involves the capability to deal with cultural differences effectively. Cultural sensitivity leads to adaptation to other cultures through knowledge of specific cultural information and the ability to address barriers to effective cross-cultural relations. Cultural competence involves greater personal skills that enable people to work effectively with other cultural groups. Cultural competence includes behaviors, attitudes, and policies that effectively address cultural effects and overcome potential problems from cultural differences at personal, interpersonal, and organization levels. Cultural sensitivity and competence require personal adaptations to manage the challenge of cultural differences. Our own personal adjustment can then be followed by development of specific intercultural relations skills to improve relations with culturally different people.

The initial step in one's response needs to be conceptualized in terms of self-assessments to determine the level of development of cultural awareness and competency and preparedness for responding effectively to cultural differences. There are many frameworks that have been employed to assess such variation in cross-cultural development. Bennett (1993; Bennett and Bennett 2004) discovered a general developmental model of intercultural sensitivity as a function of the progressive development of a worldview that allows different orientations towards cultural differences. This research has led to the creation of an Intercultural Development Inventory that has been subjected to confirmatory factor analysis, external validity assessments, and reliability assessments (see Hammer, Bennett, and Wiseman 2003) and has been a widely used measure (see Special Training issue of the *International Journal of Intercultural Relations* 27[4] 2003). This concept of a range of ethnocentric and ethnorelative stages has been the basis of my own framework for assessment of cross-cultural development (Winkelman 2005, 2009). These tools provide a determination of where one lies along a range of ethnocentric postures (ethnocentrism, denigration, universalism) or whether one has progressed to ethnorelative stages of acceptance, adaptation and bicultural integration.

This scale of intercultural development involves increasing ability to construe differences in terms of cultural factors and respond to these cultural differences in appropriate ways. These understandings in terms of cultural difference lead to a recognition that different cultures process and produce different realities. These perspectives can spur the development of communication and relations skills based on adaptation to cultural differences, adaptations which may become integrated into self and identity. The ultimate implication of cross-cultural development is personal transformation.

The ability to deal effectively with cultural issues in clinical settings is not a monolithic set of skills but one that varies by task. For instance, the skills for culturally competent administration of personnel involve a different skill set than those required for clinical assessment, and these are not the same as the skills required for cultural competence in developing appropriate and effective intervention. Even within a given ethnic group, different skills are required for sensitivity with different segments (e.g., one may be competent in relations with younger Mexican-Americans but lack sensitivity in dealing with elderly Mexican-Americans or vice versa). Social class provides another dimension of intracultural diversity as do gender and transgendered identities. While general cultural competency might be conceptualized as the ability to deal with all of these and other dimension of difference within a culture, the reality is that we may at best be able to respond to a few specialty areas (administration or clinical care) and specific segments (e.g., migrant families), applying limited cultural knowledge, cultural resources (e.g., translators, interpreters), intercultural skills, and reflective thinking to resolve difficulties presented by cultural differences.

Specific cultural competencies in regard to particular cultural groups (e.g., Mexican-Americans) require long periods of time to develop. Children take years to develop minimal competencies in their own cultures and we all know members of our own cultures whom we might consider to be incompetent within the spheres of their own culture! A true cultural competency is generally beyond the reach of providers unless they are native members of the culture or have spent long periods of time engaged with the culture in both professional relations and everyday life. Providers are generally more likely to learn how to incorporate aspects of cultural knowledge into culturally aware or sensitive care rather than develop true cultural competency and proficiency.

This plateau which falls short of true cultural competency can be conceptualized as cultural responsiveness. This involves an ability to interact with and respond to clients that is consistent with their concepts regarding appropriate care. This is based in a personal style which is cognizant of the cultural values, norms and social expectations of the client, accommodating their expectations regarding the appropriate dynamics of social relations. It also involves an ability to incorporate in the care relationship the clients worldview regarding healing and well-being, including the incorporation of the care modalities they prefer in a dynamic of complementary medicine.

The directives to develop cultural sensitivity are generally framed in humanistic terms as something that is right to do. While altruism is a good motivation for developing intercultural skills, we can recognize and engage this development trajectory for more selfish motives—our own wellbeing. Success in learning about and adaptation to other cultures provides a number of advantages, enhancing the wellbeing of providers and their clients and the effectiveness of their institutions.

Physicians exemplify a profession beset by the difficulties produced by a myriad of factors, including the challenges presented by cultural diversity. Physicians are among the professions most afflicted by addictions and suicide. "Healing the healer" can start with making the job of health service providers easier by reducing the problems presented by an inability to effectively deal with cultural differences. These cultural responses can provide personal and interpersonal benefits as well as enhanced institutional operations.

The personal benefits of developing cross-cultural competencies include increased personal awareness of unconscious cultural influences that shape one's behavior and that of others. This awareness can help to reduce the stress produced by cultural differences, allowing better adaptation to cultural differences and reduced provider frustration and burnout. Knowledge enhances coping and expands options for our own lives and behaviors with an enhanced appreciation of the value of cultural diversity. Awareness of this diversity can enhance understanding of non-verbal communication and facilitate better relations with clients.

Cross-cultural competency is ultimately about enhancing client and community relations, reducing conflict and misunderstandings and providing more effective communication with clients. This enhanced communication will result in more effective client disclosure and cooperation and a better recognition of client psychocultural dynamics and sociocultural and other environmental effects on clients, including a better understanding of client problems and community needs. These understandings can result in enhanced service delivery to clients and communities, more effective management of client resistance and reduced client dissatisfaction, non-compliance, and withdrawal/dropout by more appropriate assessment, problem solving and treatment.

Ultimately our agencies—and society in general—can be expected to function more effectively. Cross-cultural understanding will facilitate effectiveness of service delivery, enhance the effectiveness of outreach and assure better utilization of agency and community resources. Agencies will also experience better community support as they recognize the best practices for engaging diversity and empowering it to contribute to our collective wellbeing.

In the world of today this seems like wishful thinking. Instead, nationalism dominates intergroup relations at the international level, and many other "isms" produced by politics, gender, religion, ethnicity, and many other ideological orientations divide us at local levels. The egocentrism of the ethnocentric point of view is something that we do not naturally overcome. Rather it requires an effort at self-transcendence that can ultimately enable us to overcome blinders of ignorance and enhance our personal awareness and collective wellbeing. Gurung's compilation of articles here in *Multicultural Approaches to Health and Wellness* offers a step in that direction.

Michael Winkelman, MPH, PhD, Retired
Fulbright Professor, Brazil 2009
Arizona State University

References

Bennett, M. 1993. "Toward Ethnorelativism: A Developmental Model of Intercultural Sensitivity." In *Education for the Intercultural Experience,* edited by M. Paige, 21–71. Yarmouth, Maine: Intercultural Press.

Bennett, J. and M. Bennett. 2004. "Developing Intercultural Sensitivity: An Integrative Approach to Global and Domestic Diversity." In *Handbook of Intercultural Training,* edited by D. Landis, J. Bennett, and M. Bennett, 147–165. Thousand Oaks, CA: Sage.

Hammer, M., M. Bennett, and R. Wiseman. 2003. "Measuring Intercultural Sensitivity: The Intercultural Development Inventory." *International Journal of Intercultural Relations* 27(4): 421–443.

Winkelman, M. 2001. "Ethnicity and psychocultural models." In *Cultural Diversity in the United States,* edited by I. Susser and T. Patterson, 281–301. Boston: Blackwell Publishers.

Winkelman, M. 2005. *Cultural Awareness, Sensitivity and Competence.* Peosta, IA: Eddie Bowers.

Winkelman, M. 2009. *Culture and Health Applying Medical Anthropology.* San Francisco: John Wiley and Sons.

Introduction

I grew up in Bombay (now Mumbai), India, surrounded by diversity. There was religious diversity—my family was Catholic but most of my friends were Hindu, Muslim, Jain, and Buddhists; ethnic diversity—people in Bombay hail from all over India, a very diverse country; and even global diversity—as Bombay has many residents from all over the world. To make matters even more interesting, my father was intrigued by different approaches to health and read up on some of the most esoteric (and some would say outlandish) medical practices. The house was filled with books on the power of magnets, gem therapy, reiki, pyramid power, aura therapy, homeopathy, and many more. Starting from a very young age, I noticed that there are many ways to deal with illness. Whereas we frequented conventional doctors subscribing to classic western medicine, my family also used a fair share of folk remedies. We even had shamans come over to conduct spirit cleansings to combat illnesses that seemed resistant to conventional medicine. This two volume series takes a rigorous approach to shine the light on all the different approaches to health, acknowledging that people have diverse practices.

In most of the countries around the globe, health is understood using either the Western evidence-based medical approach or traditional indigenous approaches. In traditional systems, a wide range of practitioners provide help. For example, in Sub-Saharan Africa, four types of traditional healers provide health care, namely, traditional birth attendants (TBAs), faith healers, diviners and spiritualists, and herbalists. Even in the United States, health beliefs and health behaviors vary by cultural groups. Women in New Mexico and men in Chicago may have the same physical problem, but their doctors must take into account the existing differences in their patients' social systems (differences in culture, beliefs, family structure, and economic class) and their patients' expectations of health care and health care workers to cure them. Italian Americans in New York may have different traditional ways of dealing with being sick from Polish Americans in Milwaukee.

For most people basic indicators of good health include the absence of disease, injury, or illness, a slow pulse, the ability to do many physical exercises, or the ability to run fast. These all represent only one general way of being healthy, the one supported by Western medicine. In Western medical circles, health is commonly defined as the state in which disease is absent. Different societies have different understandings of health. For example, in Traditional Chinese Medicine (TCM), health is the balance of the yin and yang, the two complementary forces in the universe. Other cultures also believe that health is the balance of different qualities. Ancient Indian scholars and doctors defined health as the state in which the three main biological units, enzymes, tissues, and excretory functions, are in harmonious condition and when the mind and senses are cheerful. Ayurveda, this ancient system of medicine, focuses on the body, the sense organs, the mind, and the soul. Most of the world's cultures use a more global and widespread approach to assessing health instead of just looking at whether or not disease is absent to determine health (as the biomedical model and most Western approaches do).

There are critical cultural variations in the conceptualization, perception, health-seeking behaviors, assessment, diagnosis, and treatment of abnormal behaviors and physical sickness. This two volume set describes the variety of cultural approaches to health practiced by the diverse groups of people living in the United States of America. Volume One presents a detailed view of key factors related to different approaches to health such as immigration, acculturation, and health disparities. It also provides in-depth descriptions of the health beliefs of major cultural groups such as Latino/Latina, American Indian, and Asian American. Chapter authors unpack major world philosophies of health and wellness such as Ayurveda, Chinese Traditional Medicine, and Curanderismo. Volume Two focuses on mental health issues such as anxiety and mood disorders, and suicide. Chapters layout key demographics of the cultural group under study, the historical origins of the health beliefs, key treatments, and where possible, the scientific evidence in support of the practices. These different approaches can explain some differences in health behaviors, differences in why people get sick, and how they cope when they do. Having a better understanding of cultural variations in health and sickness provides the general reader and scholar alike with better insight into the rich diversity of the planet.

Regan A. R. Gurung

CHAPTER ONE

Cultural Competence

Larry Purnell and Sherry Pontious

The United States, like many countries throughout the world, is becoming more multicultural, making healthcare delivery more complex for patients and providers. Many times healthcare teams are multilingual and multicultural; the cultures of the patient (e.g. Mexican), of the primary healthcare provider (e.g. European American), and of the nurse (e.g. German) are increasingly diverse. In addition, each profession (medicine, nursing, social work, and physical therapy, to name a few) has its own culture. The specialties within each profession also have their own cultures (psychiatry, shock/ trauma, obstetrics, rehabilitation, oncology, etc.). Plus, different cultures exist in each organization and each organization has many subcultures. A short scenario depicting the complex issues of working on a culturally diverse healthcare team is described below. This chapter describes various terms used to describe culture, its determinants, and outcomes of cultural perspectives and includes knowledge, skills, principles and approaches healthcare professionals may use to provide culturally competent health care to multicultural patients within the increasingly divergent healthcare systems.

Elena Maria de Diaz y Cabrera, 49, arrived in the United States from Mexico five years ago to work as a housekeeper for a large hotel chain. Her husband, Juan, and their three children are living with Juan's parents in a suburb of Mexico City. Elena's employer called the paramedics to take her to the local Emergency Department because she was clutching her chest with pain and became hysterical, talking rapidly in Spanish after having an argument with another housekeeper with whom she worked.

In the Emergency Department, the intake triage nurse, Mrs. Steckler, is a registered nurse who recently immigrated from Germany. The treating physician, Dr. Stevenson, born and raised in the Midwest and noted for his acute medical-surgical clinical skills, prescribed medicine for Mrs. Cabrera's chest pain and prescribed an injectable tranquilizer to control her "hysteria." Her electrocardiogram was normal, and he could find no physical cause of her chest pain except for some mild hypertension and obesity, but she was admitted to the cardiac unit for further workup.

The cardiologist, Dr. Gupta, is an Asian Indian who is noted for prescribing a very strict Ayurvedic diet for his patients. The nurses on the admitting unit are Miss Guerrero from the Philippines and Mr. Jamison, an African American. The nutritionist, Mr. Chiang, is from China.

Later on the day of admission, Elena's landlady, Mrs. Morales, a native of Cuba, came to visit her. She asked the receptionist for Mrs. Diaz and was told that there was no patient by that name. After further search, the receptionist found Elena under the name Cabrera instead of Diaz. After speaking with Elena, Mrs. Morales told the nurse that Mrs. Diaz did not need a cardiologist, she needed a *curandero* (male) or *curandera* (female) preferably because she had *susto,* not a cardiac problem.

The day after Elena's admission, a team conference was held in which a number of issues arose, including identifying Elena's legal name, the meaning of *susto,* and who or what is a *curandero/curandera.* The nutritionist recommended against the Ayurvedic diet because Elena would not eat the foods on that diet, preferring the foods that her landlady brought in from home. (See chapter 7 on Ayurveda, chapter 10 on *curanderismo,* and chapter 11 on *susto.*) Mrs. Guerrero explained that among most Hispanic/Latino cultures that are similar to the Filipino culture, a married woman adopts her husband's surname preceded by *de,* and might elect to keep her father's surname, Cabrera, and even her mother's maiden name, especially if her mother came from a prominent family. A woman may choose any name she wishes as her legal name; the name she selected should be determined and used to keep medical records accurate.

Initiatives for Cultural Competence

Since the early 1990s, cultural competence (defined shortly) became a focal point as a result of multiple agencies elucidating increasing health disparities (inequalities) with associated higher healthcare costs to the public. An extensive review of these initiatives is not possible here; many of them are addressed in other chapters. The National Standards on Culturally and Linguistically Appropriate Services (CLAS Standards) are primarily directed at healthcare organizations; however, individual providers are encouraged to use these standards to make their practices more culturally and linguistically appropriate. The principles and activities of culturally and linguistically appropriate services should be integrated throughout an organization and undertaken in partnership with the communities being served (U.S. Department of Health and Human Services: Office of Minority Health 2007). Of the 14 standards initiated in 2001, four address language and access services and are requirements for all recipients of Federal funds.

In many reports, the Centers for Disease Control and Prevention includes culture as a component of health promotion and wellness; of illness, disease, and injury prevention; and of health maintenance and restoration (CDC Health Disparities and Inequalities Report 2011). Some additional select few reports include: Healthy People 2020 (2012), The Robert Wood Johnson Foundation (2012), the Institute of Medicine (2012), the Joint Commission (2010), The U.S. Department of Health and Human Services: Office of Minority Health (2011). Most healthcare accrediting and professional associations (e.g., nursing, medicine, physical therapy, and social work) also address the importance of culturally competent health care.

Essential Terminology Related to Cultural Competence

The professional literature from anthropology, sociology, and the health professions is replete with cultural terminology, much of which is confusing. This section defines, clarifies, and differentiates many of these terms.

The three terms cultural awareness, cultural sensitivity, and cultural competence are frequently confused and/or used synonymously. However, to healthcare providers working in culture, these terms have quite different meanings (Giger et al. 2007). *Cultural awareness* is an appreciation of the external or material signs of diversity, such as the arts, music, dress, food, religious activities or physical characteristics. *Cultural sensitivity* reflects personal attitudes and includes not saying or doing things that might be offensive to someone from a different cultural or ethnic background than that of the healthcare provider (Giger et al. 2007).

Cultural competence incorporates but goes beyond cultural awareness and sensitivity; it is often defined as using a combination of culturally appropriate attitudes, knowledge, and skills that facilitate providing effective healthcare for diverse individuals, families, groups, and communities. Cultural competence is more complex and includes the following:

- Becoming aware of one's own existence, sensations, thoughts, and environment without allowing them to unduly influence those from other backgrounds

- Demonstrating understanding of the individual's culture, health-related needs, healthcare practices and culturally specific meanings of health and illness
- Continuing to learn about additional cultures of individuals to whom one provides care
- Recognizing that primary and secondary variants of culture determine the degree to which an individual adheres to the beliefs, values, and practices of his/her dominant culture
- Accepting and respecting cultural differences in ways to facilitate individual's and family's abilities to make decisions that meet their needs and beliefs
- Recognizing the healthcare provider's beliefs and values are NOT the same as the individual's
- Resisting judgmental attitudes, such as "different is not as good"
- Desiring and being comfortable with cultural encounters
- Adapting care to be congruent with the individual's cultural beliefs, values, and practices
- Engaging in cultural competence is a conscious process, not necessarily linear
- Being accountable for one's own education in cultural competence by attending conferences, reading professional literature, and observing cultural practices (Purnell 2013)
- Being able to communicate between and among cultures while working within the individual's, family's, or community's cultural context

Culture, subculture, and ethnicity are additional terms requiring clarification. The beliefs and values of culture are primarily unconscious and powerful influences on health and illness. *Culture* is the totality of socially transmitted behavioral patterns, arts, beliefs, values, customs, lifeways, and all other products of human work and thought characteristics of a population that guide their worldview and decision-making. Health and healthcare beliefs, values, and practices are assumed in this definition. Behavioral patterns may be explicit or implicit, are primarily learned and transmitted within the family, are shared by most (but not all) members of the culture, and are emergent phenomena that change in response to global phenomena (Purnell 2013). Culture has three levels: (a) a tertiary level visible to outsiders, such as things that can be heard, worn, or otherwise observed; (b) a secondary level, known and articulated only by members such as in the rules of behavior; and (c) a primary level representing the deepest level in which all rules are known by all and observed by most implicitly, and taken for granted (Koffman 2006).

Within all cultures are subcultures and ethnic groups with different experiences who do not hold all the values of the dominant culture with which they identify. In sociology, anthropology, and cultural studies, a *subculture* is a group within a culture that differentiates them from the larger culture of which they are a part (Giger et al. 2007). Subcultures may be distinct or hidden (e.g. gay, lesbian, bisexual, or transgendered popula-tions) and include individuals who may or may not be opposed to the mainstream trends of their culture. A transgendered population may have members from the European, American, Mexican, Chinese, Thai, etc. cul-tures who come together and form a subculture. If the subculture is char-acterized by a systematic opposition to the dominant culture, then it may be described as a counterculture. Examples of subcultures are Goths, punks, and stoners, although popular lay literature might call these groups cultures instead of subcultures. A counterculture would include cults (Goffman and Joy 2006).

An *ethnic group* is a group of people within an identified culture whose values and beliefs are different from their dominant group (Giger et al. 2007). For example, Mexico, like many countries, has groups that are out-side the "dominant group" such as Mayan or any number of indigenous Indian groups. They are all considered Mexicans but have their own dis-tinct lifeways and may speak a different language from Mexican Spanish, especially at home, and have their own traditional healers.

Enculturation, acculturation, and assimilation also need to be distin-guished. *Enculturation* is the process of learning cultural beliefs, values, and practices from birth (Clarke and Hofsess 1998): first at home, then in the church and other places where people congregate, and then in educa-tional settings. Therefore, a child with Iranian Islamic heritage adopted by a French Canadian family and reared in a dominant French Canadian en-vironment will have a French Canadian worldview. However, if that child's heritage has a tendency toward genetic/hereditary conditions, they would come from the Iranian ancestry, not from French Canadian genetics.

Acculturation occurs when a person gives up the traits of his/her cul-ture of origin as a result of contact with another culture (Giger et al. 2007; see chapter 5 this volume). Acculturation is not an absolute and has varying degrees. Traditional people hold on to the majority of cultural traits from their culture of origin; this is frequently seen when people live in ethnic enclaves and get most of their needs met without mixing with the outside world, like the Amish. Bicultural acculturation occurs when an individual is able to function equally in the dominant culture and in one's own culture. People who are comfortable working in the dominant culture and return to their ethnic enclave without taking on most of the dominant culture's traits are usually bicultural. Marginal-ized individuals are not comfortable in their new culture or in their cul-ture of origin. *Assimilation* is the gradual adoption and incorporation of characteristics of the prevailing culture (Portes 2007). An example of assimilation for the Amish is that they are now forced to enter the technological era, since many of the catalogues from which they ordered material and supplies are now totally online. For them, a member of the Amish church district will have a computer and telephone in a place of business rather than in their homes.

Other terms that continue to cause discourse are stereotyping, generalization, and ethnocentrism. *Stereotyping* is having a simplified and standardized conception, opinion, or belief about a person or group. The healthcare provider who fails to recognize individuality within a group is jumping to conclusions about the individual or family and therefore, stereotyping. If one concentrates on the primary and secondary variants of culture when assessing the individual, this tendency can be ameliorated. *Generalization* begins with assumptions about the individual or family within an ethnocultural group but leads to further information seeking. For example, the Roman Catholic Church has tenets that come from the central authority, the Vatican; most Catholics adhere to some of them to some degree. However, these tenets are general characteristics and must be validated by the individual to determine his/her degree of adherence. *Ethnocentrism* is a universal tendency to believe one's own worldview is superior to another's. It is often experienced in the healthcare arena, especially when the healthcare provider's culture or ethnic group is considered superior to another. For example, healthcare providers often tell their clients to stop taking herbal remedies because they believe the medicine prescribed is much superior.

Cultural relativism, cultural imposition, and cultural imperialism are sometimes violated or not recognized by healthcare providers who are new to the field of cultural competence. *Cultural relativism* is the belief that the behaviors and practices of people should be judged only from the context of that culture's cultural system of beliefs and values. Proponents of cultural relativism argue that issues, such as, abortion, euthanasia, female circumcision, and physical punishment in child rearing should be accepted as cultural values without judgment from the outside world. Opponents argue that cultural relativism may undermine condemnation of human rights violations, and issues such as family violence cannot be justified or excused on a cultural basis (Purnell 2001, Purnell 2013).

Cultural imposition is the intrusive application of the majority group's cultural view upon individuals and families (Universal Declaration of Human Rights 2001). The practice of prescribing special diets without regard to individuals' cultural food choices or requiring hospitalized patients to drink ice water with medication for a client's perceived "cold" disease borders on cultural imposition. Healthcare providers must continually recognize that their beliefs and values may not be the same as the individual's. *Cultural imperialism* is the practice of extending policies and procedures of one organization (usually the dominant one) to disenfranchised and minority groups. Proponents appeal to universal human rights values and standards. Opponents posit that universal standards are a disguise for the dominant culture to destroy or eradicate traditional cultures through worldwide public policy (Purnell 2001, Purnell 2013).

Additional terms found in the literature are cultural humility, cultural leverage, cultural safety, and cultural brokering. *Cultural humility* focuses on the process of intercultural exchange, paying explicit attention to clarifying values and beliefs of the healthcare provider and of the client and their family, and incorporating the cultural characteristics of the healthcare provider and the individual into a mutually beneficial and balanced relationship (Trevalon and Murray-Garcia 1998). This term appears to be most popular with physicians and healthcare providers from social sciences. *Cultural leverage* is a process whereby the principles of cultural competence are deliberatively invoked to develop interventions. It is a focused strategy for improving the health of racial and ethnic communities by using their cultural practices, products, philosophies, or environments to facilitate behavioral changes of the individual and healthcare provider (Fisher et al. 2007). *Cultural safety* expresses the diversity that exists within cultural groups, such as social determinants of health, religion, and gender and is an addition to ethnicity (Nursing Council New Zealand 2008). Cultural safety is popular in Australia and New Zealand, although the term is used elsewhere. *Cultural brokering* occurs in the workforce or in community settings where a new employee or new arrival to the community is paired with someone who orients and mentors that new person and knows both the culture of the organization/community and the culture of the new employee/arrival (Purnell 2013). It is also used to describe the process of educating and negotiating with members of a multicultural team from cultures different from the client, to plan culturally acceptable and compatible treatments, education, and prescriptions for a client, family, or group. For example, negotiating with hospital administrators, doctors, nurses and cleaning staff to allow and maintain a circle of maize around a Navajo child's bed left by the medicine man to protect the child from evil spirits and to assist his/her healing. Cultural brokering requires the broker to be very knowledgeable about the beliefs, values and practices of all members of the healthcare team or organization and that of the client and his/her family.

The terms *transcultural* and *cross-cultural* are hotly debated by many in academia with a preference by discipline and/or healthcare providers.

Specific definitions of these terms vary. *Transcultural* is the comparative study of cultures to understand similarities (cultural universal) and differences (culture-specific) across human groups (Leininger 1991) whereas the term cross-cultural implies comparative interactivity between cultures. Healthcare providers need not worry about slight differences in meaning between these two terms.

Variant Cultural Characteristics

Variant cultural characteristics can theoretically be divided into primary and secondary traits of culture, although not categorically imperative. Most primary characteristics of culture are things that cannot easily be changed and if changed, a significant stigma may occur for the individual or family. Primary characteristics include age, generation, race, color, gender, and religion. Gender can be changed with reassignment surgery, but it may cause a significant stigma for the person or family. Religion for Orthodox Jews drives their communication, clothing, and nutritional practices. If an Orthodox Jew decides to change to Islam or Catholicism, a stigma for him/her or their family may result.

Secondary characteristics are things that can more easily change and include educational status, socioeconomic status, occupation, military status, political beliefs, urban versus rural residence, enclave identity, marital status, parental status, physical characteristics, sexual orientation, gender issues, and immigration status (immigrant, sojourner, or undocumented). One's educational and socioeconomic status can change, for better or for worse, resulting in a change in beliefs and practices. Marital status can change from single to married, to divorced, to remarried, resulting in some lifestyle changes. A few may change their sexual orientation, although it is probably most common among people who are incarcerated or for those in a same-sex environment for extended periods of time.

Purnell Model as an Assessment Guide

The Purnell Model for Cultural Competence has been classified as a complex and holographic theory because its organizing framework can be used in all practice settings and by all healthcare providers (Purnell and Paulanka 1998). The model is a circle with the metaparadigm concepts (global society, community, person, and family) forming rims around the model. The outlying rim represents global society, a second rim represents community, a third rim represents family, and the inner rim represents the

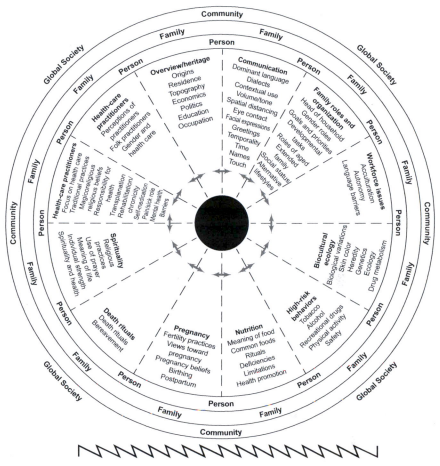

Figure 1.1 Purnell Model for Cultural Competence

person (see Figure 1.1). The interior of the circle is divided into 12 pie-shaped wedges depicting cultural domains (constructs) and their associated concepts. The dark center of the circle represents unknown phenomena. Along the bottom of the model is a jagged line representing the nonlinear concept of cultural consciousness.

Metaparadigm Concepts

The metaparadigm concepts of the Purnell model are global society, community, person, and family. Phenomena related to a global society include world communication and politics; conflicts and warfare; natural and man-made disasters and famines; international exchanges in education, business, commerce, and information technology; advances in health science; space exploration; and the expanded opportunities for people to travel around the world and interact with diverse societies. Global events that are widely disseminated by television, radio, satellite transmission, newsprint, and information technology affect all societies, either directly or indirectly. One such example is the burning of the Quran by a minister in Florida and a few members of the U.S. military. Such events may create chaos while consciously and/or unconsciously forcing people to change their lifeways.

In the broadest definition, community is a group of people having a common interest or identity that may extend beyond the physical environment. Community includes the physical, social, and symbolic characteristics that cause people to connect. Bodies of water, mountains, rural versus urban living, and even railroad tracks help people define their physical concept of community. Today, however, technology and the Internet allow people to expand their community beyond physical boundaries with social networking. Economics, religion, politics, age, generation, and marital status delineate the social concepts of community. Sharing a specific language or dialect, lifestyle, history, dress, art, or musical interest are symbolic characteristics of a community. People actively and passively interact with the community, necessitating adaptation and assimilation for equilibrium and homeostasis in their worldview. Individuals may willingly change their physical, social, and symbolic community when it no longer meets their needs.

A family is two or more people who are emotionally connected. They may, but do not necessarily, live in close proximity to each other. Family may include physically and emotionally close and distant consanguineous relatives as well as physically and emotionally connected non-blood-related significant others. Family structure and roles change according to age, generation, marital and parental status, relocation or immigration, and socioeconomic and educational status, requiring each person to rethink individual beliefs and lifeways.

A person is a biopsychosociocultural being who is constantly adapting to his or her community. Human beings adapt biologically and physiologically to the aging process; psychologically in the context of social relationships, stress, and relaxation; socially as they interact with the changing community; and ethnoculturally within the broader global society. In Western cultures, a person is a separate physical and unique psychological being and a singular member of society. The self is separate from others. This is not true for many other cultures.

The Domains and Concepts

The 12 domains and their concepts provide the organizing framework. Each domain includes concepts that need to be addressed when assessing the individual and family in various settings. In addition, healthcare providers can use these same concepts to better understand their own cultural beliefs, attitudes, values, practices, and behaviors. No single domain stands alone; they are all interconnected. Each domain has an organizing framework with extensive questions that the experienced clinician may use to complete an assessment. Space does not permit the entirety of the organizing framework to be included here but it can be obtained from the textbook, *Transcultural Health Care: A Culturally Competent Approach* (Purnell, 2013) or from *Guide to Culturally Competent Health Care* (2014). The twelve domains and their concepts follow.

Overview and heritage include concepts related to the country of origin and current residence. The topography of the country of origin and of current residence influence health beliefs, economics, politics, reasons for migration, educational status, and occupations.

Communication includes concepts related to the dominant language, dialects, and the contextual use of the language; paralanguage variations, such as voice volume, tone, intonations, inflections, and willingness to share thoughts and feelings; nonverbal communications, such as eye contact, gesturing and facial expressions, use of touch, body language, spatial distancing practices, and acceptable greetings; temporality in terms of past, present, and future orientation of worldview; clock versus social time; and the amount of formality in use of names.

Family roles and organization include concepts related to the head of the household, gender roles (a product of biology and culture), family goals and priorities, developmental tasks of children and adolescents, roles of older adults and extended family, individual and family social status in the community, and acceptance of alternative lifestyles such as single parenting, nontraditional sexual orientations, childless marriages, and divorce.

Workforce issues include concepts related to autonomy, acculturation, assimilation, and gender roles.

Biocultural ecology includes physical, biological, and physiological variations among ethnic and racial groups such as skin color (the most evident) and physical differences in body habitus; genetic, hereditary, endemic, and topographical diseases; psychological makeup of individuals; and the physiological differences that affect the way drugs are metabolized by the body. In general, most diseases and illnesses fall in three categories: lifestyle, environment, and genetics. *Lifestyle* causes include cultural practices and behaviors that can generally be controlled: for example, smoking, diet, and stress. *Environmental* causes refer to the external environment (e.g., air and water pollution) and situations over which the individual has little or no control (e.g., presence of malarial mosquitoes, exposure to chemicals, radiation and pesticides, access to care, and associated diseases). *Genetic* conditions are caused by genes.

High-risk health behaviors include substance use and misuse of tobacco, alcohol, and drugs; lack of physical activity; increased (or decreased) calorie consumption; nonuse of safety measures e.g., seat belts, helmets, safe driving and safe sex practices.

Nutrition is more than satisfying hunger. It includes the meaning of food, commonly used foods and their preparation, and rituals; nutritional deficiencies and food limitations; and the use of food for health promotion and restoration, and illness and disease prevention. For example, in many Hispanic cultures, vegetables are used minimally even though they are easily available.

Pregnancy and childbearing practices include culturally sanctioned and unsanctioned fertility practices; views on pregnancy; and prescriptive, restrictive, and taboo practices related to pregnancy, birthing, and the postpartal period.

Death rituals include how the individual and the society view death and euthanasia, rituals to prepare for death, burial practices, and bereavement behaviors. Death rituals are slow to change.

Spirituality includes formal and informal religious beliefs related to faith and affiliation and the use of prayer, behavior practices that give meaning to life, and individual sources of strength.

Healthcare practices include the focus of healthcare (acute versus preventive); traditional, magicoreligious, and biomedical beliefs and practices; individual responsibility for health; self-medicating practices; views on mental illness, chronicity, and rehabilitation; acceptance of blood and blood products; and organ donation and transplantation.

Health care practitioners include the status, use, and perceptions of traditional, magicoreligious, and biomedical healthcare providers, priority order of use of healthcare providers, and the gender of the healthcare provider.

Individualism versus Collectivism

The degree to which a person/culture is oriented on the individualism versus collectivism continuum is one of the least understood yet very powerful primary traits of culture that influences cultural worldviews; it is an important factor influencing how individuals/families/communities act, communicate, and make decisions. Cultural competence requires the healthcare professional to understand the individualistic/collectivistic beliefs of each patient, family, and healthcare provider to provide culturally competent care. Guidelines for working with patients/families/communities from different individualistic/collectivistic orientations are provided to enhance the healthcare provider's use of culturally appropriate behaviors and communication approaches to improve culturally competent care.

The individualism versus collectivism primary cultural trait continuum of values includes orientation to self or group, decision-making, knowledge transmission, individual choice, personal responsibility, the concept of progress, competitiveness, shame and guilt, help-seeking, expression of identity, and interaction/communication style (Hofstede 1991, Hofstede 2001, Hofstede and Hofstede 2005, Purnell 2013). Elements of and some degree of individualism and collectivism exist in every culture. People from an individualist culture will more strongly identify with the values at the individualistic end of the scale. Moreover, individualism and collectivism fall along a continuum, and some people from an individualistic culture will, to some degree, align themselves towards the collectivistic end of the scale and vice versa. The degree of acculturation and assimilation and the variant characteristics of culture determine the degree of adherence to traditional individualistic and collectivist cultural values, beliefs, and practices (Hofstede 1991, Hofstede and Hofstede 2005, Purnell 2013).

Communicating, assessing, counseling, and educating a person from an individualistic culture where the most important person in society is the individual, may require different techniques than for a person in a collectivist culture where the needs and wishes of the group is seen as more important than those of the individual (Hofstede and Hofstede 2005, Purnell 2013). The healthcare provider must not confuse *individualism* with *individuality*. *Individuality* is the sense that each person has a separate and equal place in the community and where individuals who are considered 'eccentrics or local characters' are tolerated (Purnell 2010).

Some highly individualistic cultures include traditional European American (USA), British, Canadian, German, Norwegian, and Swedish. Some examples of collectivist cultures include traditional Arabic, Amish, Chinese, Filipino, Haitian, Indian, Korean, Japanese, Mexican, American Indians and most indigenous groups, Taiwanese, Thai, Turks, and Vietnamese. Far more world cultures are collectivistic than are individualistic, which can be problematic for a healthcare provider from a highly collectivist culture to communicate with patients and staff in highly individualistic cultures, such as the United States and Germany, or vice versa (Hofstede and Hofstede 2005, Purnell 2011b, 2013).

Cultures differ in the extent to which health and information is explicit or implicit. In low-context or individualistic cultures, great emphasis is placed on the verbal mode and many words are used to express a thought. In high-context or collectivistic cultures, much of the information is implicit where fewer words are used to express a thought, resulting in more of the message being in the nonverbal mode. Great emphasis is placed on personal relationships and others' perceptions of the person or family (Hofstede 1991, Hofstede 2001, Purnell 2011a, 2013).

Consistent with individualism, *individualistic cultures* encourage self-expression. Adherents to individualism freely express personal opinions, share many personal issues, and ask personal questions of others to a degree that may be seen as offensive to those who come from a collectivistic culture. Direct, straight-forward questioning with the expectation that answers will be direct is usually appreciated with individualism; however, small talk before getting down to business is not appreciated. The healthcare provider should take cues from the patient before this immediate, direct, and intrusive approach is initiated. Individualistic cultures usually tend to be more informal and frequently use first names. Ask the patient by what name she/he prefers to be called. Questions that require a yes or no answer are usually answered truthfully from the patient's perspective. In individualistic cultures with values on autonomy and productivity, one is expected to be a productive member of society and responsible and accountable for one's actions (Purnell 2011b, 2013).

Individualistic cultures expect all to follow the rules and hierarchical protocols, and each person is expected to do their own work and to work until the job is completed. Thus, young people are often expected to become more responsible at a younger age and have more independence and self-expression. Decisions are made by those with the highest status or position in the family or group, usually after consulting with the group. However, in situations where the group makes decisions, each member has an equal right to express their opinions, and opinions differ greatly, enhancing the chance the decision is better than one person's decision would be. The expectation is that all will follow the decisions made.

In *collectivistic cultures,* decisions are made in groups when consensus is attained; this is often a time-consuming, informal process with many passive or silent members who will not challenge the oldest or most senior members on the team. The collectivistic cultural members' perception is that this is a very democratic, team-driven process. Rules are known; however, they are frequently bent, broken, or ignored. In addition, collectivistic members perceive they have a lower workload and less stress when working with team members who are very supportive and help each other.

Among collectivistic cultures, people with a mental or physical disability are *more likely* to be hidden from society to save face. The cultural norms and the values of collectivistic families mean that care of all immediate and extended family members is provided by the family at home (Purnell 2010). In collectivist cultures, it is absolutely imperative to include the family, and sometimes the community, for effective counseling; otherwise, the treatment plan will not be followed. For many indigenous populations (e.g., American Indian) the fact that one member of the tribe or clan is ill means that the tribe or clan is sick, resulting in one or more members becoming ill. Thus, healing rituals and treatments or counseling should be provided to the whole tribe or clan, not just to those individuals with signs and symptoms of illness. Among many Middle Eastern and other collectivistic cultures, people with a mental or physical disability are sometimes hidden from the public because "their pollution" may mean that other children in the family will not be able to obtain a spouse if the condition is known. For example, those with tuberculosis will be relegated to sleeping on the back porch and not allowed in their home in the Haitian American culture. In many Orthodox and conservative Jewish communities, children with "weak eyes" (vision problems) are not given glasses to allow that child and their siblings to attract spouses with "strong eyes" or those from highly valued families, for the reasons given above. For other impairments, such as ones resulting from HIV, the conditions may be kept hidden, not because of confidentiality rights but for fear that news of the condition may spread to other family members and the community (Colin and Paperwalla 2013). In addition, in many cultures, spiritual healers (e.g., curandero/curandera, root-worker, voodoo priest/priestess, medicine man/woman) are typically consulted first for all illnesses but especially for those cultural illnesses such as *susto* or those caused by the evil-eye, curses, or bad spirits entering the person. The greater the cultural stigma and the more the culture values spiritual or magicoreligious healers, the more likely will be a delay in seeking healthcare and counseling, resulting in the condition being more severe at the time of treatment (Purnell 2013). For example, children with asthma from the Mexican culture are frequently first taken to the eldest family female, than to a *paterna,* then a *curandera,* then a *pharmacia,* and then to a Western medical clinic, by which time the asthma attack may be severe (see chapter 11 this volume).

In individualistic cultures, a person's identity is based mainly on one's personal accomplishments, career, and challenges. A high standard of living supports self-efficiency, self-direction, self-advocacy, and independent living. Decisions made by elders and people in hierarchal positions may be questioned or not followed, because the ideal is that all people are equal and expect, and are expected, to make their own decisions about their lives. Moreover, people are personally responsible and held accountable for their decisions and even for their own health and wellbeing. For example, those who are obese with or without current health problems are held responsible for losing the weight to improve their health and to minimize the cost of their healthcare to society. Improving self, doing "better" than others (frequently focused on material gains), and making progress on a community or national level are expected. If one fails, the blame and shame are on "self" (Purnell 2013).

In collectivistic cultures, people are socialized to view themselves as members of a larger group, family, school, church, educational setting, work, etc. They are bound through the expectations of loyalty and personal and familial lifetime protective ties. Children are socialized where priority is given to connections and interrelationships with others as the basis of psychological well-being. Older people, and those in hierarchal positions, are respected, and people are less likely to openly disagree with them. Individuals are not seen as equal; those seen as not as good as others are left behind. Parents and elders may have the final say in their children's careers and life partners. The focus is not on the individual but on the needs of the group and what is best for the group as a whole (Purnell 2013).

Collectivism is characterized by not drawing attention to oneself and people are not encouraged to ask questions. When one fails, shame may be extended to the family; external explanations, spiritual forces, superiors, or fate, may be given as causes of the health problem. To avoid offending someone, people practice smooth interpersonal communication by not openly disagreeing and are evasive with negative issues. For example, when one of the authors, Pontious asked questions perceived by the Chinese hosts in China as potentially negative toward their political system, the hosts changed the subject until this line of questioning stopped. In collectivistic cultures that primarily use oral history, the healthcare provider should not take notes. Taking notes is perceived as the healthcare provider being stupid or rude, not being able to listen well, or not being interested enough to remember what the individual, family, or community is saying.

Among most collectivist cultures, to disagree or to answer the healthcare provider with a negative response is considered rude; asking questions is seen as disrespectful and causes the elder/or respected healthcare provider to lose face since teaching was not clear or understood. In fact, in some languages a word for "no" does not exist. Do not ask the patient if s/he knows what you are asking, understands you, or knows how to do something, because the only option that a person would have is to answer "yes." Yes, could mean (a) I hear you but I do not understand you, (b) I understand you, but I do not agree with what has been said, (c) I agree with you but I may not necessarily follow recommendations due to cost, or what you are asking is culturally unacceptable. Nodding is a sign of respect, not agreement. Repeating what is prescribed does not ensure understanding; instead ask for a demonstration, the place they will purchase the medication and times they will give it or from whom they will receive the treatments or some other response that is more likely to determine understanding (Purnell 2013). Healthcare providers need to be especially careful to know the herbs and remedies commonly used by the individual and family and ensure medications and treatments prescribed do not contradict, counteract, or enhance the effects of herbs or cultural remedies used, since undesirable side and toxic effects will be perceived to be due to the unfamiliar medications/treatments resulting in them not being used. For example, in the Mexican culture, Ma Huang tea is used to help breathing; it contains naturally occurring ephedrine. Thus, when children with asthma from this culture are prescribed ephedrine or epinephrine in combination with other medications, the dose of these drugs should be lowered depending on the amount and intensity of Ma Huang they drink in order to prevent the child becoming hyperactive, having a rapid pulse, and being unable to sleep. Otherwise, the family will stop the prescribed medication, and it is likely this child will be readmitted with an exacerbated asthma attack or status asthmaticus.

Evidence-Based Practice and Culture

To improve safety and enhance quality outcomes for patients, evidence-based practice (EBP) must be used especially to attain culturally competent care. We can no longer rely on "opinion-based" healthcare that was primarily grounded in the healthcare provider's intuition, clinical experience/expertise, and/or pathophysiological rationale (Swanson, Schmitz, and Chung 2010). The "opinion-based" culture often led to healthcare provided based on stereotypes, generalizations, and ethnocentrism; all of which frequently resulted in patients' and family's misunderstandings, inability or unwillingness to follow the recommended care treatments. A cultural shift is required; we must change to an EBP culture in which there is conscientious, explicit, and judicious use of current best evidence in making shared (among healthcare providers and patients) decisions about healthcare to match the appropriate care with multicultural individuals' and groups of patients' preferences. This is especially true if we are to provide EBP culturally competent healthcare. Large cultural qualitative studies are scarce or nonexistent in culture resulting in less research evidence to inform decision-making in culturally competent care. Evidence-based practice includes the best evidence from the literature, clinical expertise, patient preferences and values, and clinical context (Kitson 2002). Moreover, the weight given to each component varies according to the clinical situation (Melnyk et al. 2009).

With more than 1500 new articles and 55 new clinical trials per day, staying current with all of the conditions and situations that patients present is impossible. Healthcare providers must recognize these limitations and reflect on their practice to determine upon what evidence they can rely. They must ask why things are being done as they are, if there is evidence supporting the approach, what the evidence suggests may be best in this clinical situation, and if there is likely to be cultural considerations that necessitate examining evidence specific to the cultural group (Salmond 2007).

Locating Best Evidence from the Literature

An evidence-based perspective requires asking clinical questions and searching for the evidence to guide practice. Ask focused questions, which is especially important in culture. Who is your population of interest? What is the intervention or phenomenon of interest? What is the outcome in which you are interested? Consider that your broad interest is severe mental illness. Determine whether you want evidence for a particular culture or subculture and specify this population by using key words (e.g. Mexican, lesbian). Narrow the clinical area of interest (palliative care, stigma), and educational and support programs in palliative care. Finally, for quantitative studies, select an outcome that defines how you will measure success of the program (e.g., professional and/or family interventions). Ask if a structured support program will impact the acceptance of and satisfaction with palliative care for this patient, family, or interprofessional team.

The goal is to search for the "best" evidence that is usually found in clinically relevant research conducted using sound methodology (Sackett

2000). Haynes (2006) suggests beginning with sources where the clinician can access "filtered" evidence that has already been critically appraised and determined to be of sufficient rigor to be considered for application into practice. These include systematic reviews, critically appraised guidelines, and critically appraised individual articles.

By using a systematic review, the clinician can generally rely on the fact that there: (a) was a comprehensive search for all available information and (b) the information was screened for relevance to the clinical question and appraised for the rigor of the research. Sources for systematic reviews include the Agency for Healthcare Research and Quality, Cochrane Collaboration, Campbell Collaboration, and Joanna Briggs libraries. Bibliographic databases should also be searched.

Practice guidelines translate research findings into systematically developed statements to assist healthcare providers and patients in making decisions about healthcare for specific clinical circumstances and cultures. Guidelines are not cookbooks where recipes must be followed. Sources for guidelines include: Agency for Healthcare Research and Quality, guideline. gov website, and the Guidelines International Network. Guidelines can be specific to a disease condition such as exercise induced asthma, or can address broader program and intervention issues such as mental health and substance abuse, literacy interventions and outcomes, alcohol consumption and cancer risk (AHRQ 2012).

In the absence of systematic reviews or practice guidelines, search for single studies using bibliographic databases. There are many evidence-based journals (*Evidence-Based Nursing, Evidence-Based Medicine, and Evidence-Based Mental Health*) that provide filtered literature–synopses of primary research providing a summary, an appraisal, and recommendations for translation into practice. Begin your single search with these journals by adding the journal in your key word search to review filtered literature.

If you have still not found the answer to your cultural question after searching the filtered literature, search for primary studies (non-filtered) by searching the bibliographic databases. If you know of journals that commonly carry articles related to your topic, include the journal title in your electronic search or manually search the hard copy of the journal. The *Journal of Transcultural Nursing* may be a helpful source for information on culture for nurses and other health professionals.

Articles retrieved from non-filtered sources need to be critically appraised to determine scientific rigor prior to use in practice. This requires determining whether the best or strongest design was used for the particular questions and whether the study design was rigorous. For questions of intervention (e.g., What is the best psychotropic dosage for

Chinese with bi-polar disorder?), randomized controlled trials are the best type of design, followed by cohort studies, case-controlled studies, case series, and descriptive studies. For questions about meaning or understanding an experience (e.g., What is the experience of marginalization in new Mexican immigrants?), qualitative studies are the best design. Reviewing the article for its adherence to design principles assesses rigor. There are many tools to assist in this process such as CASP International (2012) that has a tool for the different study design types.

Another source of evidence that provides valuable information about culture is grey literature—material that is not formally published by commercial publishers or peer reviewed journals. It includes technical reports, fact sheets, state-of-the-art reports, conference proceedings, culturally competent simulation scenarios; other documents from institutions, organizations, and government agencies; internet-based materials, and other forms of media (newspapers, films, published photographs). The grey non-peer reviewed literature is an important source for information on culture as there are few peer-reviewed publications on specific diseases and cultural implications of diseases or management among the culturally and linguistically diverse. It is important that grey literature be authenticated as reliable and accurate as far as this can be assessed (Purnell and Salmond 2013).

The New York Academy of Medicine obtains and adds grey literature to the catalog (Gray 1998), resulting in the New York Academy of Medicine's *Grey Literature Report,* a bi-monthly online report targeting researchers, practitioners, students, and the lay public who are interested in public health, health and science policy, health of minorities, vulnerable and special populations (children, women, uninsured, elderly) and those areas of general medicine and disease in which the Academy has research interests. Other key grey literature sites are the World Health Organization, Family Health International, Kaiser Family Foundation, United Nations Educational, Scientific, and Cultural Organization, Scirus for Scientific Information, and Culture Link Network. Examples of valuable grey literature reports relevant to understanding the impact of culture on health decision making or reporting on cultural health issues include *Cross-Cultural Considerations in Promoting Advance Care Planning in Canada* and *Culture and Mental Health in Haiti: A Literature Review* (WHO/PAHO 2010).

Evidence from Clinical Expertise

Drawing from best evidence is important; by itself it cannot direct practice because of the lack of quality evidence on some topics, such as true evidence of social and cultural influences on health and health outcomes.

There has been an historical dearth of studies including ethnic minority groups; challenges continue in recruiting ethnic minority groups to participate in research (Hulme 2010). In addition, there is a poor fit between our patients in actual practice and those studied in research. Most studies control for one or two variables whereas in practice patients' problems are very complex and their value systems are very different. Mosley articulates that we spend most of our lives in the gray area with only somewhat adequate evidence. Navigating this gray area requires clinicians to use their practical knowledge, professional knowledge or practical 'know how' (Rycroft-Malone et al. 2004).

Healthcare providers rely on their clinical judgment and expertise to thoroughly assess the patient and differentiate nuances that influence treatment perspectives. Unfortunately in healthcare, emphasis is on assessing the biophysical domain with much less attention to psychological, cultural, and social factors that clearly affect health behaviors and outcomes. Clinical expertise must be holistic and recognize the social and cultural determinants of health (McMurray 2004). Evidence requires an inclusive skill set requiring a comprehensive model for a cultural assessment, of which the Purnell Model is just one example. Healthcare providers must use their clinical expertise to determine whether there are intervening biophysical, psychological, social, or cultural considerations that could be influencing outcomes and make necessary adjustments (Shah and Chung 2009).

Patient Values and Preferences

Critics of evidence-based practice posit that there is too great an emphasis on empirical evidence and clinical expertise; the reality is that evidence-based practice that integrates all four components is complementary to patient-centered care. The clinician must recognize the uniqueness of the patient and family and value the patient as a co-decision maker in selecting interventions and approaches towards their improved health.

The individual's or group's beliefs about health and illness must be understood if one is to design interventions that are likely to impact their health behavior. Their definition of health, their perceptions of the importance of health states and commonly used healthcare practices, and traditional practitioners are important to determine and incorporate in their plan of care. These values influence both recommendations and patient decisions. Failure to consider these patient preferences or practicing primarily from a medical model value system leads to "unintentional biasing" toward a professionals' view of the world (Kitson 2002). It is critical to assure that the users of the knowledge, the patients, become "active shapers" of knowledge and action (Clough 2005). Clinicians must be prepared to make "real-time" adjustments to their approach to care based on patient feedback.

When designing counseling and prevention programs for communities and populations, it is important to understand that best practices do not automatically translate intact across cultural lines (Giihert, Harvey, and Belgrave 2009). What is effective in an African American community will likely not fit in an Arab or Mexican community. *Cultural translation,* adapting evidence-based guidelines or best practice to be congruent with selected populations of interest is required (Purnell and Salmond 2013).

Integrating patient values and beliefs requires attention to ethnocultural factors, such as beliefs, values, language, traditions, common healthcare practices used, and traditional practitioners. Developing a relationship with the patient; listening to the patient's expectations, concerns, and beliefs; and informing the patient of the evidence is the beginning of establishing trust and making the patient central to the decision-making process. In shared decision-making, the healthcare provider contributes technical expertise while the patient is the expert on his or her own needs, situations, and preferences. Bringing the two together advances the goal of the decision-making process to match care with patient preferences and to shift the locus of decision-making from solely the healthcare provider towards the patient (Johnson, Kim, and Church 2010).

Shared decision-making is called for when there is no clearly indicated "best" therapeutic option or in preference-sensitive situations or situations where the best choice depends on the patients' values or their preferences for the benefits, harms, and scientific uncertainties of each option (Godolphin 2009). Examples of preference-sensitive situations include the following:

1. Should I take herbal and traditional therapies with professional prescriptions?
2. Should I see traditional practitioners along with Western practitioners?

Healthcare providers need to partake in shared decision making with all patients and be willing to discuss options congruent with culture.

Evidence-based patient decision aids (PtDAs) have been developed (Godolphin 2009). They aid people in making specific and deliberative choices among options by providing information about the options and outcomes that are relevant to a person's health status. In randomized trials, PtDAs improved patient knowledge, improved the proportion of patients with realistic perceptions of the chances of benefits and risks, reduced decisional conflict/uncertainty, and prevented overuse of options that informed patients do not value (O'Connor et al. 2004). They are different from traditional patient education material because they present balanced, personalized information about options in enough detail and in appropriate language for patients to make informed judgments about the personal value of the options (O'Connor et al. 2007). They are designed to complement rather than replace counseling from a healthcare provider.

Clinical Context

The clinical context encompasses the setting in which practice takes place or the environment in which the proposed change is to be implemented. Drennan (1992) argues that culture, or "the way things are done around here" at the individual, team, and organizational levels creates the context for practice and change. Organizational culture is a paradigm and has its own belief system, paradigms, customs, and language. The medical culture values objectivity, cause and effect, biophysical care, and, in many cases, the power of their own expertise and status. These cultures may be resistant to new paradigms calling for evidence-based practice. Additionally these values may be in opposition to patient values, creating clashes between providers and patients often resulting in patients being "non-compliant."

Currently a largely unexplored disparity exists between the beliefs and expectations of healthcare providers and patients, particularly when there is also a disparity between the cultures/ethnicity of the two (Enarson and Ait-Khaled 1999, Walker et al. 2005). Viewing biomedicine as a culture in itself, such that interactions between patients and healthcare providers become a communication between cultures or transactions between worldviews, appears to be a necessary process in establishing a trusting and effective partnership and thus improving the health outcomes of patients.

The clinical context also includes the environment in which health behaviors are enacted and includes the traditional healthcare organizational setting, the home, residential care setting, the neighborhood, and the broader community. However, evidence on which interventions work in specific contexts is not readily available.

Clearly more research is needed that focuses on the contextual realities of implementation. It is believed that better attention to context will result in testable approaches to facilitate translating knowledge into action in real world settings. Innovative approaches have been developed and can serve as models for clinicians. Three examples include: the CDC's DEBI (Diffusion of Effective Behavioral Interventions, 2001) project, the RE-AIM framework, and the HealthCare Innovations Exchange.

The abundance of new evidence that has *not* been successfully translated into practice is a critical reminder of the importance of context and the strength of the existing culture. Difficult questions need to be grappled with. What should be done with clinicians who cannot or will not adapt to EBP? How will lack of interdisciplinary collaboration be approached? How will it be handled if long-standing treatment approaches show no evidence of fostering improvement? What is the individual's responsibility, as compared with the organization's and community's responsibility, in assuring readiness for EBP? What are the best approaches for facilitating knowledge translation in different contexts? Knowing the answer to some of these questions will influence outcomes of getting knowledge into practice (Purnell and Salmond 2013).

Conclusion

Culture embodies a way of living, a worldview targeting our beliefs about human nature; interpersonal relationships; relationships of people to nature, time or the temporal focus of life; and ways of living one's life (activity). Providers armed with culture-general knowledge are more open to multiple ways of being; culture-general knowledge serves as a framework for building culture-specific knowledge. Understanding factors that an individual from one cultural group perceives to lead to different types of illnesses and the culture-specific remedies to treat the illness are important to understand.

Given the complexity of the multicultural mosaic in which we live, healthcare providers are in a unique position to decrease disparities and improve the overall health of our citizens. To accomplish this, providers need to (a) be open and comfortable with cultural encounters, (b) use a framework/model for cultural assessment of each client, family or group, (c) critically reflect on their own cultures to decrease ethnocentrism and stereotyping, (d) learn as much as possible about the aggregate variant cultural characteristics of the populations they care for, and (e) employ the four components of evidence-based practice. Through these avenues, patient and provider satisfaction with care will increase. Being familiar with individualistic and collectivistic cultural attributes is one method to learn about cultures from a broad perspective. Healthcare providers will always come across patients from cultures with which they are not familiar. Combining knowledge of a cultural model and individualistic and collectivistic cultural attributes is a good starting point for an assessment.

References

Agency for Healthcare Research and Quality. 2012. "A to Z Guide." http://www.ahrq.gov/clinic/epcquick.htm#Mtopics

CASP International. 2012. www.caspinternational.org/

CDC Health Disparities and Inequalities Report. 2011. http://www.cdc.gov/mmwr/pdf/other/su6001.pdf

Clarke, L., and L. Hofsess. 1998. "Acculturation." In *Handbook of Immigrant Health*, edited by S. Loue, 37–59. New York, NY: Plenum Press.

Clough, E. 2005. "Foreword." In *Researching Health Care Consumers, Critical Approaches*, ix–xi. Basingstoke, UK: Palgrave (MacMillan).

Colin, J. and G. Paperwalla. 2013. "People of Haitian Heritage." In *Transcultural Health Care: A Culturally Competent Approach*, edited by L. Purnell and B. Paulanka. Philadelphia: F.A. Davis.

Drennan, D. 1992. *Transforming Company Culture.* London: McGraw-Hill.

Enarson, D.A., N. Ait-Khaled. 1999. "Cultural Barriers to Asthma Management." *Pediatric Pulmonology* 28: 297–300.

Evidence-Based Medicine. 2011. BMJ Publishing Group Ltd. http://ebn.bmj.com/

Evidence-Based Mental Health. 2012. BMJ Publishing Group Ltd. http://ebn.bmj.com/

Evidence-Based Nursing. 2012. BMJ Publishing Group Ltd. http://ebn.bmj.com/

Family Health International. 2010. "Evidence-Based Guidelines for Youth Peer Education." http://www.fhi.org/NR/rdonlyres/einc2hb5no52blspygp6gksckcgdvpa6b76gfevo7k537fzyc53zrangjrhxisliwsagwqjeju7kfn/peeredguidelines.pdf

Fisher, T.L., D. L. Burnet, E. S. Huang, T. L. Chin, and K. A. Cagney. 2007. "Cultural Leverage: Interventions Using Culture to Narrow Racial Disparities in Health Care." *Medical Care Research Review* 64(5 suppl.): 243S–282S.

Foggs, M.B. 2008. "Guidelines Management of Asthma in a Busy Urban Practice." *Current Opinions in Pulmonary Medicine* 14(1): 46–56.

Giger, J., R. Davidhizar, L. Purnell, J. Taylor Harden, J. Phillips, and O. Strickland. 2007. "American Academy of Nursing Expert Panel Report: Developing Cultural Competence to Eliminate Health Disparities in Ethnic Minorities and Other Vulnerable Populations." *Journal of Transcultural Nursing* 18(2): 95–102.

Giihert, D.J., Á. R. Harvey, and F. Z. Belgrave. 2009. "Advancing the Africentric Paradigm Shift Discourse: Building Toward Evidence-Based Africentric Interventions in Social Work Practice with African Americans." *Social Work* 54(1): 243–252.

Godolphin, W. 2009. "Shared Decision Making." *Healthcare Quality* 12: 186–190.

Goffman, K., and D. Joy. 2006. *Counterculture through the Ages.* NY: Random House and Villard Books.

Gray, B. 1998. "Sources Used in Health Policy Research and Implications for Information Retrieval Systems." *Journal of Urban Health* 75(4): 842–852.

Grey Literature Report. New York Academy of Medicine. 2011. http://www.nyam.org/library/online-resources/grey-literature-report/

Haynes, R. B. 2006. "Of Studies, Syntheses, Synopses, Summaries and Systems: The '5S' Evolution of Information Services for Evidence-Based Health Care Decisions." *American College of Physicians (ACP) Journal Club* 145(3): A8-A9.

Healthy People 2020. 2012. www.healthpeople.gov/

Hofstede, G. 1991. *Cultures and Organizations: Software of the Mind.* NY: McGraw-Hill.

Hofstede, G. 2001. *Culture's Consequences: Comparing Values, Behaviors, Institutions, and Organizations across Nations* (2nd ed.). Thousand Oaks, CA: Sage.

Hofstede, G. and J. Hofstede. 2005. *Cultures and Organizations: Software of the Mind* (2nd ed.). New York, NY: McGraw-Hill.

Hulme, P. A. 2010. "Cultural Considerations in Evidence-Based Practice." *Journal of Transcultural Nursing* 21(3): 271–280.

Institute of Medicine. 2012. www.iom.edu/

International Journal of Evidence Based Healthcare. 2011.Wiley-Blackwell. http://www.wiley.com/bw/journal.asp?ref=1744-1595

Johnson, S. L., Y. W. Kim, K. Church. 2010. "Towards Patient-Centered Counseling: Development and Testing of the WHO Decision-Making Tool." *Patient Education and Counseling 81*: 355–361.

Joint Commission. 2010. "Advancing Effective Communication, Cultural Competence, and Patient and Family Centered Care: A Roadmap for Hospitals." http://www.jointcommission.org/assets/1/6/aroadmapforhospitalsfinalversion727.pdf

Kaplan, J. E., C. Benson, K. H. Holmes, J. T. Brooks, A. Pau, H. Masur. 2009. "Centers for Disease Control and Prevention (CDC), National Institutes of Health, HIV Medicine Association of the Infectious Diseases Society of America. Guidelines for Prevention and Treatment of Opportunistic Infections in HIV-Infected Adults and Adolescents: Recommendations from CDC, the National Institutes of Health, and the HIV Medicine Association of the Infectious Diseases Society of America." *MMWR Recommendation Report 10*(58) (RR-4): 1–207.

Kitson, A. 2002. "Recognizing Relationships: Reflections on Evidence-Based Practice." *Nursing Inquiry 9*(3): 179–186.

Koffman, J. 2006. "Transcultural and Ethical Issues at the End of Life." In *Stepping into Palliative Care,* edited by J. Cooper, 171–186. Abington, UK: Radcliffe Publishing Ltd.

Leininger, M. 1991. Madeleine Leinger's Culture Care: Diversity and Universality Theory. In M. Leininger *Culture Care Diversity and Universality: A Worldwide Nursing Theory.* Sudbury, MA: Jones & Bartlett.

Leininger, M. and M. McFarland. 2006. *Culture Care Diversity and Universality: A Worldwide Theory.* CT: Jones and Bartlett.

McCormack, B., A. Kitson, G. Harvey, J. Rycroft-Malone, A. Titchen, and K. Seers. 2002. "Getting Evidence into Practice: The Meaning of 'Context.'" *Journal of Advanced Nursing 38*(1): 94–104.

McMurray, A. 2004. "Culturally Sensitive Evidence-Based Practice." *Collegian* 11: 14–18.

Melnyk, B. M, E. Fineout-Overholt, S. B. Stillwell, and K. M. Williamson. 2009. "Igniting a Spirit of Inquiry: An Essential Foundation for Evidence-Based Practice." *American Journal of Nursing 109*(11): 49–52.

Mosley, C. 2009. "Evidence-Based Medicine: The Dark Side." *Journal of Pediatric Orthopedics* 29(8): 839–843.

National Assessment of Adult Literacy. 2003. http://nces.ed.gov/naal/.

New World Encyclopedia. 2006. Murdock, George Peter. http://www.new worldencyclopedia.org/entry/George_Peter_Murdock

Nursing Council New Zealand. 2008. Guidelines for Cultural Safety. http://www .nursingcouncil.org.nz/index.cfm/1,54,0,0,html/Guidelines

O'Connor, A. M., H. A. Llewellyn-Thomas, and A. B. Flood. 2004. "Modifying Unwarranted Variations in Health Care: Shared Decision Making Using Patient Decision Aids." *Health Affairs* 23(11): 63–72. http://content.healthaffairs.org/ content/early/2004/10/07/hlthaff.var.63.citation.

O'Connor, A. M., J. E. Wennberg, F. Legare, H. A. Llewellyn-Thomas, B. W. Mouton, K. R. Sepucha, A. G. Sodano, J. S. and King. 2007. "Toward the 'Tipping Point': Decision Aids and Informed Patient Choice." *Health Affairs* 26(3): 716–725.

O'Connor, A.M., D. Stacey, V. Entwistle, H. Llewellyn-Thomas, D. Rovner, M. Holmes-Rovner, V. Tait, J. Tetroe, V. Fiset, M. Barry, and J. Jones. 2004. "Decision Aids for People Facing Health Treatment or Screening Decisions." *Cochrane Review, Issue 1.* Chichester, UK: John Wiley and Sons, Ltd.

Portes, A. 2007. "Migration, Development and Segmented Assimilation: A Conceptual Review of Evidence." *Annals of American Academy of Political and Social Science 610*: 73–97.

Purnell, L. 2001. "Cultural Competence in a Changing Health-Care Environment." In *The Nursing Profession: Tomorrow and Beyond,* edited by N. L. Chaska, 451–461. Thousand Oaks, CA: Sage Publications.

Purnell, L. 2010. "Cultural Rituals in Health and Nursing Care." In *Diversiteit in de Verpleeg-kunde [Diversity in Nursing],* edited by P. Esterhuizen and A. Kuckert, 130–196. Amsterdam: Bohn Stafleu van Loghum.

Purnell, L. 2009. *Guide to Culturally Competent Health Care.* Philadelphia: F.A. Davis.

Purnell, L. 2011a. "The Purnell Model for Cultural Competence." In *Interventions in Mental Health – Substance Use,* edited by D. B. Cooper, 29–50. NY: Radcliffe Publishing.

Purnell, L. 2011b. "The Purnell Model for Cultural Competence." In *Application of Transcultural Theory to Mental – Substance Use in an International Context,* edited by D. B. Cooper, 51–68. NY: Radcliffe Publishing.

Purnell, L. 2012. "Application of Transcultural Theory to Practice." In *Palliative Care within Severe Mental Health,* edited by D. Cooper and J. Cooper. London: Radcliffe Publishing.

Purnell, L. 2013. *Transcultural Health Care: A Culturally Competent Approach* (4th ed). Philadelphia: F. A. Davis Co.

Purnell, L. and J. Paulanka. 1998. "Transcultural Diversity and Health Care." In *Transcultural Health Care: A Culturally Competent Approach,* edited by L. Purnell and B. Paulanka, 1–7. Philadelphia: F.A. Davis Co.

Purnell, L. and S. Salmond. 2013. "Individual Cultural Competence and Evi-dence-Based Practice." In *Transcultural Health Care: A Culturally Competent Ap-proach,* edited by L. Purnell, 45–60. Philadelphia: F. A. Davis Co.

Robert Wood Johnson Foundation. 2012. www.rwjf.org/

Rycroft-Malone, J., K. Seers, A. Titchen, G. Harvey, A. Kitson, and B. McCormack. 2004. What Counts as Evidence in Evidence-Based Practices. *Journal of Advanced Nursing* 47(1): 81–90.

Sackett, D. 2000. *Evidence-Based Medicine: How to Practice and Teach EB.* Amsterdam, The Netherlands: Churchill Livingstone.

Salmond, S. 2007. "Advancing Evidence-Based Practice: A Primer." *Orthopaedic Nursing* 26(2): 114–123.

Shah, H.M. and K. C. Chung. 2009. "Archie Cochrane and His Vision for Evidence-Based Medicine." *Plastic and Reconstructive Surgery* 124(3): 982–988.

Swanson, J. A., D. Schmitz, and K.C. Chung. 2010. "How to Practice Evidence-Based Medicine." *Plastic and Reconstructive Surgery* 126(1): 286–294.

Trevalon, M. and J. Murray-Garcia. 1998. "Cultural Humility Versus Cultural Competence." *Journal of Health Care for the Poor and Underserved* 9(2): 117–125.

Universal Declaration of Human Rights. 2001. www.un.org/en/documents/udhr/

U.S. Department of Health and Human Services: Office of Minority Health. 2011. "National Standards on Culturally and Linguistically Appropriate Services." http://minorityhealth.hhs.gov/templates/browse.aspx?lvl=2andlvlID=15.

U.S. Department of Health and Human Services: Office of Minority Health. 2011. "Think Cultural Health." https://www.thinkculturalhealth.hhs.gov/

Walker, C., A. Weeks, B. McAvoy, E. Demetriou. 2005. "Exploring the Role of Self-Management Programs in Caring for People from Culturally and Linguistically Diverse Backgrounds in Melbourne, Australia." *Health Expect* 8: 315–323.

WHO/PAHO. 2010. *Culture and Mental Health in Haiti: A Literature Review.* Geneva: WHO. http://www.who.int/mental_health/emergencies/culture_mental_health_haiti_eng.pdf

CHAPTER TWO

The Complexity of Culture: Culture's Impact on Health Disparities

Lauren Brinkley-Rubinstein
and Abbey Mann

There has been increasing awareness of the macro and micro structures that affect health and exacerbate health disparities. Health disparities are "differences in health outcomes between groups that reflect social inequalities" (Frieden 2011, 3). Culture, while an often explicitly acknowledged contributor to many facets of social and personal life, has been overlooked as an important factor contributing to health or the lack thereof. While the exact definition is debated, it is popularly defined as the shared beliefs and values among a specific group that have been "transmitted intergenerationally through child-rearing, folklore, art, interpersonal interactions, ceremonies, and the structure of community institutions" (Trickett 2009, 257). However, increasing levels of globalization and immigration have led to a more complex meaning of culture and changed the many ways in which it can manifest (Trickett 2009).

Additionally, the cultural norms that permeate the social structures in society are defined by the dominant classes (Bourdieu 1984). Patricia Hill Collins (2006) further conceptualizes culture as a political space in which social inequities are reproduced. Therefore, adhering to the dominant classes' conceptualizations of culture is marginalizing to those outside the ruling majority group. This means that cultural milieus that are beyond that of dominant norms lead to inequality and can exacerbate health inequality within vulnerable groups.

Therefore, culture affects health disparities via mechanisms particular to marginalization caused by not conforming to dominant ideologies. These mechanisms can take the form of culturally-infused customs such as methods of communication, doctor-patient relationships, the experience of illness, and individual health care outcomes or access to health care services. Thus, in this chapter we will briefly examine the health disparities that affect immigrant and minority populations, provide a theoretical and empirical background relevant to intersectionality and social ecological frameworks, and illustrate how the blending of a social ecological and intersectional approach may guide interventions, practical programmatic application, and research efforts that seek to stem immigrant health disparities.

Immigrant Health Disparities

Minorities and immigrant populations, or those who do not represent groups that largely determine cultural norms, often bear a disproportionate burden of disease. Additionally, from 1990 to 2000 the number of individuals living in the United States who were foreign born has increased exponentially and is now 36 million (Derose et al. 2009). Certain immigrant populations suffer a higher incidence of depression and other mental health illnesses, have higher cancer mortality rates, and experience a decrease in health status in each generation (Kim et al. 2005). Research has explored the underlying macro and micro causes for the exacerbation of disease within minority and immigrant populations. The mechanisms by which health disparities are exacerbated for immigrant groups fall into four major categories: concentrated disadvantage, policy level changes, quality of care, and access to care.

Concentrated Disadvantage

In comparison to other groups, immigrants have disproportionately low levels of education and lower levels of income than native-born populations. Abundant research in this area has demonstrated the link between low socioeconomic status and poorer health outcomes. For immigrant populations, lower levels of education and income leads to lack of access to and availability of healthcare and is often compounded by other barriers to health care access and quality of healthcare once connected to a healthcare provider. These barriers include acculturation, linguistic barriers, and fear of deportation (Elder 2003). Cultural and language barriers may lead to subpar health care, due to limited ability of the medical provider to comprehend the patient and the symptoms they are experiencing, and, subsequently, produce an untenable progression of treatment from the patient's perception (Waddell 1998). Additionally, undocumented immigrants may obtain less health care than actually needed due to restricted access or due to distress surrounding the possibility of deportation (Siddharthan and Ahern 1996).

Access to Care

Decreased access to care due to unavailability of healthcare insurance has been consistently shown to be a salient issue for immigrant populations. Additionally, children born in the United States who come from low income families and who have a non-citizen parent are significantly less likely to have health insurance (Alker 2004, Ku and Matani 2001, Waidmann and Rajan 2000). However, there are distinct differences in health insurance rates between certain immigrant groups and there are also important within-group disparities for most immigrant populations. For instance, immigrants from Western Europe often have much higher rates of health insurance than individuals who migrated from Latin America. In addition, elderly populations and those who migrated within the last five years are much more likely to lack healthcare insurance (Carrasquillo, Carrasquillo, and Shea 2000).

Quality of Care

Healthcare quality also acts as a mechanism via which immigrant health is negatively affected. Foreign born populations report receiving a low level of care and being less satisfied with their healthcare as compared to their U.S.-born counterparts (Lasser, Himmelstein, and Woolhandler 2006). Exploration into why immigrants report being less satisfied with their healthcare has revealed that patient-physician relationship, communication and language barriers, and provider discrimination often undergird and predict higher levels of dissatisfaction (Lasser, Himmelstein, and Woolhandler 2006).

Policy Level Changes

Policy reform resulting from the Personal Responsibility and Work Opportunity Reconciliation Act of 1996 (PRWORA) also has negatively affected immigrants' eligibility for public insurance programs (e.g. Medicaid) and ability to access affordable care via legislation that limits their ability to utilize healthcare services. Previous research has found that PRWORA is correlated with a significant number of immigrants losing access to public insurance that has led to a restriction of immigrants' access to routinized healthcare and has led to less immigrant populations seeking care. Additionally, PRWORA affected different individuals more or less severely. PRWORA has disproportionately affected foreign-born individuals who also fall into the following categories: those with less education, single women (when compared with U.S.-born single women), and single immigrant mothers (Kaushal and Kaestner 2007). Researchers have also investigated the individual level effects of the policy and have found that its enactment led to fear and alienation among immigrant populations and, subsequently, led to a decreased enrollment in safety net programs whose main aim is to cover individuals who are the most likely to have gaps in healthcare access (Derose et al. 2009).

These policy, community, family, and individual-level differences within and among immigrant populations suggest a need to focus on strengthening interventions targeting individual-level change. Additionally, there is a need to also consider the intersection of multiple inequalities, in combination with a concentration on the policy level and environmental factors that affect certain marginalized populations. Furthermore, from a systems perspective, attention must be paid to the influence of culture on a macro-scale and how the societal conceptualization of culture affects an individual's construction of culture and its manifestations. Lastly, the interaction between individual and societal norms and productions of culture must be better understood in order to more comprehensively address the means through which culture intensifies health disparities.

An Intersectional Approach to Understanding the Implications of Culture on Health

Intersectional approaches seek to explain how social and cultural classifications interact to contribute to inequality (McCall 2005). These social categories can include gender, race, class, ability, and other axes upon which individuals build their identity. Additionally, intersectionality posits that these multiple forms of identity do not act independently of one another and instead compound increasing the risk of multiple macro and micro level inequalities and creating a system of oppression that mirrors the intersection of multiple forms of discrimination (Andersen and Collins 1998). According to Collins, *intersectionality* is a model describing the social structures that create social positions. Second, the notion of intersectionality describes micro-level processes—namely, how each individual and group occupies a social position within interlocking structures of oppression described by the metaphor of intersectionality. Together they shape oppression (1995, 492).Therefore, cultural tapestries of oppression are not only interrelated but compound and impacted by the intersectional systems that make up a neighborhood, a community or a society as a whole (Collins 2000).

Intersectional theory was spurred into existence formerly via the feminist movement of the late 1960s and was led, primarily, by women of color (Collins 2000, Hooks 1984). One of the main tenets of the movement was that women's lived realities and experiences of oppression were not homogeneous and instead impacted women differently. For example, white, middle class women experienced different forms of oppression than their black, poor, or disabled counterparts. Therefore, a cornerstone of intersectional theory is understanding the ways in which race, class, gender, and other attributes on which individuals build their identities interconnect and combine to impact well-being (McCall 2005). This compounding effect suggests that an individual's social location is impacted by incongruent, multiple forms of oppression that combine to highlight experience (Collins 1990, Berger 2004).

Intersectional theorists, while paying close attention to the impact of race, class, and gender, have also examined the intersection of other forms such as labor, violence, and parenthood. Intersectional theory has been used in recent years as a viable alternative to either/or approaches (Berger 2004). Viewing inequality as multiplicative rather than additive (as is the case with binary approaches) allows one to understand how multiple types of oppression and occupying many overlapping social positions can simultaneously affect individuals positively or negatively (Collins 1990, Berger 2004, Stephens 1994). Therefore, intersectionality is important to understanding the ways in which immigrant populations are subject to health disparities in that it attempts to address the experiences of those who are subjected to multiple forms of oppression within a particular society including health-related issues such as health care access and quality of care received.

Anchored by Bourdieu's (1984) and Collins's (2006) conceptualization of culture, theories of intersectionality are rooted in feminist traditions that stress the importance of the interaction of multiple inequalities. Due to the inherently entangled essence of inequity, multiple inequalities interact with and augment one another (Veenstra 2011). This leads to a compounded experience of inequality in which one form cannot be disentangled from another and emphasizes the power structures that create roles of domination and subordination (Rogers and Kelly 2011, Veenstra 2011). Individuals who experience multiple forms of domination are marginal-ized in all aspects of society, including health status and the delivery of health care (Rogers and Kelly 2011). Thus, it is important to understand the influence of the interaction of these characteristics and inequalities, and how this manifests at the individual level, in order to understand the true impact of culture on individual health and on the exacerbation of health disparities.

Intersectionality and Health

Increasingly in health research, intersectional frameworks have been used in the analysis of the compounding effects of marginalization. In addition, researchers have conceptualized models of intersection that also include quantifiable inequalities such as poverty, stigma, lack of education and, most importantly, culture. Research has been conducted that specifically examines the impact of intersectionality on many facets of health. For instance, Veenstra (2011) investigated the intersection of race, gender, class, sexual orientation, and self-rated health and found that intersectionality was a suitable framework to use to better understand health disparities. Additionally, research on harm reduction strategies found that individuals seeking mental health and substance abuse treatment were likely to have a number of compounding social determinants of drug use. These findings stressed the intersectional nature of historical, socio-cultural, and political forces that impact mental illness and substance use and abuse and suggest the need for intersectional approaches to harm reduction (Smye et al. 2011). Furthermore, attempts have been made to integrate intersectional and biomedical approaches to understanding and eliminating health disparities (Kelly 2009). An intersectional approach to health disparities research also adheres to and may expand upon the principles of autonomy, beneficence, non-maleficence, and justice which are foundational ethical values in health related research and service delivery (Rogers and Kelly 2011).

Intersectional approaches stress the multiplicity of inequality rather than the additive effect. This is key to understanding how inequality compounds to affect health of especially vulnerable groups. Therefore, research considering health disparities or health care approaches specifically designed for multicultural or immigrant groups must take into consideration the accumulation of multiple inequalities that result from macro-level and micro-level cultural differences that lead to marginalization and negatively affect health. Health disparities that disparately affect immigrant groups are often a result of exposure to negative social conditions that have a deleterious effect on health. Immigrant groups are often subjected to substandard housing, decreased access to transportation, and decreased access to federal, state, and local subsidies; they often have decreased educational opportunities and increased exposure to violence and victimization (Tillet 2006, Mermin 2006) In addition, immigrants find themselves at the axis of multiple non-dominant intersections such as lack of English language proficiency which may, in turn, impact the ability to access healthcare and, once healthcare access is attained, the quality of care received. Thus, social norms of the privileged (those who are white, male, middle class) become the accepted normative standard bearers for marginalized groups such as immigrants (Johnson 2006, Kendall 2006). These social norms are reflected in healthcare, health interventions and programs aimed at improving health outcomes. Therefore, culturally sensitive, multidimensional programs and approaches are needed for immigrant populations. However, to fully understand the implications of culture on the intensification of health disparities, the inclusion of social ecological perspectives on the impact of culture must be examined.

A Social Ecological Approach to Understanding Health Disparities

Social ecological models of health have a focus extending beyond individuals, taking a crucial stance that shifts responsibility for reducing health inequalities away from individuals onto the environmental factors and systems in which they are situated. In addition, social ecological models provide complex, comprehensive, and multi-level contexts for describing and explaining the mechanisms involved in creating health disparities. These models explicitly focus on environmental factors that influence health rather than individuals' behavior and characteristics. Using social ecological models to analyze health disparities can illuminate the ways in which multiple levels act and interact within a system to result in asymmetrical health outcomes among groups.

In 1979, Urie Bronfenbrenner put forth a theory of human development that used an ecological framework to better understand the systems in which humans exist, the factors at each level of those systems, and the ways in which the levels and factors interact and affect the individual of interest.

In recent years, several authors have created social ecological models that specifically address health outcomes, many of which explicitly include culture. Daniel Stokols (1992) elaborated a model for health promotion that included cultural influences on health such as religious practices, health messages in the media, and access to health care and health insurance. McLeroy et al. (1988) addressed the way that power dynamics within a community can operate in a way that fails to direct resources towards those with the poorest health outcomes. Deborah Cohen and colleagues (2000) outlined a health behavior model that includes social structures, such as policy and legal influences on health, in addition to cultural and media influences, such as health-related news and media messages. Each of these authors adds to our increasingly sophisticated understanding of the multi-level cultural mechanisms affecting health disparities and contributes to the compelling case for the inclusion of cultural factors in empirical work addressing these disparities.

Despite inherent challenges in testing complex and comprehensive models, several researchers have employed multi-level models to examine cultural factors at work in disparities in poor birth outcomes (Alio et al. 2010, Aronson et al 2007, Koenen, Lincoln, and Appleton 2006) reproductive health (Reeve and Basalik 2011), inequality in access to dental care (Kim 2005), discrepancies in nutritional outcomes (Robinson 2008), and other health disparities. This research makes apparent a need for a consistent set of operational definitions of cultural influences on health, as well as larger scale, longitudinal research on the multi-level cultural mechanisms that contribute to pervasive and obstinate health disparities.

Theoretical Approaches to Understanding Health Disparities: A Long History of the Use of Ecological Frameworks

In *The Ecology of Human Development* (1979), a seminal text on ecological models, Urie Bronfenbrenner defines four levels of environmental settings in which we exist. The microsystem, the mesosystem, the exosystem, and the macrosystem are nested within one another "like a set of Russian dolls" (Bronfenbrenner 1979, 3). Bronfenbrenner's logic about a multisystem, time-sensitive approach can, and has been, applied to health research. There is a preponderance of research that seeks to isolate variables within systems of health in the hope of finding a statistically significant tie among factors. If x causes y, while holding a though m constant, than changing x will help us tackle the all-important problem y. Although this may be true, as Bronfenbrenner notes in *The Ecology of Human Development*, a truly comprehensive study of x and y (taking a through m into account, of course), must include an understanding of x and y in the microsystem, x and y in the mesosystem, x and y in the exosystem, and macrosystem implications for x and y. Employing approaches from a number of fields (including Public Health, Epidemiology, Anthropology, Sociology, and Psychology) can shed light on a number of important factors within, across, and among these systems.

Bronfenbrenner's framework is not the only relevant theoretical approach in this context as a number of ecological models have been applied to a number of health issues. All of these models explicitly or implicitly include cultural influences on health and health behaviors. Most models include individual-level factors and structural factors that affect health as well as a conceptualization of interactions among factors and levels. What ecological models provide, in a unique way, is a shift in focus to the influence of structural and environmental factors *in addition* to individual level-factors. Models that focus only on the individual can result in theoretical frameworks that place responsibility, and possibly even blame, on the person with poor health outcomes. Disregarding the influence of numerous culturally-bound factors on health status paints an incomplete and erroneous picture of the causes of health and mental health issues, and can lead to the development of ineffective or even harmful interventions. However, researchers and practitioners must also beware of interventional approaches that focus primarily on top-down solutions, which can result in paternalism rather than coming to a consensus with a community in which a health need exists (McLeroy et al. 1988).

In recent years, a number of authors have described ecological models of health, outlining ways in which individuals interact with their environments to produce certain health outcomes. Many of these models go beyond the concentric circles framework to reflect and attempt to explain complex relationships among individuals, families, communities, and cultures. Stokols (1992) outlined essential assumptions and elements integral to creating a social ecological model of health promotion that takes into account the complex and multifaceted relationship between the environment and health outcomes. The author explicitly stated that the goal of his focus on the role of the environment in health promotion was to shift responsibility away from individual behaviors. In addition, he explained important assumptions of environments and social ecological models of health. Among them were that health is influenced by environmental, social, behavioral, and biological factors simultaneously in a complex and dynamic way; environments themselves are complex and can be described in many different ways; environments can be examined on many different levels (e.g. individuals, groups, communities, or cultures); and lastly, environmental factors at different levels influence one another simultaneously and it is important to take their interdependence into account. Stokols noted that a truly comprehensive ecological model of health promotion must be interdisciplinary. Not only, he pointed out, do different disciplines tend to focus on different levels, but they take different factors into account at various levels. Stokols' all-encompassing set of guidelines for a thorough ecological approach to health promotion set a high standard for thoughtful practitioners and researchers striving to include an ecological approach in research or interventions.

Hancock (1993) proposed three models of health, human develop-ment, and the social ecosystem, including a model of sustainable health in the community which focuses on the community, the environment, and the economy. The community, Hancock posits, needs to be convivial, while the environment needs to be viable, and the economy must be ade-quate. Furthermore, in this model, each of these three spheres overlaps with the other two. At the intersection of community and environment is the built environment, which the author suggests needs to be livable. At the intersection of community and economy is the ideal that economic wealth be evenly distributed in the economy. Finally, the in-shared space between economy and environment is sustainability. Hancock's model stressed a broad, holistic approach to understanding the impact of the social ecosystem on health, rather than explicitly identifying separate lev-els of influence on individuals or community health itself. The dynamic and complex relationships that exist among the intersecting influences and disciplines of community, economy, and environment can operate and intersect at different levels.

Authors have taken varied approaches to depicting the multidimen-sional characteristics of social ecological models of health, however, one that differs significantly from the traditional concentric-and-overlapping-circle approach is The Hoop and the Tree framework (Hoffman 1998). The author imagined two axes: the horizontal axis—the hoop—representing relationships between persons and the environment, and the vertical axis—the tree—representing development over time. Though Hoffman did write about the relationship between the tree and general health, the metaphor serves more saliently as a model for development of a healthy person which relied heavily on one's environment and psychological well-being. This model is unique due to its focus on form rather than defini-tions of model elements and breaks from the traditional ecological form. The hoop and tree can each take on different psychological, developmen-tal, and environmental factors, but the form remains constant.

One group of researchers with a more practical approach to examining the environment's impact on the health-related behaviors of individuals identified four distinct but related structural factors (Cohen et al. 2000). The first of these factors is access to consumer goods that can have either positive or deleterious effects on one's health, such as healthful foods or firearms, cigarettes, or alcohol. Not only did the authors posit that access to these products will lead to higher rates on individuals using them, but that in communities in which there is greater access to these goods, using them becomes a normative behavior. The second factor the authors outlined was the quality and appearance of the built environment, which is often affected by decisions made at a policy level. A healthful built environment is evidenced by clean streets, adequate housing, green space, and other psychical structures that can have a positive effect on the health of groups and individuals. Another policy-level factor the authors cited was what they referred to as "social structure" or the presence of laws that pertain to individual health-related behaviors and their enforcement. Finally, the last of the four factors the authors examined was another macro-level factor: the influences of messages in the media that can affect the wellbeing of individuals through the creation of cultural norms.

This model of the relationship between individual or community health and structural or environmental factors is one that is more easily testable or applicable than some other social ecological models. Its focus is clearly limited to known and observable systems and phenomena that are known to have a direct impact on health outcomes, as opposed to some other models which take many more variables into account and strive to incorporate more of the complex relationship between individuals and multiple environmental factors.

The last decade has brought a more nuanced understanding of ecology and health. With growing focus on large-scale environmental changes and the growing obesity epidemic sweeping across the United States, scholars have begun to build upon the foundation laid by previous scholars and looked at not just practical implications of social ecological models, but expanded and shifted their scopes to include pertinent issues. One such model reflects the recent effects of globalization by expanding the definition of environment to include not just green space in the built environment, but the effects of current trends in recreation and tourism (Dustin, Bricker, and Schwab 2010). The authors suggest that the trend away from outdoor recreation in the United States is an important, multifaceted and environmentally-bound factor negatively influencing physical health status, citing not just a shift towards sedentary occupational habits, but a more urbanized and less active lifestyle driven by recent economic changes. The authors' focus on globalization, as well as their practical and interdisciplinary framework, builds on the work of former theorists connecting concentric and overlapping environmental factors to health outcomes and in line with more pragmatic and applicable models.

Social Ecological Models: From Theory to Practice

The challenge of applying these complex models has been undertaken by many researchers in recent years and has addressed a variety of multi-level issues. A focus on the practicality of applying social ecological models of health itself is the focus of recent literature. Four examples in which researchers applied ecological models to disparities in health outcomes are examined in the *Journal of Professional Nursing* (Reifsnider, Gallagher, and Forgione 2005). The authors focus on the ability of researchers to focus on particular pieces of models posed by theorists such as Bronfenbrenner, to isolate the influence of particular social ecological characteristics on health outcomes of both communities and individuals. They stress the importance of examining multiple factors of influence on health outcomes with a high prevalence among minority individuals and communities.

Research over the last decade has followed the developmental trajectory outlined in the current work and has begun to take a multi-level social ecological view into account in both examination of health outcomes and development and implementation of interventions. Recent studies have taken an ecological framework and applied it to examining the impact of sexual assault on women's mental health (Campbell, Dworkin, and Cabral 2009), increasing consumption of fruit and vegetables (Robinson 2008), examining disparities in birth outcomes (Alio et al. 2010), and how multiple systems within a hospital work together to affect outcomes in patient satisfaction (Moore, Wright, and Bernard 2009).

One rich illustration of the application of an ecological framework was performed by researchers who examined the use of substance abuse programs by adolescents who rely on Tennessee's Medicaid program (Jones, Heflinger, and Saunders 2007). Researchers apply a model, explicitly influenced by Bronfenbrenner, which includes broader social factors, community and service system characteristics, and individual factors as predictors of both service use and clinical outcomes. Using hierarchical linear modeling, an approach that is both well-suited for and popular in examination of multi-level predictors inherent in the application of ecological models, researchers were able to isolate the predictive values of independent factors at the community and individual level, revealing important information about service use that can inform practitioners and policy makers.

Health-related social ecological models' definitions of culture lie in cultural factors that influence health status. Culture is the setting, or is comprised of multiple settings in which health-influencing factors exist. Cultural norms at large both influence and are influenced by one another, at multiple levels, and work together to impact the health of individuals, families, neighborhoods, communities, societies, and the environment. The main challenge facing researchers today is not only how to define culture within ecological frameworks but how to go about examining pieces of these frameworks and putting them together to create a comprehensive picture of the many environmental and cultural factors influencing health at a given time.

Examining the Complex Impact of Culture: The Need for a Dynamic Ecological and Intersectional Strategy for Combatting Health Disparities

Those who belong to non-dominant groups and who are at the intersection of multiple inequalities are more likely to experience greater health disparities. Immigrant populations have a unique set of barriers that deleteriously affect their overall health, access to health care services, and the quality of care they receive (Mermin 2006). Additionally, theory and empirical literature demonstrate that macro-structural and ecological apparatuses including systems-level understandings of culture affect individual, group, and community health dynamics. Negative reactions to different cultural milieus as expressed by dominant groups can lead to oppression and can exacerbate health disparities experienced by vulnerable populations. Therefore, in order to properly prevent, address, and stem health disparities experienced by immigrant populations, a framework that combines intersectional and social ecological approaches is necessary.

There are some important distinctions between the two types of frameworks. Ecological theories implicitly touch on intersections among factors and levels, though not always explicitly, whereas intersectional models focus mainly in the relationships between factors, while not explicitly addressing levels. However, as mentioned previously, important health-related variables such as race, class, gender, ethnicity, and sexuality exist on multiple levels. Context makes a difference when considering these important categories. For example, one's experience of gender is not the same across contexts such as family, neighborhood, society. One's experience of race is also contextually based. Similarly, ethnicity, and nationality have cultural and contextual manifestations across settings that can act as a barrier of buffer to health care interventions. Therefore, an approach that takes both ecological and intersectional models into account is necessarily neither only top-down or bottom-up. Due to the focus of each of these frameworks on either the multi-level or the multi-faceted nature of health, an intervention that takes into account each framework cannot take into account both the individual and the structural apparatuses that may exacerbate or ameliorate health disparities.

Intersectional theories have their roots in feminist theory, standpoint, black feminist thought and sociological approaches to health that take into account population-level disparities in health outcomes. Social ecological models have their roots in ecology, psychology, systems theory, and environmental work. Both attend to the multi-faceted, mutli-level, and complex relationships among a wide range of factors that influence health. Immigrant populations are situated at the intersection of a number of factors associated with health status. In addition, social factors such as immigration policy, community economies, neighborhood characteristics and the built environment influence the health of immigrants in particular and specific ways.

A blended theoretical framework of intersectionality and social ecological perspectives should pay particular attention to the effect of culture on the (re)production of health disparities specifically for immigrant and minority populations. Additionally, multi-level, interdisciplinary interventions are necessary to address the various issues that affect health negatively. Multilevel, community-based, culturally-oriented interventions utilize the ecological impact on the neighborhood setting, demonstrate a guarantee to collaborative partnerships with organizations and groups that are invested in the local community, and provide an understanding of how interventions are positioned in and influenced by micro-level culture and context (Trickett 2009). Changes at the individual level may be challenging to sustain without also addressing the environmental context within which the individual resides (Campbell 2000; Campbell, Nair, and Maimane 2007). Multilevel interventions should answer the question of how to best create social environments that are the most supportive of sustaining individual-level change. Utilizing a multilevel approach encourages the development of programs and policies that are in line with community priorities and are responsive to both individuals and communities (Green, Daniel, and Novick, 2001). Multilevel interventions should include, integrate, and coordinate with community-based organizations that are currently providing services to individuals and create opportunities for individuals to utilize services that are outside of existing organizations and should be attuned to larger policy issues that affect individuals at the macro, meso, and micro level.

Additionally, public health entities alone cannot mediate the negative effect of social conditions on immigrant populations. Cross-sector collaboration is needed among various entities, agencies, and community-based organizations (Stokols 2006). These organizations may include those working on issues related to a number of social and medical issues such as refugee and immigration, housing, transportation, linguistics, legal services, criminal justice, and many others. Additionally, interventions should take into account the multiple intersections of identity and inequality that affect immigrant populations. A one-size-fits-all intervention that is targeted in general toward immigrant populations is unlikely to succeed due to the within-group differences regarding individual experiences and behaviors. Therefore, we posit that in order to best address the health disparities that affect immigrant

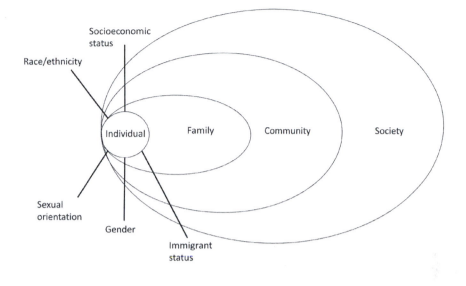

Figure 2.1   A Blended Model of Intersectionality and Social Ecology

populations, multilevel and multi-sector interventions that also address individual identity intersections must be used. Figure 2.1 above visually demonstrates the framework on which these interventions should be built.

Context makes a difference when considering the compounding intersections that people identify with and are affected by. For example, an individual's experience of gender is not the same across contexts such as family, neighborhood, society just as an individual's experience of "being an immigrant" is also contextually based. Race, ethnicity, and nationality have cultural and contextual implications across settings that can act as barriers to health care interventions that do not take cultural differences into account, further justifying the need for multilevel, ecologically based interventions that also focus on individual level intersections of identity and manifestations of inequality.

Practical Applications of This Approach

Creating effective interventions to address health disparities based on complex, culturally-competent, and comprehensive models poses some inherent challenges. It may be necessary in most instances to prioritize some elements of both the social ecological or intersectional models as well as the health issues that they are used to address.

Action-oriented and community-based participatory interventions and approaches may be effective avenues for the application of intersectional and social ecologically-influenced multilevel models. Social action oriented research and interventions focus on the inclusion of the community during the conception, design, and administration of intervention efforts, lend voice to individuals to determine which issues they think are the most pertinent to address, and enable communities to seek answers to their own solutions according to their own concerns (Cornwall and Jewkes 2010, Rahman and Fals-Borda 1991). With its focus on social, structural, and physical contributors to health disparities, participatory approaches in public health facilitate active involvement of community members, organizational representatives, and researchers (Israel et al. 2001). Engaging the community via participatory approaches can lead to more effective program implementation and design as well as inform relevant policy decisions that may minimize the impact of socially-determined, intersecting health disparities (Choudhry et al. 2002; Ganann 2012). Participatory action research approaches have increasingly been used to examine the social determinants of health, yielding critical insight into the development of interventions that are culturally relevant, and providing a meaningful approach to addressing immigrant health disparities (Savage et al. 2006). Additionally, research has shown that reduction in health disparities through participatory approaches fosters individual and community empowerment (Baum, MacDougall, and Smith 2006, Travers 1997). Thus, participatory, action oriented approaches that include researcher-community dialogue, collaborative data collection and analysis can lead to the creation and implementation of a plan of action to address community identified issues with the intention of improving conditions within communities (Craig 2009; Ozer, Ritterman, and Wanis 2010).

Holistic approaches to health intervention that are focused on the social determinants of wellbeing may also appropriately use the model characteristics put forth herein. These interventions should focus on the structural determinants that affect individuals on each level (micro, meso, and macro) and, thus, ideally must also be multidisciplinary and include partnerships across sectors. There must also be a focus on the ways in which these structural barriers manifest in intermediary psychosocial functioning and behaviors. These types of interventions may not be primarily intended to directly affect health and instead affect the social conditions that have been demonstrated to indirectly affect health such as the built environment, transportation, or urban planning.

Conclusion

Immigrant populations often experience a disproportionate burden of disease. Cultural norms defined by dominant groups permeate societal institutions informally and formally, negatively affect the medical and social service arena, and affect policy that results in limited access to health care services and resulting lack of quality care. Research has indicated that intersecting forms of identity and inequalities that manifest at the individual level can lead to negative health outcomes. These intersections of identity and inequality are further compounded by structural forms of inequality that affect the social conditions in which immigrant populations work and reside. In order to address and prevent further exacerbation of health disparities among immigrants, multilevel, multidisciplinary approaches must be used, blending frameworks that focus on the impact of the social environment and intersecting forms of identity and inequality, and the intermediary manifestation of structural conditions.

Participatory approaches and those that take a holistic view of health and incorporate cross sector partnerships provide avenues to apply the blended social ecological and intersectional frameworks. These types of approaches have been shown to increase individual empowerment and ameliorate the deleterious effects of traditional power dynamics that exist in traditional research-driven interventions by including and giving power to the affected population at every step of the intervention.

References

Alio, A. P., A. R. Richman, H. B. Clayton, D. F. Jeffers, D. J. Wathington, and H. M. Salihu. 2010. "An Ecological Approach to Understanding Black-White Disparities in Perinatal Mortality." *Maternal and Child Health Journal* 14(4): 557–566.

Alker, J.C. 2004. *Immigrants and Health Coverage: A Primer.* Washington, DC: Kaiser Commission on Medicaid and the Uninsured.

Andersen, M. L., and P. H. Collins. 1998. *Race, Class, and Gender: An Anthology* (3rd ed.). Belmont, CA: Wadsworth Pub. Co.

Aronson, R. E., A. B. Wallis, P. J. O'Campo, and P. Schafer. 2007. "Neighborhood Mapping and Evaluation: A Methodology for Participatory Community Health Initiatives." *Maternal and Child Health Journal* 11(4): 373–383.

Baum, F., C. MacDougall, and D. Smith. 2006. "Participatory Action Research." I *Journal of Epidemiology and Community Health* 60(10): 854–857.

Berger, M. T. 2004.*Workable Sisterhood: The Political Journey of Stigmatized Women with HIV/AIDS.* Princeton, N.J.: Princeton University Press.

Bourdieu, P. 1984. *Distinction: A Social Critique of the Judgement of Taste.* Cambridge, Mass.: Harvard University Press.

Campbell, C. 2000. "Selling Sex in the Time of AIDS: The Psycho-Social Context of Condom Use by Sex Workers in a Southern African Mine." *Social Science & Medicine* 50(4): 479–494.

Campbell, C., Y. Nair, and S. Maimane. 2007. "Building Contexts that Support Effective Community Responses to HIV/AIDS: A South African Case Study." *American Journal of Community Psychology* 39(3-4): 347–363.

Campbell, R., E. Dworkin, and G. Cabral. 2009. "An Ecological Model of the Impact of Sexual Assault on Women's Mental Health." *Trauma, Violence, and Abuse* 10(3): 225–246.

Carrasquillo, O., A. I. Carrasquillo, and S. Shea. 2000. "Health Insurance Coverage of Immigrants Living in the United States: Differences by Citizenship Status and Country of Origin." *American Journal of Public Health* 90(6): 917–923.

Choudhry, U. K., S. Jandu, J. Mahal, T. Singh, R., H. Sohi-Pabla, and B. Mutta. 2002. "Health Promotion and Participatory Action Research with South Asian Women." *Journal of Nursing Scholarship* 34(1): 75–81.

Cohen, D. A., R. A. Scribner, and T. A. Farley. 2000. "A Structural Model of Health Behavior: A Pragmatic Approach to Explain and Influence Health Behaviors at the Population Level." *Preventive Medicine: An International Journal Devoted to Practice and Theory* 30 (2): 146–154.

Collins, P. H. 1990. *Black Feminist Thought: Knowledge, Consciousness, and the Politics of Empowerment* (2nd ed.). New York: Routledge.

Collins, P. H. 2006. *From Black Power to Hip Hop: Racism, Nationalism, and Feminism.* Philadelphia: Temple University Press.

Cornwall, A., and R. Jewkes. 2010. "What is Participatory Research?" *Social Science & Medicine,* 41(12): 1667–1676.

Craig, D. V. 2009. *Action Research Essentials.* San Francisco: Josesy-Bass.

Derose, K. P., B. W. Bahney, N. Lurie, and J. J. Escarce. 2009. "Immigrants and Health Care Access, Quality, and Cost." *Medical Care Research and Review* 66(4): 355–408.

Dustin, D. L., K. S. Bricker, and K. A. Schwab. 2010. "People and Nature: Toward an Ecological Model of Health Promotion." *Leisure Sciences* 32(1): 3–14.

Elder, J. P. 2003. "Reaching out to America's Immigrants: Community Health Advisors and Health Communication." *American Journal of Health Behavior* 27 (Suppl. 3): S196–S205.

Frieden, T. R. 2011. "CDC Health Disparities and Inequalities Report—United States, 2011." *Morbidity and Mortality Weekly Report* 60: 3–4.

Ganann, R. 2013. "Opportunities and Challenges Associated with Engaging Immigrant Women in Participatory Action Research." *Journal of Immigrant and Minority Health* 15(2): 341.

Green, L., M. Daniel, and L. Novick. 2001. "Partnerships and Coalitions for Community-Based Research." *Public Health Reports* 116: 20–31.

Hancock, T. 1993. "Health, Human Development and the Community Ecosystem: Three Ecological Models." *Health Promotion International* 8(1): 41–47.

Hoff, E. 2003. "The Specificity of Environmental Influence: Socioeconomic Status Affects Early Vocabulary Development Via Maternal Speech." *Child Development* 74(5): 1368–1378.

Hoffman, C. 1998. "The Hoop and the Tree: An Ecological Model of Health." *The Humanistic Psychologist. Special Issue: Humanistic Psychology and Ecopsychology* 26(1-3): 123–154.

Hooks, B. 1984. *Feminist Theory from Margin to Center.* Boston, MA: South End Press.

Israel, B. A., A. J. Schulz, E. A. Parker, and A. B. Becker, A. B. 2001. "Community-Based Participatory Research: Policy Recommendations for Promoting a Partnership Approach in Health Research." *Education for Health: Change in Learning & Practice* 14(2): 182–197.

Johnson, A. G. 2006. *Privilege, Power, and Difference* (2nd ed.). Boston, Mass.: McGraw-Hill.

Jones, D. L., C. A. Heflinger, and R. C. Saunders, R. C. 2007. "The Ecology of Adolescent Substance Abuse Service Utilization." *American Journal of Community Psychology* 40(3-4): 345–358.

Kaushal, N., and R. Kaestner, R. 2007. "Welfare Reform and Health of Immigrant Women and Their Children." *Journal of Immigrant and Minority Health* 9(2): 61–74.

Kelly, U. A. 2009. "Integrating Intersectionality and Biomedicine in Health Disparities Research." *Advances in Nursing Science* 32(2): E42–E56.

Kendall, F. E. 2006. *Understanding White Privilege: Creating Pathways to Authentic Relationships across Race.* New York: Routledge.

Kim, M.T., H. R. Han, H. S. Shin, K. B. Kim, and H. B. Lee. 2005. "Factors Associated with Depression Experience of Immigrant Populations: A Study of Korean Immigrants." *Archives of Psychiatric Nursing* 19(5): 217–225.

Kim, Y. O. R. 2005. "Reducing Disparities in Dental Care for Low-Income Hispanic Children. *Journal of Health Care for the Poor and Underserved* 16(3): 431–443.

Koenen, K. C., A. Lincoln, and A. Appleton. 2006. "Women's Status and Child Well-Being: A State-Level Analysis." *Social Science & Medicine* 63(12): 2999–3012.

Ku, L. and S. Matani. 2001. "Left Out: Immigrants' Access to Health Care and Insurance." *Health Affairs, 20*(1): 247–256.

Lasser, K. E., D. U. Himmelstein, and S. Woolhandler. 2006. "Access to Care, Health Status, and Health Disparities in the United States and Canada: Results of a Cross-National Population-Based Survey." *American Journal of Public Health* 96(7): 1300–1307.

McCall, L. 2005. "The Complexity of Intersectionality." *Signs* 30(3): 1771–1800.

McLeroy, K. R., D. Bibeau, A. Steckler, and K. Glanz. 1988. "An Ecological Perspective on Health Promotion Programs." *Health Education Quarterly* 15(4): 351–377.

Mermin, L. S. P. 2006. *Living in America: Challenges Facing New Immigrants and Refugees.* Washington, DC: Robert Wood Johnson Foundation.

Moore, S. D., K. B. Wright, and D. R. Bernard. 2009. "Influences on Health Delivery System Satisfaction: A Partial Test of the Ecological Model." *Health Communication* 24(4): 285–294.

Ozer, E. J., M. L. Ritterman, and M. G. Wanis. 2010. "Participatory Action Research in Middle School: Opportunities, Constraints, and Key Processes." *American Journal of Community Psychology* 46: 152–166.

Rahman, M. A., and O. Fals-Borda, O. 1991. "A Self-Review of P.A.R. in Action and Knowledge: Breaking the Monopoly with Participatory Action Research." In *Action and Knowledge: Breaking the Monopoly with Participatory Action-Research,* edited by M. A. Rahman and O. Fals-Borda, 24–36. New York: The Apex Press.

Reeve, C. L., and D. Basalik. 2011. "A State Level Investigation of the Associations among Intellectual Capital, Religiosity, and Reproductive Health." *Intelligence* 39(1): 64–73.

Reifsnider, E., M. Gallagher, and B. Forgione. 2005. "Using Ecological Models in Research on Health Disparities." *Journal of Professional Nursing* 21(4): 216–222.

Robinson, T. 2008. "Applying the Socio-Ecological Model to Improving Fruit and Vegetable Intake among Low-Income African Americans." *Journal of Community Health: The Publication for Health Promotion and Disease Prevention* 33(6): 395–406.

Rogers, J., and U. A. Kelly. 2011. "Feminist Intersectionality: Bringing Social Justice to Health Disparities Research." *Nursing Ethics* 18(3): 397–407.

Savage, C. L., Y. Xu, R. Lee, B. L. Rose, M. Kappesser, and J. S. Anthony. 2006. "A Case Study in the Use of Community-Based Participatory Research in Public Health Nursing." *Public Health Nursing* 23(5): 472–478.

Siddharthan, K., and M. Ahern. 1996. "Inpatient Utilization by Undocumented Immigrants Without Insurance." *Journal of Health Care for the Poor and Underserved* 7(4): 355–363.

Smye, V., A. J. Browne, C. Varcoe, and V. Josewski. 2011. "Harm Reduction, Methadone Maintenance Treatment and the Root Causes of Health and Social Inequities: An Intersectional Lens in the Canadian Context." *Harm Reduction Journal* 8(17): 1–12.

Stephens, B. 1994. "The Civil Lawsuit as a Remedy for International Human Rights Violations against Women." *Hastings Women's Law Journal* 5(2): 143.

Stokols, D. 1992. "Establishing and Maintaining Healthy Environments: Toward a Social Ecology of Health Promotion." *American Psychologist* 47(1): 6–22.

Stokols, D. 2006. "Toward a Science of Transdisciplinary Action Research." *American Journal of Community Psychology* 38(1-2): 63–77.

Tillet, T. 2006. "Public Health: Inadequate Housing May Put Immigrant Farmworkers at Risk." *Environmental Health Perspectives* 114(8): A467.

Travers, K. D. 1997. "Reducing Inequities through Participatory Research and Community Empowerment." *Health Education & Behavior* 24(3): 344–356.

Trickett, E. J. 2009. "Multilevel Community-Based Culturally Situated Interventions and Community Impact: An Ecological Perspective." *American Journal of Community Psychology* 43(3-4): 257–266.

Veenstra, G. 2011. "Race, Gender, Class, and Sexual Orientation: Intersecting Axes of Inequality and Self-Rated Health in Canada." *International Journal for Equity in Health* 10(3): 1–11.

Waddell, B. 1998. "United States Immigration: A Historical Perspective." In *Handbook of Immigrant Health,* edited by S. Loue. New York: Plenum, 2011.

Waidmann, T. and S. Rajan. 2000. "Race and Ethnic Disparities in Health Care Access and Utilization: An Examination of State Variation." *Medical Care Research Review* 57(1): 55–84.

CHAPTER THREE

Health Disparities and Immigrants

*Ayşe Çiftçi, Laura Reid-Marks,
and Lamise Shawahin*

Today, there are approximately 40 million immigrants in the United States (U.S. Census 2011) with over 1 million immigrants arriving every year (U.S. Immigration and Naturalization Service 1999). Twenty-five percent of children in the United States have a parent who was born outside of the United States (Mather 2009). The number of immigrants (i.e., persons who are not born U.S. citizens) is estimated to be 40 million (approximately 13 percent) of the population (U.S. Census 2012). Approximately one-third of this population came to the United States in 2000 or later. Mather (2009) reported that there are about 16 million children living in immigrant families, and that these children, "defined as people under age 18 who are foreign born or who live with at least one foreign-born parent, are the fastest-growing segment of America's youth and are leading a racial/ethnic transformation of the U.S. population" (1). Thus, the immigrant population is increasing and altering the demographics of the United States.

The percentage of children in immigrant families has increased from 13 percent of all U.S. children in 1990 to 22 percent in 2007. In addition, there are estimates that as many as 11 million immigrants are undocumented (Hoefer et al. 2009) living in the United States without legal authorization. There is no question that the increasing immigrants are changing the current structures in the United States. Compared to the total population with 84.5 percent covered by private health insurance, only 65 percent of the immigrant population in the United States is covered by health insurance. There are also significant discrepancies within the immigrant community with foreign born immigrants from Latin America, who have the least coverage (51 percent). In this chapter, we focus on health disparities among immigrants by providing current literature, discussing factors contributing to health disparities among immigrants, and focusing on specific immigrant communities (e.g., Caribbean, Latin American, Middle Eastern, Asian) with recommendations for psychologists working with immigrants to close the disparities gap.

Health Disparities among Immigrants

In the past decades, we have witnessed significant advancements and scientific discoveries, leading to improved health and better quality of life. However, not everyone who lives in the United States (U.S.) has benefitted from these advancements and discoveries. Immigrants are sometimes placed in a disadvantaged position when compared to other groups in the U.S. Health disparities refer to differences in health outcomes among individuals based on social groups and inequalities. For example, breast cancer leads as the major cause of cancer deaths among Latinas in the United States. Moreover, disparities exist in cancer prevalence depending on Latina women's place of birth. Research has found that women from Mexico and Central America are less likely to have ever completed a mammogram, whereas Mexican women were less likely to indicate having completed a mammogram recently (Rosales and Gonzalez 2013).

Although, the incidence of tuberculosis has been declining in the United States for decades, this disease disproportionally affects immigrants. Abraham, Winston, Magee, and Miramontes (2013) assessed the case rates of tuberculosis using the *U.S. National Tuberculosis Surveillance System*. They found that in 2009, the case rate among African born immigrants living in the United States was three times higher compared to other immigrant groups and 27 times higher compared to U.S.-born individuals. Furthermore, not only is the tuberculosis rate highest among Africans living in the United States, but this group is more likely to be HIV-positive and to be affected by extrapulmonary tuberculosis. Choi (2012) utilized the 2003 New Immigrant Survey (NIS) to determine the prevalence rates of overweight and obesity of recent immigrants to the United States. This study found that more than 45 percent of recent immigrants to the United States are either overweight or obese, and the highest prevalence of both overweight and obesity was found in immigrants from Latin American and the Caribbean, and those immigrants who lived longest in the United States. Bharmal and Chaundry (2012) assessed weight and body fat for Vietnamese immigrants and found that in a sample of 703 Vietnamese immigrants, this group was more likely to be overweight and to have high waist-height ratio when compared to non-immigrants.

Undocumented immigrants are becoming an increasingly large percentage of the immigrant population in the United States. In 2009, the Pew Hispanic Center (2009) estimated that in the United States more than 11 million immigrants were undocumented and that this number continues to grow, with the majority of these immigrants coming from Mexico (59 percent), Central America (11 percent) and Asia (11 percent). Undocumented immigrants may be less likely to seek medical attention when they are ill because they fear being reported to the authorities. Consequently, they might wait too long before they seek help for their ailments, which can lead to a poorer quality of life and a shorter life expectancy. The stigmatization of undocumented immigrants and language barriers may lead to a lower quality of care.

Additionally, undocumented immigrant workers often do not have health insurance. These immigrants are often paid low wages under the table. Low wages, coupled with no health insurance, means seeking help from a healthcare provide could be too costly for many undocumented immigrants. Often they seek assistance from community health agencies or emergency rooms when they are in dire need of services. Frequently these providers are too overwhelmed with large numbers of patients and transitional staff; therefore, they cannot provide the immigrant with the care they may need for long-term healthy living, including mental health care services to address stress.

Stress from being undocumented can also lead to negative health outcomes. Joseph Smith (2010) found in her qualitative study that undocumented immigrants from Brazil reported difficulties that arose from their undocumented status, including being exploited in the workplace, concern over deportation and an overall sense of nervousness living in the United States. If an individual is constantly concerned about being deported, the state of perpetual fear will have a harmful effect on his or her physical and mental health outcomes. Moreover, if one stands out based on their race/ethnicity, as is the case with some undocumented immigrants, further uneasiness can arise.

An immigrant's race/ethnicity can have a strong influence on how they are treated by others in their new community, and ultimately impact health outcomes. White Europeans, who colonized the Americas, settled in the United States with relative ease until restrictions on immigration were put in place in the early 1900s (Yakushko 2008). Legislation on immigration privileged northern European immigrants and early non-white immigrants did not have the right to become naturalized citizens until 1952 (Yakushko 2008). However, after the Civil Rights movement of the 1960s, ethnocentric immigration policies were overturned which resulted in the majority of contemporary immigrants hailing from Mexico, Asia, and Central America

(Yakushko 2008). Individuals from these countries are often visible minorities in the United States. By being a visible minority they can never "blend in" and may thus never truly feel at home in their host country. Many immigrants were members of the dominant group in their home country and are unaccustomed to being visibly different, or speaking a different language in the host country. As a result of their visible and sometimes invisible differences, many of these immigrants face racism and discrimination.

Factors Contributing to Health Disparities in Immigrants

Acculturation

Acculturation is an adjustment process that occurs when persons from one culture come in to contact with persons from another culture (Berry 1997). Upon migration to a new country, immigrants experience an acculturative process that occurs as a result of differences between their home culture and the culture of their host country (Chun, Chesla, and Kwan 2011). These differences can include language, religion, gender roles, and other cultural aspects. Acculturation has received a significant amount of attention in the scholarly literature because of the impact it can have on immigrant health (see Bernstein et al. 2011; Huh, Prause, and Dooley, 2008; Leu, Walton, and Takeuchi 2010). The way in which an immigrant acculturates has been found to be a significant determiner of their physical and mental health outcomes.

There are multiple theories that have had a strong impact in acculturation research (Berry 1997, Searle and Ward 1990). Berry's (1997) acculturation model proposed four different acculturation strategies: assimilation, separation, integration, and marginalization (see chapter 5 this volume). Although there is usually one preference over the other, there may be variations according to the individual's location. For example, an individual can be more separated (seeking cultural maintenance) depending on whether he/she is living at home or with extended family. Furthermore, individuals may utilize different acculturation strategies during their acculturation process. Although there is no sequential strategy used according to age or gender, there may be changes throughout the process.

Searle and Ward (1990) identified two dimensions of acculturation as *psychological adjustment* (emotional/affective) and *socio-cultural adaptation* (behavioral). *Psychological adjustment* refers to an individual's psychological well-being and is based on stress and coping models. *Socio-cultural adaptation* refers to learning culturally appropriate skills and has been rooted in social learning models. Although these two dimensions are related to each other, they are explained by different factors. Psychological adjustment is related to life changes, coping styles, personality, and social support. Socio-cultural adaptation is influenced by social skills acquisition and culture learning (e.g., length of stay in the new culture, degree of interaction with host nationals, language fluency, and acculturation strategies).

The various acculturation models (Berry 1997, Searle and Ward 1990) have received some criticisms (Schwartz et al. 2010). Hermans and Kempen (1998) criticized the traditional dichotomy models of acculturation (i.e., "individualism versus collectivism" and "egocentric versus sociocentric") as linear in nature. They argued that acculturation and identity issues should be considered as "mixing and moving" instead of a linear relationship from culture A to culture B. Bhatia and Ram (2001) criticized Berry's model because individuals moving from different countries or continents will have different acculturation processes. For instance, an individual moving from Europe will have a different acculturation process than an individual moving from Africa. They also criticized Berry's model for suggesting that integration seemed to be the ultimate goal; however, the model does not include any way to reach that goal or address how other socio-political factors might play a role in the acculturation process.

From as early as the 1980s, Angel and Worobey (1988) found that Latinos who had lower acculturation levels reported lower health ratings than their more acculturated counterparts. More recently, research on Type II Diabetes and acculturation has indicated that acculturative experiences impact the management of this chronic disease and perceived health status in Chinese American immigrants (Chun, Chesla, and Kwan 2011). Today in the literature, numerous factors have been and continue to be measured as dimensions of acculturation and a plethora of researchers have found these factors to be related to health outcomes. These dimensions of acculturation include language fluency, immigration status and race/ethnic identity.

Immigrants often speak a different language than members of their host country and this language barrier can cause them significant stress (Ding and Hargraves 2009). Language fluency can negatively impact access to preventative and remediation healthcare services, the quality of care received, and physical and mental health outcomes. Ding and Hargraves (2009) utilized data from the CTS Household Survey, where they analyzed information from 29,510 individuals, concluding that immigrants' health is heavily impacted by stress and the language barrier. Furthermore, although, many immigrants are found to be initially healthier than their U.S.-born peers, this *immigrant paradox* is less likely to be found in immigrants with low English language fluency (Ding and Hargraves 2009). The negative health outcomes that accompany low language fluency might be the result of stress due to the inability to find a job, lack of understanding of others in the dominant culture and thus less understanding of the culture itself, and/or the inability to communicate and find the services one might need. For all of these reasons and others, an immigrant who does not speak the language of the dominant culture might experience *acculturative stress.* Moreover, the burden of language fluency might be exacerbated in immigrants who are concerned about their legal status in their new home.

Duration of time spent in the host country is also a factor that has been identified as contributing to overall health disparities in immigrant communities. For immigrants, less time spent in the United States has been found to be related to a lower likelihood of utilizing mental health care services (Keyes et al. 2011). At the same time, immigrants who have been in the United States for a shorter amount of time report better self-rated mental health than immigrants who have been in the United States for a longer amount of time (Zhang and Ta 2009). Furthermore, increased time spent in the United States puts immigrants at a higher risk for mental health disorders such as anxiety and depression (Cook et al. 2009). Scholars speculate that health disparities associated with longer residences in the United States for immigrants may be due to family culture conflict and routine experiences of discrimination (Cook et al. 2009, Dolly et al. 2012). Interventions aimed at addressing difficulties with cultural conflicts between their host country and country of origin as well experiences with discrimination will likely benefit immigrants' mental health outcomes.

Racism, Discrimination, and Xenophobia

Immigration is one of the most significant issues in any debate around economy, politics, and social issues in the United States. Immigrants have been typically blamed for overpopulation, the suffering economy, increased violence, drained social resources (e.g. medical), and terrorism and also perceived as poor, violent, uneducated, and criminal (Yakushko 2009). Xenophobia, racism, and discrimination have been found to impact the mental and physical health of immigrants living in the United States. In 2001, the World Health Organization asserted that racism is a significant and widespread problem around the globe that may negatively impact the health of racial and ethnic minorities. Furthermore, researchers have found that discrimination takes place along multiple dimensions that are not specifically related to race, such as language fluency and accents, clothing, and religious practices (Yoo, Gee, and Takeuchi 2009). Even though racism and xenophobia share commonalities, they are quite distinct in that they have different historical realities and that one does not always imply the other.

Most recently, Paradies (2006) reported in a review of the literature that included 138 studies that 72 percent of the studies found a significant association between self-reported racism and mental health. In the same review, Paradies (2006) found that 62 percent of the studies found a significant association between self-reported racism and physical health.

Bernstein, Park, Shin, Cho and Park (2011) assessed acculturation, discrimination, language proficiency, and depression in 304 Korean immigrants in New York City and found that perceived discrimination and self-reported lower English language fluency was related to higher depression. Interestingly, in this same study, Bernstein, Park, Shin, Cho, and Park (2011) found a stronger relationship between perceived discrimination and depressive symptoms than acculturative stress and depressive symptoms, indicating that stress originating from discrimination might be more potent that stress originating from acculturation. Other studies on self-reported discrimination and physical health found that there was a negative association between perceived discrimination and physical health in a sample of Latino immigrants (Ryan, Gee, and Laflamme 2006).

Ahmad and Szpara (2003) found in their study that Muslim students in New York City experienced pervasive misconceptions and negative stereotypes of Islam. Evidence from studies of Muslim-American adults indicates that perceived discrimination may be related to mental health problems (Abu-Ras and Abu Badr 2008; Abu-Ras and Suarez 2009, Ghaffari and Çiftçi 2010, Hassouneh and Anahid 2007, Padela and Heisler 2010). Studies of the effects of discrimination on U.S. minority groups, including African American, Latino, East Asian, and South Asian adolescents, suggest that discrimination distress was negatively correlated with psychological and physical health (Fisher, Wallace, and Fenton 2000).

Poverty and Inequality

In 1995, the World Health Organization affirmed that, "The World's most ruthless killer and the greatest cause of suffering on the earth is extreme poverty." Almost one in every five foreign born is living below the poverty line (U.S. Census 2012). Half of the children in immigrant families are low-income compared to 36 percent of the children in U.S.-born families. Poverty leads to unemployment, underemployment, lack of health insurance and lack of food availability and is strongly related to mental and physical health outcomes (Sue and Sue 2008). Poverty and socio-economic status are both factors that have a significant influence on the quality of life of immigrants in the United States.

In recent years, the face of immigration has changed, causing different experiences based on immigrant's race, country of origin, cultural distance, religion, etc. For example, one out of every four U.S. physicians, scientists, and engineers with a bachelor's degree and one out of every two scientists with doctorates are immigrants (Portes and Rumbaut 2006). However, many of these immigrants have extreme difficulty finding a job when they move to the United States initially. Immigrants may have a wide range of occupations in their country of origin resulting in different expectations and perceptions of their environment. In their discussion on social class and immigrants, Çiftçi, Broustovetskaia, and Reid-Marks (2013) presented the complexity of social class among immigrants as "Middle social class professionals from El Salvador may work as day laborers and janitors after migration and identify as part of the working social class due to hostile experiences with discrimination and racism" (Baker-Cristales 2004). In addition, Albanian women employed as domestic workers in Greece experience exploitation, shame about their place of origin, marginalization, and social distancing from their employers even if they may possess more education and a higher standing at home (Hantzaroula 2008).

Numerous research findings have documented the negative impact that poverty has on physical and mental health outcomes. In their chapter, entitled "Poverty, Social Inequality, and Mental Health," Murali and Oyebode (2010) bring readers' attention to the profound impact that poverty and social inequality can have on mental health. Their findings can be expanded to immigrants who belong to a nation's poorer classes. Additionally, other researchers have found a link between poverty and physical health concerns. In the United States, low-income immigrants experience a higher incidence of Type II Diabetes when compared to their White same aged counterparts. Chaufan, Davis, and Constantino (2011) conducted a study on Latino immigrants who received services from a non-profit organization. They interviewed six staff members of non-profit organizations, conducted focus groups with 15 immigrants, collected information on issues such as income, housing, immigration experience life quality, etc., and surveyed local groceries, convenience stores, supermarkets, local Farmers' markets, and a local Flea Market to estimate food prices and food resources. Their findings suggested that nine out of 15 participants lived at or below the poverty line. The majority of the participants (11 out of 15) "reported that they had access to the [food] amount, yet not the quality, of food they desired (73.3 percent), or that they frequently did not have enough food (13.3 percent)" (Chaufan, Davis, & Constantino, 2011, p. 1036). Their findings indicated that the concurrence of Type II Diabetes and poverty was high in a community of immigrants. It makes sense that poverty would be related to lower health outcomes. Poverty leads to the inability to afford proper foods, healthcare, and preventative measures. Those who are living in poverty tend to work longer hours in more physically strenuous jobs that have long-term negative health consequences. Many immigrants tend to hold manual labor jobs and for some this is an unwelcome shift in profession and socioeconomic status.

Some immigrants suffer stress as a result of shifts in their socioeconomic status when they enter their host country (Dow 2011). Sometimes these shifts are objective changes in social class, where the immigrant makes less money or lives in a smaller house. Other times the change in social class is subjective, where the immigrant might feel less valued than they did when they were in their home country (Liu 2002). Many immigrants from higher social classes are distraught when they arrive in their new homes, only to find that their professional certifications are not valued and they have to take employment in a less prestigious job than they had when they were in the country of their birth (Dow 2011). Many resist this change refusing to take jobs as manual laborers and in other professions which they deem "beneath them," thus adding to the unemployment rate in their new home. On the contrary, immigrants from lower social classes who are accustomed to manual labor often find their shift in social class more pleasant and welcome the opportunity to work in professions similar to those in which they worked back in their home country. Often these immigrants are able to live at a higher standard than they did before migration. However, they still experience poor health outcomes that may be impacted by their lack of education surrounding their own health.

According to APA task force on socio-economic status (SES) (APA 2007), there are four broad categories in which socioeconomic status impacts health: (a) differential access to health care, (b) differential exposure to environmental hazards, (c) health behaviors (e.g., smoking, poor diet, lack of exercise), and (d) differential exposure to stress. One can argue that immigrants are a marginalized group who are at-risk and have limited access to health care, higher exposure to environmental hazards (considering over half of the immigrants live in metropolitan areas), poor health behaviors and higher levels of exposure to stress. Specifically, of the last two paths, psychosocial issues are most relevant to psychologists to develop interventions to reduce health risk behaviors and reduce the stress in immigrants' environment.

Health Education

Many immigrants live in poverty and are not educated on disease prevention and healthy living. Often as a result of poverty, immigrants do not have access to health education services, which can ultimately lead to an improved quality of life and higher life expectancy. Furthermore, an immigrant who does not speak the dominant language is unlikely to find health education services spoken in their native tongue. To combat the higher incidence of negative health outcomes in immigrant populations, many researchers and organizations have begun developing health education programs to assist with closing the health disparity gap. For example, Grigg-Saito et al. (2010) report the beneficial results of the Lowell Community Health Center's whole community approach (e.g., emphasizing physical, psychosocial, spiritual needs) to address health disparities in Cambodian immigrants and refugees. Utilizing this community approach, the Lowell Community Health Center noticed that all 50 of their diabetic patients showed improvement and patients reported teaching their family members about condom use and HIV and themselves utilizing condoms more. Studies such as these show the beneficial role that health education can have on closing the immigrant health disparities gap.

Other Structural Factors

In addition to acculturation, poverty, inequality, racism, xenophobia, discrimination and health education, Tucker et al. (2007) discussed biological and social and environmental factors such as health care quality and access to health care factors that contribute to health disparities. More specifically, additional factors that contribute to health disparities among immigrant populations are: (a) different beliefs about what health means and how symptoms are expressed, (b) lack of culturally sensitive health services for immigrants, (c) language barriers, (d) lack of knowledge about the health care system, and (e) lack of cultural competence among health care providers.

Health Disparities in Specific Immigrant Groups

Caribbean Immigrants

In 2009, there were over 3.5 million Caribbean born immigrants living in the United States, with the majority originating from Cuba, Haiti, Jamaica, the Dominican Republic, and Trinidad and Tobago. These numbers account for approximately nine percent of the total immigrant population and two percent of undocumented immigrants in the United States (Migration Information Source 2011). Despite these significant numbers, the majority of health research with Caribbean immigrants has been conducted in countries outside the United States. In the United States, research on Caribbean immigrant health disparities is often grouped with other ethnic minorities, making it more difficult to ascertain the potentially unique struggles that this group may face

(Read, Emerson, and Tarlov 2005). However, Wheeler and Mahoney (2008) asserted that Caribbean born immigrants encounter a plethora of barriers when it comes to utilization and access to health care services, including immigration status, health beliefs, lack of insurance, and practices, as well as stigma related to mental health services. These barriers are also applicable to physical healthcare and health outcomes.

Research in the literature on Caribbean immigrants is sparse and often only black Caribbean immigrants have been studied. Given that the majority of Caribbean population is of African origin this trend makes logical sense; however, other races, especially mixed individuals, deserve more attention in the literature. Several studies have utilized national data sets to examine health outcomes in Caribbean immigrants. Jackson, Neighbors, Torres, Martin, Williams, and Baser (2007) assessed mental health outcomes in Black Caribbean immigrants utilizing the *National Survey of American life*. These researchers found that in regards to formal mental health services, a significant dissimilarity in rates and sources of use, relative satisfaction, and perception of helpfulness depended on when migration occurred, as well as generational status of Caribbean Black immigrants. Hamilton and Hummer (2011) found that black Caribbean immigrants are in general good health in the Caribbean upon migration but experience a health decline after living in the United States for 20 years. In summary, Caribbean immigrants are a group which scholars have generally neglected. However, like other immigrant groups, they experience disparities when it comes to health and wellbeing. The factors which account for these changes are being studied widely in the health disparities literature (see section on *Factors Contributing to Health Disparities in Immigrants*).

Latin American Immigrants

Immigrants from Central and South America account for the majority of immigrants in the United States today, with the largest number of immigrants migrating from Mexico (57 percent). This large percentage of Mexican immigrants has led to much controversial discussion about policy on how immigrants from Mexico should be treated, especially undocumented Mexican immigrants living in the United States. According to the Center for Immigration Statistics (Camarota 2012) there were over 140,000 Mexican immigrants who became legal immigrants of the United States in 2011. This number does not include the many undocumented Mexican immigrants living and working in the United States, often in low wage jobs with no health insurance. Consequently, the same health disparities that affect other ethnic minorities affect Latin America immigrants.

There is a plethora of data available on the Latino population and the diseases that disproportionately affect this population. Immigrants from Latin America have the highest incidence of chronic liver disease and cirrhosis among all racial/ethnic groups (Hayes-Bautista 2002). Latinos account for 20 percent of people in the United States living with HIV and/or Aids, while accounting for approximately 13 percent of the U.S. population (Centers for Disease Control and Prevention 2011). In the Latino immigrant population the incidence of Type II Diabetes is two to three times higher than in whites. Latino immigrants are also more likely than whites to be overweight or obese, putting them at a higher risk for Type II Diabetes (Vega and Amaro 2002). This finding is likely due to the adoption of a more sedentary American lifestyle, with lack of exercise and an emphasis on cheaper fast food. These statistics are frightening considering that initially, when compared to their U.S.-born counterparts, Latino immigrants fare well in regard to their mental and physical health. However, over time this immigrant paradox dissipates and they are affected with the health concerns above (Cook, Alegria, Lin, and Guo 2009).

This paradox can be seen more clearly by other data. Among Mexican immigrants, the rate of low baby birth weight increases from first to subsequent generations, indicating an association with acculturation and other factors (Scribner and Dwyer 1989). Alcohol use in this population tends to increase with time, which possibly accounts for the larger incidence of liver disease mentioned above. Drug use also tends to increase with time spent in the United States (Amaro et al. 1990). In particular, many immigrants do not smoke until their after their migration to the United States (Pérez-Stable et al. 2001). Both alcohol and drug use might be linked to the stresses of migration and living in the United States. The factors which account for these changes are being studied widely in the health disparities literature (see section on *Factors Contributing to Health Disparities in Immigrants*).

Middle Eastern Immigrants

Middle Easterners are an immigrant group that is quickly increasing in the United States, and the current population is estimated to be close to 2.5 million (Nasseri and Moulton 2011). Middle Eastern immigrants typically live in urban areas with large populations in the Midwest and East Coast. Individuals who are immigrants from the Middle East typically arrive from the Levant, North Africa, Turkey, and Iran, and adhere to Christianity or Islam. Research on the specific barriers experienced by Middle Eastern immigrants have typically focused on the greater Detroit area, namely Dearborn, which has one of the highest populations of Middle

Eastern immigrants. However, this population is not necessarily representative of the entire Middle Eastern immigrant population, as it represents a disproportionate amount of lower income Middle Easterners and Muslims (Ghazal Read, Amick, and Donato 2005). Ghazal Read et al. (2005) suggested that disadvantage in health outcomes and profiles is not as uniform as prior research suggests, and noted that, unlike other immigrant groups, length of stay in the United States does not sufficiently explain the association between health outcomes and acculturation. Iranian and Turkish immigrants are underrepresented in research on Middle Eastern health disparities. However, researchers have noted disparities in terms of health outcomes, health profiles (Ghazal Read et al. 2005), and underutilization of preventative care due to cultural norms and stigma (Abdoul-Enein and Abdoul Enein 2010).

Notable health problems faced by Middle Eastern immigrants that have been documented include tobacco use, hypertension, diabetes, and psychological wellbeing. Middle Eastern immigrants have higher rates of tobacco use than other minority groups in the United States with estimates of usage ranging from 12 percent to 40 percent with Middle Eastern immigrant adolescents exhibiting greater tobacco usage than their non-Middle Eastern counter parts (Aswad 2001, El Sayed and Galea 2009, Jamil et al. 2008). El Sayed and Galea (2009) synthesized literature regarding the health of Arab-Americans and noted that the hypertension rate is between 13–20 percent. The percentage of Arab-Americans with diabetes is estimated to be between 16–33 (El Sayed and Galea, 2009). Recent spikes in discrimination against Middle Eastern Americans account for high rates of psychological distress in this population (Abu-Ras and Abu Bader 2009). In terms of health education, Arab-Americans tend to be less informed about HIV/AIDS than the general population (Kulwicki and Cass 1994). Ghazal Read and Reynolds (2012) examined a national dataset from 2000–2007 comparing health outcomes and gender differences among immigrant groups and found that Middle Eastern immigrants are not as likely as their U.S.-born White counterparts to utilize health care services and that women were even less likely to do so. Aboul-Enein and Aboul-Enein (2010) speculate that increased cultural awareness among practitioners can help bridge the gaps in health care utilization and outcomes among Middle Eastern Immigrants.

Asian Immigrants

The number of new Asian immigrants to the United States has recently surpassed that of new Latino/Hispanic immigrants (Pew 2012). The majority of Asian-American adults (74 percent) were born overseas and the majority of recent immigrants (61 percent) from Asia have a bachelor's degree or higher (Pew 2012). The U.S. Asian population is primarily comprised of individuals with roots in China, the Philippines, India, Vietnam, Korea, and Japan and is estimated to be roughly 17 million (Pew 2012). The U.S. Asian population is comprised of individuals from diverse religious and cultural backgrounds and differences exist in terms of what health disparities are more prevalent in various populations. Although numerous intergroup differences exist among various Asian populations, Yu, Huang, and Singh (2004) found that among all Asian American (e.g., Chinese, Indian, Filipino, and other Asian/Pacific Islander) children missing school due to illness or injury and learning disabilities were less prevalent compared to non-Hispanic whites.

Health profiles differ greatly among various Asian American populations. Jonnalagadda and Diwan (2005) found in a sample of Asian Indian immigrants that 41 percent were vegetarian, 55 percent exercised regularly, and 5 percent used tobacco. However, hypertension (31 percent) and diabetes (18 percent) were found to be a common problem in this population. Parikh, Fahs, Shelly and Yerneni (2009) found that among Chinese immigrants, 66 percent exercised regularly while 14.1 percent used tobacco. More health disparities are found in the children of Asian American immigrants, but not those of U.S.-born Asian Americans (Huang et al. 2012). For example, Southeast Asian children of immigrants experience higher rates of overweight than any other group of Asians, including U.S.-born Asians (Huang et al. 2012). In addition, Huang et al. (2012) found that Asian children have more difficulties with interpersonal relationship skills and exhibit more internalizing problems than their U.S.-born white and Asian counterparts.

Recent research on health disparities faced by Asian Americans has challenged previous misconceptions about their health profiles. Previous research indicated that breast cancer was not a major concern among Asian Americans. However, a recent study examining breast cancer rates among Asian immigrants (e.g., Chinese, Japanese, Filipina, Korean, and South Asian) found that among some Asian American populations, like Chinese Americans, breast cancer rates were higher for U.S.-born Chinese Americans—whereas for Japanese Americans, the cancer rates were the same regardless of birth place (Gomez et al. 2010). In some Asian-American populations (e.g., Filipina), the breast cancer rate exceeds that of white women (Gomez et al. 2010). As research continues to expand on Asian American immigrants the unique issues that affect this group and their etiology will become clearer.

Recommendations for Psychologists Working with Immigrants to Close the Disparities Gap

1. Psychologists need to consider our roles in training or consulting other health care providers to become culturally competent professionals. Psychology has been a pioneer in multiculturalism and cultural competencies. Consistent with our commitment to multiculturalism and social justice, we can develop interventions for other health care providers to raise awareness and provide training/consultation about issues specific to immigrants.
2. Psychologists can advocate and raise awareness in the public. Due to social responsibility, psychologists have a role in advocating policy change, specifically policies that will impact marginalized groups such as immigrants.
3. Psychologists should work with the communities. In most cases, immigrants similar to other minority groups have limited knowledge (and stigma) about health services. Psychologists can reach out to the communities, identify the leaders/respected figures and *work with* them for prevention or other health access related issues.
4. Psychologists should incorporate diverse research methodologies (e.g., community-based participatory research, mixed-methods, longitudinal) as well as investigate the applicability/adaptation of evidence-based interventions for the immigrant populations.
5. Psychologists need to consider our training standards and guidelines to train our students to become competent in working in interdisciplinary settings with other health care professionals. We need to implement "interdisciplinary competencies" as training goals in our programs.

References

Abraham, B. K., C. A. Winston, E. Magee, and R. Miramontes. 2013. Tuberculosis Among Africans Living in the United States, 2000–2009. *Journal of Immigrant and Minority Health* 15(2): 381–389. doi: 10.1007/s10903-012-9624-4

Aboul-Enein, B. H., and F. Aboul-Enein, 2010. "The Cultural Gap Delivering Health Care Services to Arab American Populations in the United States." *Journal of Cultural Diversity* 17(1): 20–23.

Abu-Ras, W., and S. Abu-Bader. 2008. "The Impact of the September 11, 2001 Attacks on the Wellbeing of Arab Americans in New York City." *Journal of Muslim Mental Health* 3(2): 217–239.

Abu-Ras, W., and S. Abu-Bader. 2009. "Risk Factors for Depression and Posttraumatic Stress Disorder (PTSD): The Case of Arab and Muslim Americans Post-9/11." *Journal of Immigrant & Refugee Studies* 7(4): 393–418. doi: 10.1080/15562940903379068

Abu-Ras, W. M., and Z. E. Suarez. 2009. "Muslim Men and Women's Perception of Discrimination, Hate Crimes, and PTSD Symptoms Post 9/11." *Traumatology* 15(3): 48–63.

Ahmad, I., and M. Y. Szpara. 2003. "Muslim Children in Urban America: The New York City Schools Experience." *Journal of Muslim Minority Affairs* 23: 295–301.

Amaro, H., R. Whitaker, G. Coffman, and T. Heeren. 1990. "Acculturation and Marijuana and Cocaine Use: Findings from HHANES 1982–84." *American Journal of Public Health* 80(12): 54–60.

American-Arab Anti-Discrimination Committee. 2008. "2003–2007 Report on Hate Crimes and Discrimination against Arab Americans (Rep.)" Washington DC.

American Psychological Association, Task Force on Socioeconomic Status. 2007. *Report of the APA Task Force on Socioeconomic Status.* http://www.apa.org/pi/ses/resources/publications/task-force-2006.pdf

Angel, R., and J. Worobey. 1988. "Acculturation and Maternal Reports of Children's Health: Evidence from the Hispanic Health and Nutrition Examination." *Social Science Quarterly* 69(3): 707–721.

Aswad, A. 2001. *Health Survey of the Arab, Muslim, and Chaldean American Communities in Michigan.* Lansing: Michigan Department of Community Health.

Baker-Cristales, B. 2004. "Salvadoran transformations: Class Consciousness and Ethnic Identity in a Transnational Milieu." *Latin American Perspectives* 31: 15–33.

Bernstein, K., S. Park, J. Shin, S. Cho, and Y. Park. 2011. "Acculturation, Discrimination and Depressive Symptoms among Korean Immigrants in New York City." *Community Mental Health Journal,* 47(1): 24–34. doi:10.1007/s10597-009-9261-0

Berry, J. W. 1997. "Immigration, Acculturation, and Adaptation." *Applied Psychology: An International Review* 46: 5–34. doi:10.1080/026999497378467

Bharmal, N., and S. Chaudhry. 2012. Preventive health services delivery to South Asians in the United States. *Journal of Immigrant and Minority Health* 14(5), 797–802. doi: 10.1007/s10903-012-9610-x

Bhatia, S., and A. Ram. 2001. "Rethinking 'Acculturation' in Relation to Diasporic Cultures and Postcolonial Identities." *Human Development* 44: 1–18.

Camarota, S. 2012. "Immigrants at Mid-Decade: A Snapshot of American's Foreign-Born Population in 2005." *Center for Immigration Studies.* Retrieved from http://www.cis.org/articles/2005/back1405.html

Centers for Disease Control and Prevention. 2011. "CDC Health Disparities and Inequalities Report," U.S. Dept. of Health and Human Services. http://www.cdc.gov/mmwr/pdf/other/su6001.pdf

Centers for Disease Control and Prevention. 2012. *Office of Minority Health and Health Equity Fact Sheet.* http://www.cdc.gov/minorityhealth/about/OMHHE.pdf

Chaufan, C., M. Davis, and S. Constantino. 2011. "The Twin Epidemics of Poverty and Diabetes: Understanding Diabetes Disparities in a Low-Income Latino and Immigrant Neighborhood." *Journal of Community Health* 36(6): 1032–1043. doi:10.1007/s10900-011-9406-2

Choi, J. Y. 2012. Prevalence of overweight and obesity among US immigrants: Results of the 2003 New Immigrant Survey. *Journal of Immigrant and Minority Health* 14(6), 1112–1118.

Chun, K. M., C. A. Chesla, and C. L. Kwan. 2011. "So We Adapt Step by Step: Acculturation Experiences Affecting Diabetes Management and Perceived Health for Chinese American Immigrants." *Social Science & Medicine* 72(2): 256–264, doi:10.1016/j.socscimed.2010.11.010

Çiftçi, A., A. Broustovetskaia, and L. Reid-Marks (in press). International Issues, Social Class and Counseling. In W. M. Liu (Ed.), *The Oxford Handbook of Social Class in Counseling Psychology.* New York, NY.

Cook, B., M. Alegria, J. Y. Lin, and J. Guo. 2009. "Pathways and Correlates Connecting Latinos' Mental Health with Exposure to the United States." *American Journal of Public Health* 99: 2247–2254.

Ding, H., and L. Hargraves. 2009. "Stress-Associated Poor Health among Adult Immigrants with a Language Barrier in the United States." *Journal of Immigrant & Minority Health* 11(6): 446–452. doi:10.1007/s10903-008-9200-0

Dolly, J. A., A. B. de Castro, D. P. Martin, B. Duran, and D. T. Takeuchi. 2012. "Does an Immigrant Health Paradox Exist among Asian Americans? Associations of Nativity and Occupational Class with Self-Rated Health and Mental Disorders." *Social Science & Medicine* 75(12): 2085–2098. doi: 10.1016/j.socscimed.2012.01.035, 2012.

Dow, H. D. 2011. "An Overview of Stressors Faced by Immigrants and Refugees: A Guide for Mental Health Practitioners." *Home Health Care Management and Practice* 23(3): 210–217. doi:10.1177/1084822310390878

El-Sayed, A. M., and S. Galea. 2009."The Health of Arab-Americans Living in the United States: A Systematic Review of the Literature." *BMC Public Health* 9(1): 272. doi: 10.1186/1471-2458-9-272

Fisher, C. B., S. A. Wallace, and R. E. Fenton. 2000. "Discrimination Distress during Adolescence." *Journal of Youth and Adolescence* 29: 679–695.

Ghaffari, A. and A. Çiftçi. 2010. "The Religiosity and Self-Esteem of Muslim Immigrants to the United States: The Moderating Role of Perceived Discrimination." *International Journal for the Psychology of Religion* 20: 14–25.

Ghazal-Read, J. G., B. Amick, and K. M. Donato. 2005. "Arab Immigrants: A New Case for Ethnicity and Health?" *Social Science & Medicine* 61(1): 77–82. doi: 10.1016/j.socscimed.2004.11.054

Ghazal-Read, J., and M. M. Reynolds. 2012. "Gender differences in immigrant health: The case of Mexican and Middle Eastern immigrants." *Journal of Health and Social Behavior* 53(1): 99–123. doi: 10.1177/0022146511431267

Gomez, S. L., T. Quach, P. L. Horn-Ross, J. T. Pham, M. Cockburn, E. T Chang, and C. A. Clarke. 2010. "Hidden Breast Cancer Disparities in Asian Women: Disaggregating Incidence Rates by Ethnicity and Migrant Status." *American Journal of Public Health* 100(S1): S125–S131. doi: 10.2105/AJPH.2009.163931

Grigg-Saito, Toof, Silka, Liang, Sou, Najarian, Peou and Och. 2010. "Long-term Development of a 'Whole Community' Best Practice Model to Address Health Disparities in the Cambodian Refugee and Immigrant Community of Lowell, Massachusetts." *American Journal of Public Health* 100(11): 2026–2029. doi:10.2105/AJPH.2009.177030

Hamilton, T. G. and R. A. Hummer. 2011. "Immigration and the Health of U.S. Black Adults: Does Country of Origin Matter?" *Social Science & Medicine* 73(10): 1551–1560. doi:10.1016/j.socscimed.2011.07.026

Hantzaroula, P. 2008. "Perceptions of Work in Albanian Immigrants' Testimonies and the Structure of Domestic Work in Greece." In *Migration and Domestic Work: A European Perspective on a Global Theme,* edited by H. Lutz, 61–74. Burlington, VT: Ashgate.

Hassouneh, D. M., and K. Anahid. 2007. "Mental Health, Discrimination, and Trauma in Arab Muslim Women Living in the U.S.: a Pilot Study." *Mental Health, Religion and Culture* 10(3): 257–262.

Hayes-Bautista, D. E. 2002. "The Latino Health Research Agenda for the Twenty-first Century." In *Latinos: Remaking America,* edited by M. M. Suarez-Orozco and M. Paez, 215-235.

Hermans, H. J. M., and H. J. G. Kempen. 1998. "Moving Cultures." *American Psychologist* 53: 1111–1120.

Hoefer, M., N. Rytina, and B. C. Baker. 2009. *Estimates of the Unauthorized Population Residing in the United States: January 2009. Population Estimates.* Washington, DC: Department of Homeland Security.

Huang, K., E. Calzada, S. Cheng, and L. M. Brotman. 2012. "Physical and Mental Health Disparities among Young Children of Asian Immigrants." *The Journal of Pediatrics 160*: 331–336. doi: 10.1016/j.jpeds.2011.08.005

Huh, J., Jo Prause, and C. Dooley. 2008. "The Impact of Nativity on Chronic Diseases, Self-Rated Health and Comorbidity Status of Asian and Hispanic Immigrants." *Journal of Immigrant and Minority Health* 10(2): 103–118.

Jackson, J. S., H. W. Neighbors, M. Torres, R. Baser, L. A. Martin, and D. R. Williams. 2007. "Use of Mental Health Services and Subjective Satisfaction with Treatment among Black Caribbean Immigrants: Results from the National Survey of American Life." *American Journal of Public Health* 97(1): 60–67. doi:10.2105/AJPH.2006.088500

Jamil, H., Fakhouri, M., F. Dallo., T. Templin, R. Khoury, and H. Fakhouri. 2008. "Disparities in self-reported diabetes mellitus among Arab, Chaldean, and Black Americans in Southeast Michigan." *Journal of Immigrant and Minority Health* 10(5): 397-405. doi: 10.1007/s10903-007-9108-0

Jonnalagadda, S. S. and S. Diwan. 2005. "Health Behaviors, Chronic Disease Prevalence and Self-Rated Health of Older Asian Indian Immigrants in the U.S." *Journal of Immigrant Health* 7: 75–83. doi: 10.1007/s10903-005-2640-x

Joseph, T. D. 2011. "'My Life Was Filled with Constant Anxiety': Anti-Immigrant Discrimination, Undocumented Status, and Their Mental Health Implications for Brazilian Immigrants." *Race and Social Problems* 3(3): 170–181. doi:10.1007/s12552-011-9054-2

Keyes, K. M., S. S. Martins, M. L. Hatzenbuehler, C. Blanco, L. M. Bates, and D. S. Hasin. 2011. "Mental Health Service Utilization for Psychiatric Disorders among Latinos Living in the United States: The Role of Ethnic Subgroup, Ethnic Identity, and Language/Social Preferences." *Social Psychiatry and Psychiatric Epidemiology* 47: 383–389. doi: 10.1007/s00127-010-0323-y

Kulwicki, A. D. and P. S. Cass. 1994. "An Assessment of Arab American Knowledge, Attitudes, and Beliefs about AIDS." *Journal of Nursing Scholarship* 26(1): 13–17. doi: 10.1111/j.1547-5069.1994.tb00288.x

Leu, J., E. Walton, and D. Takeuchi. 2011. "Contextualizing Acculturation: Gender, Family, and Community Reception Influences on Asian Immigrant Mental Health." *American Journal of Community Psychology* 48(3/4): 168–180. doi:10.1007/s10464-010-9360-7

Liu, W. M. 2002. "The Social Class-Related Experiences of Men: Integrating Theory and Practice." *Professional Psychology: Research and Practice* 33(4): 355–360. doi:10.1037/0735-7028.33.4.355

Mather, M. 2009. *Children in Immigrant Families Chart New Path.* Washington, DC: Population Reference Bureau. http://www.prb.org/pdf09/immigrantchildren.pdf

Migration Information Source. 2011. "Caribbean Immigrants in the United States." Migration Policy Institute. Retrieved from http://www.migrationpolicy.org/article/caribbean-immigrants-united-states/.

Murali, V. and F. Oyebode. 2010. "Poverty, Social Inequality, and Mental Health." In *Clinical Topics in Cultural Psychiatry,* edited by R. Bhattacharya, S. Cross, D. Bhugra, 84–99. London England: Royal College of Psychiatrists.

Nasseri, K. and L. H. Moulton. 2011. "Patterns of Death in the First and Second Generation Immigrants from Selected Middle Eastern Countries in California." *Journal of Immigrant and Minority Health* 13: 361–370. doi: 10.1007/s109 03- 009-9270-7

National Institutes of Health. 2010. *Fact Sheet: Health Disparities.* http://report.nih.gov/nihfactsheets/Pdfs/HealthDisparities(NIMHD).pdf

Padela, A. I. and M. Heisler. 2010. "The Association of Perceived Abuse and Discrimination after September 11, 2001, with Psychological Distress, Level of Happiness, and Health Status among Arab Americans." *American Journal of Public Health* 100(2): 284–291.

Paradies, Y. C. 2006. "Defining, Conceptualizing and Characterizing Racism in Health Research." *Critical Public Health* 16(2): 143–157. doi:10.1080/09581590600828881

Parikh, N. S., M. C. Fahs, D. Shelley, and R. Yerneni. 2009. "Health Behaviors of Older Chinese Adults Living in New York City." *Journal of Community Health* 34: 6–15. doi: 10.1007/s10900-008-9125-5

Pérez-Stable, E. J., A. Ramirez, R. Villareal, G. A. Talavera, E. Trapido, L. Suarez, and A. McAlister. 2001. "Cigarette Smoking Behavior among U.S. Latino Men and Women from Different Countries of Origin." *American Journal of Public Health* 91(9): 1424–1430. doi:10.2105/AJPH.91.9.1424

Pew Hispanic Center 2009. *A Portrait of Unauthorized Immigrants in the United States.* /http://www.pewhispanic.org/2009/04/14/a-portrait-of-unauthorized-immigrants-in-the-united-states/.

Pew Research Center. 2007. *Muslim Americans: Middle Class and Mostly Mainstream.* Unpublished technical report retrieved from http://www.pewresearch.org

Pew Research. 2012. *Hispanics Trend Project.* Retrieved from http://www.pewhispanic.org/

Portes, A., and R. G. Rumbaut. 2006. *Immigrant America: A Portrait*. Berkeley, CA: University of California Press.

Read, J., M. Emerson, and A. Tarlov. 2005. "Implications of Black Immigrant Health for U.S. Racial Disparities in Health." *Journal of Immigrant Health* 7(3): 205–212. doi:10.1007/s10903-005-3677-6

Rippy, A. and E. Newman. 2006. "Perceived Religious Discrimination and Its Relationship to Anxiety and Paranoia among Muslim Americans." *Journal of Muslim Mental Health* 1: 5–20.

"The Rise of Asian Americans." 2012. *Pew Social and Demographic Trends*. http://www.pewsocialtrends.org/2012/06/19/the-rise-of-asian-americans/

Rosales, M., and P. Gonzalez. 2013. Mammography screening among Mexican, Central-American, and South-American women. *Journal of Immigrant and Minority Health* 15(2), 225–233. doi: 10.1007/s10903-012-9731-2.

Ryan, A. M., G. C. Gee, and D. F. Laflamme. 2006. "The Association between Self-Reported Discrimination, Physical Health, and Blood Pressure: Findings from African Americans, Black Immigrants, and Latino Immigrants in New Hampshire." *Journal of Health Care for the Poor and Underserved* 17(2 Suppl): 116–132.

Schwartz, S. J., J. B. Unger, B. L. Zamboanga, and J. Szapocznik. 2010. "Rethinking the Concept of Acculturation." *American Psychologist* 65: 237–251.

Scribner, R. and J. H. Dwyer. 1989. "Acculturation and Low Birth Weight among Latinos in the Hispanic HANES." *American Journal of Public Health* 79(9): 1263–1267.

Searle, W., and C. Ward. 1990. "The Prediction of Psychological and Sociocultural Adjustment during Cross;-Cultural Transitions." *International Journal of Intercultural Relations* 14: 449–464.

Smith, J. 2010. *Brazil and the United States: Convergence and Divergence*. University of Georgia Press.

Sue, D. W. and D. Sue. 2008. *Counseling the Culturally Diverse: Theory and Practice* (5th ed.). Hoboken, NJ: Wiley.

Tucker, C. M., et al. 2007. "The Roles of Counseling Psychologists in Reducing Health Disparities." *The Counseling Psychologist* 35: 650–678.

United States Immigration and Naturalization Services. 1999. *Immigration Statistics*. http://www.ins.usdoj.gov/graphics/publicaffairs/newsrels/98Legal.pdf.

U.S. Census Bureau. 2011. *Selected Population Profile in the United States: Selected Characteristics of the Native and Foreign-Born Populations. 2010 American Community Survey 1-year estimates*. http://factfinder2.census.gov/faces/tableservices/jsf/pages/productview.xhtml?pid=ACS_10_1YR_S0501andprodType=table

U.S. Census Bureau. 2012. *The Foreign-Born Population in the United States: 2010. American Community Survey Reports*. http://www.census.gov/prod/2012pubs/acs-19.pdf.

Vega, W. A., and H. Amaro. 2002. "Latino outlook: Good health, uncertain prognosis." In *Race, ethnicity, and health – A public health reader*, edited by T. A. LaVeist, 47–75. San Francisco, CA: Jossey-Bass.

Wheeler, D. P. and A. M. Mahoney. 2008. "Caribbean Immigrants in the United States—Health and Health Care: The Need for a Social Agenda." *Health and Social Work* 33(3): 238–240.

Yakushko, O. 2008. "Xenophobia: Understanding the Roots and Consequences of Negative Attitudes toward Immigrants." *The Counseling Psychologist* 37: 36–66.

Yoo, H., G. C. Gee, and D. Takeuchi. 2009. "Discrimination and Health among Asian American Immigrants: Disentangling Racial from Language Discrimination." *Social Science and Medicine* 68(4): 726–732. doi:10.1016/j.socscimed.2008.11.013

Yu, S. M., Z. J. Huang, and G. K. Singh. 2004. "Health Status and Health Services Utilization among U.S. Chinese, Asian Indian, Filipino, and Other Asian/Pacific Islander Children." *Pediatrics* 113: 101–107. doi: 10.1542/peds.113.1.101

Zhang, W. and V. M. Ta. 2009. "Social Connections, Immigration-Related Factors, and Self-Rated Physical and Mental Health among Asian Americans." *Social Science and Medicine* 68(12): 2104–2112. doi: 10.1016/j.socscimed.2009.04.012

CHAPTER FOUR

Health Disparities among Latina/os

*Leticia Arellano-Morales
and Rocio Rosales Meza*

Understanding and eliminating health disparities is a national health priority (U.S. Department of Health and Human Services [USDHHS] 2000) but the origins of these disparities are complex and poorly understood (see chapter 2 on complexity of culture). Scholars suggest that these disparities result from a combination of individual and social factors (Shelton et al. 2011). Unfortunately, it is well documented that health disparities are common among economically disadvantaged and ethnic minority groups, such as Latina/os (USDHHS 2000). For example, Latina/os are at greater risk of stroke, hypertension, and cardiovascular disease than their European American/White counterparts (National Council of La Raza [NCLR] 2010). They also have high incidence of stomach, cervical, and liver cancer (Buki, Salazar, Pitton 2009; Buki and Selem 2009). Thus, the purpose of this chapter is to identify health disparities among Latina/os. In particular, the current chapter will provide a brief demographic overview of various Latina/o subgroups to highlight the diversity among this heterogeneous group. Second, the health beliefs of Latina/os and social factors that create health disparities are discussed. Lastly, recommendations to eliminate these disparities are presented.

Demographic Overview of Latina/os

Latina/os are a heterogeneous group and include Mexican Americans, Puerto Ricans, Cubans, Central Americans, South Americans, Dominicans, and other Latina/o cultures, regardless of race. They represent individuals of

Native American, African, Asian, and European ancestry, and originate from more than 25 countries in Central and South America, and the Caribbean (Borrell and Crawford 2009). Thus, their heterogeneity is evidenced within their ethnicity, physical appearance, traditions, cultural practices, and Spanish language dialects (Gallardo, 2012; Santiago-Rivera, Arredondo, & Gallardo-Cooper, 2002). Among Latina/o subgroups within the United States, Mexicans are the largest subgroup (63 percent), followed by Central and South Americans (14 percent), Puerto Ricans (9 percent), Cubans (4 percent) and the remaining 7.5 percent are persons of other Latina/o origins (U.S. Census Bureau 2011).

Various terms are used to describe Latina/os and no single referent is used universally. While the term *Hispanic* is often used to describe Latina/os, this term is often rejected and controversial. For instance, this term was originally imposed by the U.S. Census Bureau as an umbrella term that emphasized a White European colonial heritage while excluding other important heritages, such as indigenous, mestizo, slave, non-European and non-Spanish-speaking heritages of these Latina/o subgroups (Delgado-Romero, Galvan, Hunter, and Torres 2008). In addition, the term *Latina/o* is often used as an umbrella term to emphasize roots in Latin American countries, but debate also exists regarding this term. For instance, because Brazilians were conquered by the Portuguese, and Spanish is not their primary language, they are not considered Hispanic. Thus, preferences for terminology are often associated with regional forms of self-identification, such as *Mexican American* or *Puerto Rican,* or sociopolitical views, such as *Chicano/a* or *Boricua* (Delgado-Romero et al. 2008, Gallardo 2012).

Latina/os are currently the largest ethnic minority group within the United States. Within the past decade, they accounted for more than half of the growth within the U.S. population. Census data suggest that 50.5 million Latina/os currently reside within the United States and comprise 16 percent of the total population (U.S. Census Bureau 2011). As the fastest-growing ethnic group, they are expected to represent 25 percent of the total U.S. population by 2050. Their projected growth is based upon their fertility rates and younger age. Census data also indicate that Latina/os are the youngest ethnic minority group, with a median age of 27.5 years compared to 36.9 among the general population (Motel 2012).

Life Expectancy among Latina/os

According to the National Center for Health Statistics (2011), 2,423,712 deaths were reported for Latina/os in 2007 (Miniño et al. 2011). Among those deaths, the ten leading causes of death among Latina/os included the following: heart disease, cancer, stroke, chronic lower respiratory diseases, unintentional injuries, Alzheimer's disease, diabetes, influenza and pneumonia, kidney disease, and septicemia. Gender differences were observed within 2007, with higher rates of suicide deaths among Latino men, while higher rates of Alzheimer's disease-related deaths were reported among Latinas. The overall life expectancy of Latina/os in 2007 was 80.9 but rates were higher for Latinas (83.4) than Latinos (78.2). Latinas also demonstrated higher life expectancy than their European American/white (80.8) and African American (76.8) counterparts (Miniño et al. 2011). In 2008, the infant mortality rate for Latina/o infants was 5.66 deaths per 1,000 live births, while the mortality infant rate for European American/white infants was 5.63. Among Latina/o subgroups in 2008, the infant mortality rate was 7.88 per 1,000 live births among Puerto Ricans, 5.99 for Mexican Americans, 4.73 for Cubans, and 3.13 for Central and South Americans (Miniño et al. 2011). However, caution is warranted when interpreting these rates given the health disparities of Latina/os.

There is significant evidence of increased morbidity and mortality burden among U.S.-born Latina/os compared to their foreign–born counterparts. The primary differences between these groups are attributed to variations within social resources, socialization, and human experiences (Vega, Rodriguez, and Gruskin 2009). Moreover, the factors underlying these issues are complex and there are various controversies in estimating health disparities among Latina/os. While Latina/o immigrants may experience significant stressors, recent Latina/o immigrants show better health outcomes than their U.S.-born counterparts. These outcomes are regarded as the *Latina/o Health Paradox,* because their health outcomes are better than expected due to their low educational attainment and high poverty levels (Yang, Qeadan, and Smith-Gagen 2009). For instance, foreign-born Latina/os have 45 percent lower mortality risks than U.S.-born Latina/os. However, this advantage does not apply to all Latina/os, as it is specific to foreign-born Mexican Americans and older groups of Mexican Americans (Vega et al. 2009).

It is suggested that these differences may be due to acculturation and assimilation, resulting in subsequent dietary and lifestyle changes, such as greater consumption of fat, sugar, and processed foods. Longer duration of U.S. residence is associated with greater risk of obesity and hypertension due to poor dietary habits as well as greater use of drugs and alcohol. Conversely, increased acculturation can also contribute to positive behavior, such as use of preventive services and increased leisure-time physical activity. However, acculturation alone cannot adequately explain health outcomes, as mixed effects are observed (Vélez, Chalela, and Ramirez 2008). Researchers suggest that health disparities are attributed to income, education, and access to health care, rather than cultural differences (Vega et al. 2009; Vélez et al. 2008).

Socioeconomic Status of Latina/os

Unfortunately, Latina/os live in poverty and economic disparities are also observed within Latina/o subgroups. Census data indicate that in 2010, 15.3 percent of the U.S. population lived below the poverty line. Among ethnic groups, African Americans had the largest percentage of individuals living below the poverty line (26.9 percent), followed by Latina/os (24.7 percent), Asian Americans (12.2 percent), and European Americans (10.6 percent) (Motel 2012). Among Latina/o subgroups, Hondurans (27 percent) had the largest percentage of persons living below the poverty line, while Peruvians had the smallest percentage (12 percent). In 2009 the median household income for Latina/os was $38,039 but the median household income for the U.S. population was significantly higher at $49,777 during the same year (U.S. Census Bureau 2010). Among Latina/o subgroups, Dominicans reported the lowest median household income ($35,000), while Ecuadorians reported the highest median household income ($50,700) in 2009 (Pew Hispanic Center 2012).

Educational disparities also exist among Latina/os. For instance, 28.2 percent of the total U.S. population earned a Bachelor's degree or higher in 2010. However, disparities were observed among ethnic groups, as the percentage of Asian Americans was the highest (50.2 percent), followed by European Americans (31.4 percent), and African Americans (17.9 percent). Regrettably, Latina/os had the lowest percentage of adults who earned a Bachelor's degree or higher (13.1 percent) (Motel 2012). Significant differences were also observed among Latina/o subgroups within 2009. Peruvians reported the highest percentage of educational attainment, as 29 percent earned a high school diploma and 30 percent earned a Bachelor's degree or higher. Conversely, Guatemalans earned the lowest percentage of educational attainment, as only 21 percent reported earning a high school diploma and 8 percent earned a Bachelor's degree or higher (Pew Hispanic Center 2012).

Similar trends were observed among Latina/os in terms of health insurance. Census data indicate that in 2010, Latina/os comprised the highest percentage of uninsured persons within the United States (31.2 percent), surpassing that of the total uninsured population (15.8 percent), and all ethnic/racial groups, including African Americans (19 percent), Asian Americans (15.5 percent), and European Americans (11 percent) (Motel 2012). Vast disparities were also observed among Latina/o subgroups, as Hondurans demonstrated the largest percentage of uninsured persons (52 percent) while Puerto Ricans demonstrated the smallest percentage (15 percent) (Pew Hispanic Center 2012). It is speculated that although 62 percent of Latina/os 16 years of age and older are employed, they lack health insurance due to their occupations. For instance, only 7 percent are employed in management or business positions (Motel 2012) but are twice as likely as non-Latina/os to be employed within the service sector.

Geographical Locations and Immigration Experiences of Latina/os

Extensive diversity exists among Latina/os due to their national origin, geographic region, education, income, acculturation, and other salient factors (Betancourt and Flynn 2009). In addition, their diversity is amplified by genetic, cultural, political, and religious influences (Gans et al. 2002). Statistical profiles from the Pew Hispanic Center (2012) indicate that 47 percent of immigrants were Latina/os and 29 percent of Latina/o immigrants were naturalized citizens in 2009. Among foreign born Latina/os, 29.9 percent were born in Mexico and 23.3 percent were born in Latin America. Geographically, most Latina/os (76 percent) reside within nine states, including Arizona, California, Texas, Colorado, Florida, Illinois, New Mexico, New Jersey, and New York (Pew Hispanic Center 2012). In addition, 50 percent of Latina/os reside within three states alone, including California, Texas, and Florida. Additionally, the largest Mexican populations are observed within Los Angeles, Chicago, Houston, San Antonio and Phoenix, while the largest Puerto Rican populations are found within New York, Chicago, and Philadelphia. Large concentrations of Cuban are found within Hialeah, Miami, New York, Tampa, and Los Angeles. The largest Central American populations are observed within Los Angeles, New York, Houston, Miami, and San Francisco, while the largest South American populations are found within New York, Los Angeles, Chicago, and Miami (Vélez et al. 2008).

Geographical distinctions among Latina/o subgroups are often due to their distinct immigration experiences. Although significant numbers of Latina/os immigrated within the past decade, they are not a newly arrived group within the United States, as noted by Vélez et al. (2008), "millions of Latina/os in the United States never left their homeland; they simply found themselves within the redrawn boundaries of the country" (192).

Mexican Americans have unique patterns of immigration because like Native Americans, Mexicans were native to what is currently regarded as the Southwest. The indigenous history of Mexico predates the arrival of Spanish conquistadores during the 15th century and is exemplified by a history of colonization and genocide. The admixture of Europeans and indigenous persons resulted in racially mixed Mexicans, known as *mestizos*. Because of their close proximity and the United States' need for cheap labor, a significant number of Mexicans immigrated to the United States within the past century. For instance, the labor shortage during WWII resulted in the importation of Mexicans for agricultural labor through the *Bracero Program*. Between 1942 and 1964, approximately five million braceros entered the United States from Mexico as laborers (Organista 2007). However, due to the large number of immigrants entering the United States, anti-Mexican hysteria also resurfaced and under the directives of the U.S. Immigration Service, *Operation Wetback* was developed. Approximately 3.8 million individuals of Mexican descent, including U.S.-born Latina/o children were deported (Organista 2007). Unfortunately, similar sentiments remain, such as the passage of Arizona Senate Bill 1070. This law has generated considerable controversy as one of the strictest anti-illegal immigration laws within the United States, and allows for the racial profiling of Latina/os and the deportation of undocumented immigrants.

The history of Puerto Rico is also manifested by a legacy of conquest. Spanish conquistadors landed on the island of Puerto Rico (originally known as Boriquen), in 1493 and subsequently conquered the indigenous Tainos. The demise of the Tainos resulted in the importation of African slaves and the admixture of African slaves, Spaniards, and Tainos created the rich composition of Puerto Ricans (Organista 2007). Four centuries later, Puerto Rico became a U.S. territory in 1898 due to the brief Spanish-American War. Lopez and Carrillo (2001) suggest that there were various explanations for their immigration to the mainland, including encouragement from the island government, island overpopulation, and low airfares to the United States. The establishment of the commonwealth resulted in the arrival of a large number of Puerto Ricans within New York City between 1900 and 1945 but the largest numbers of Puerto Ricans (887,000) settled in New York, New Jersey, Connecticut, Chicago, Pennsylvania, and other areas between 1946 and 1964 (Lopez and Carrillo 2001, Organista, 2007). The third wave, known as the *revolving-door migration*, began in 1965 and is characterized by fluctuating immigration patterns and greater dispersal into other areas of the United States.

Unlike the immigration histories of Mexican Americans and Puerto Ricans, the immigration experiences of Cubans were quite distinct. According to Organista (2007), Cuban Americans are regarded as the Latina/o model minority, due to their success within the United States, and their predominately elite composition. The onset of the Cuban Revolution resulted in the first wave of affluent and well-educated White Cuban immigrants who settled in south Florida. As political refugees they were provided with unprecedented refugee support and aid by the U.S. government and private sectors (Organista 2007). The second and third waves of immigrants included relatives of the prior exiles between 1960 and 1970. However, the fourth wave of immigrants in 1980 significantly differed from the prior waves of immigrants. Regarded as "Marielitos" because they sailed from the Port of Mariel, these working-class Cuban exiles were not well-received unlike their previous counterparts. Similarly, in 1994 numerous Cuban "boat people" attempted to enter the United States and this initiated a rapid change in U.S. policy. These changes resulted in the refusal of additional Cuban refugees (Galarraga 2007).

The Dominican Republic is largely comprised of three major ethnic groups, including Indians, Europeans, and Africans, although Dominicans are largely racially mixed. Like Puerto Rico, the Dominican Republic was under Spanish rule. In fact, Christopher Columbus first colonized the Dominican Republic in 1492. Due to the demise of the indigenous Caribitaino and Arawak, African slaves were imported (Lopez and Carrillo 2001). Immigrants from the Dominican Republic began to enter the United States due to the political turmoil of the 1960s and the assassination of President Trujillo. The civil war and subsequent U.S. intervention led to a large influx of immigrants who settled in the New York area. According to Lopez and Carrillo (2001), statistics about their migration are imprecise, but approximately one million Dominicans have immigrated to the United States since the 1950s.

Immigrants from Central and South America came to the United States before the 1970s, and many arrived with permanent visas or permanent resident status (Lopez and Carrillo 2001). However, immigration patterns changed thereafter, as a significant number entered the United States as political asylum applicants or without legal documentation. After the 1970s, political turmoil and economic threats created the first large waves of immigrants from Central America, beginning with Salvadorans, followed by Guatemalans in the early 1980s, as well as Nicaraguans and Hondurans in the mid-1980s (Lopez and Carillo 2001, Organista 2007). More than a million Central Americans fled to the United States to escape guerilla warfare, violence, and other traumatic events. In addition, these countries are characterized by extreme poverty and high mortality rates and vast disparities exist between the poor and wealthy. However, despite these hardships, the United States fails to grant them political asylum and government assistance as political refugees because they are often unable to prove their political persecution.

Health Beliefs and Practices among Latina/os

Chong (2002) suggests that views regarding health and disease among Latina/os are based upon a combination of Native American, African, Asian, and European influences. Thus, there are various aspects that influence the health beliefs of Latina/os, as well as the meaning of health. However, it is important to acknowledge that we can speak solely in generalities regarding these health beliefs and practices, as many within-group differences exist due to socioeconomic status, generational level, acculturation, and other demographic variables (Gallardo 2012). The meaning of health varies among Latina/os but religious and supernatural components are often evident within traditional definitions of health and illness (Spector 2009). Moreover, Ruiz (1994) suggests that Latina/os do not distinguish between illness and disease. For instance, disease is generally perceived as a malfunction of a biological-physiological process, while illness comprises personal, interpersonal, and environmental elements. Therefore, beliefs are influenced by a holistic view of the human person, and interconnections among the body, mind, and spirit (Ortiz, Davis, and McNeill 2008; see chapter 10 in this volume on *Curanderismo*).

Moreover, a conception of illness among Latina/os reflects a holistic view of health and illness that does not differentiate between psychological and physical health (Penn et al. 2000). Conceptions of illness may be attributed to psychological states (envy, anger, fight, family turmoil, etc.), supernatural causes (punishment from God, bad luck, malevolent spirits, enemies), or environmental conditions (bad air, germs, bad food, dust, etc.) (Falicov 1995, Giachello 1996). For an in-depth discussion of illnesses that are attributed to psychological states and traditional folk illnesses, see Chapter 11 regarding *susto*. Although variation exists regarding health beliefs of Latina/os, the literature suggests that they typically include two categories of beliefs, an anthropological view pertaining to hot/cold theories of illness, and traditional folk illnesses that may also include supernatural influences (Chong 2002, Falicov 1995, Spector 2009).

Hot/Cold Theories of Illness

The theory of hot and cold was taken to Mexico by Spanish priests and integrated within Aztec and other indigenous beliefs. This theory was based upon a Hippocratic theory of disease and the four body humors. The body's imbalance is expressed as either hot and cold or wet and dry. The four humors contained within the body include blood (hot and wet), yellow bile (hot and dry), phlegm (cold and wet), and black bile (cold and dry) (CDC 2010, Chong 2002, Spector 2009). Accordingly, when all four humors are balanced, the body is healthy, while any imbalance results in illness. To correct an imbalance, individuals consume food or herbs with the opposite quality. Hot conditions are treated with cold medications. For instance, a patient with a cold may find relief in drinking warm fluids, such as hot tea or a bowl of hot chicken soup (Chong 2002).

Another view regarding balance suggests that after an extremely hot experience, one should avoid extreme exposure to a cold environment to prevent illness. For instance, after extensive ironing and exposure to continuous heat, a person should avoid going outside into the cold air to avoid becoming ill and experiencing *pasmo*. *Pasmo* is described as paralysis of the face or limbs due to the disruption of the hot-cold balance (Spector 2009). However, it is important to note that not all Latina/os endorse hot/cold theories of illness, due to increased acculturation and acceptance of Western theories of health and illness (Falicov 1995). In addition, even less acculturated Latina/os may not demonstrate familiarity with this perspective. For instance, in their qualitative study examining health beliefs and diabetes among Mexican Americans from El Paso, Texas, Poss and Jezewski (2002) observed that not a single participant was familiar with hot and cold disease etiologies. Even after intense probing and questioning, participants did not reveal familiarity with this concept. Instead, conceptualizations of their diabetes included both biologically-based causes, such as poor diet, obesity, and heredity, as well as cultural explanations, such as susceptibility due to *susto*. Similarly, although they used traditional folk remedies in combination with their prescribed medication, they did not utilize humoral treatment for their *susto*. Thus, a hot-cold disease etiology was not supported by this study. Furthermore, Poss and Jezewski (2002) suggest that Mexican Americans demonstrate a synthesis of both biomedical and cultural perspectives.

Also focusing on illness beliefs, Santos, Hurtado-Ortiz, and Sneed (2009) examined diabetes illness beliefs of Latina/o college students who were at risk for Type II diabetes. They identified four factors that included emotional (anger, stress, or anxiety), folk beliefs (bad blood, cold/drafts, germs/infection), punitive (sinful or excessive behavior), and genes/heredity factors (family history). Within-group differences were observed, as less assimilated participants scored higher on the emotional factor, while traditional college-age students (18–24 years) scored higher on emotional and folk belief factors than their older non-traditional college-age peers. Given the limited empirical data to support the endorsement of hot/cold etiologies among Latina/os, it is important for researchers and clinicians to continue to understand this perspective and how Latina/os reveal the nature of their illness.

Health Practices among Latina/os

Lack of insurance and health costs are significant barriers that prevent Latina/os from accessing formal health care, and curanderos and other folk practitioners often serve as primary sources of help that enable Latina/os to address their health needs (Viladrich 2010). An in-depth discussion of folk healing practitioners is provided within the *curanderismo* chapter in this volume. The distrust of medical providers or modern health practices also contributes to their health-related practices (Giachello 1996). For instance, Latina/os may believe that medications cause someone to become worse, such as antidepressants (Penn et al. 2000). Formal medical care may function as a last resort when self-treatment and folk healing practices prove unsuccessful (Giachello 1996). Regrettably, the lack of health insurance and delayed treatment contributes to the lack of early detection of chronic diseases or a poor prognosis for recovery (Penn et al. 2000).

Penn et al. (2000) suggest that Latina/os may also engage in self-diagnosis, particularly Latina/os who reside along the U.S.-Mexico border. Because of their inability to pay for medical care, they may consult with local pharmacists regarding potential treatment. In addition, they may access prescription medications through non-medical sources such as *tiendas* (grocers), *bodegas* (convenience store), *botánicas* (stores that sell an array of health-related products), flea markets, and other businesses geared towards Latina/os (Song et al. 2012). *Botánicas* also serve as unique settings that provide a wide array of health care products, such as herbs, plants, and roots, as well as religious icons from multiple traditions. They also provide access to informal health services within their premises, or provide referrals to informal and formal health care providers (Viladrich 2010).

Contributing Factors of Health Disparities among Latina/os

Myths and Misperceptions Regarding Cancer and Chronic Illness among Latina/os

The literature suggests that a higher proportion of Latina/os demonstrate erroneous beliefs regarding cancer and other chronic beliefs that impact their screening behaviors (Buki and Selem 2009, Fernández-Esquer et al.2003, Ramirez et al. 2000, Shelton et al. 2011). Latina/os are more likely to believe that because they feel healthy they do not require preventive screening procedures. However, they are also less likely to recognize that bloody breast discharge and breast cancer lumps can indicate breast cancer (Ramirez et al. 2000). In addition, Latina/os are likely to possess medically inaccurate information regarding breast cancer, such as the belief that breast trauma and negative behaviors are risk factors (Ramirez et al. 2000). Latinas also demonstrate the belief that it is difficult to prevent breast and cervical cancer, and that it is a death sentence since cancer is incurable (Austin, McNally, and Stewart 2002). Myths regarding pap smears and cervical cancer are also observed. For instance, the belief that pap smears are expensive and that cancer treatment is worse than the disease is observed among low acculturated Latinas (Buki and Selem 2009, Fernández-Esquer et al. 2003). Many Latina/os are unfamiliar with colorectal cancer. Research supports that Latina/os also demonstrate misperceptions or poor knowledge regarding colorectal cancer (Diaz et al. 2011, Goldman, Diaz, and Kim, 2009). For instance, Latina/os believe that rectal sex is a risk factor for colorectal cancer due to the misperception that rectal sex is often associated with gay sexual behavior. In addition, factors such as bad food, constipation, and strained bowel movements are regarded as causal factors of colorectal cancer (Diaz et al. 2011, Goldman et al. 2009).

Latina/os also appear to lack adequate information regarding chronic diseases. For instance, Christian, Rosamond, White, and Mosca (2007) evaluated nine-year (1997-2006) trends associated with cardiovascular disease among a nationally represented sample. They found that awareness among Latinas was lower than European Americans (29 percent vs. 68 percent). Latinas felt least informed about heart disease, perceived it as unpreventable, and were uncomfortable discussing heart disease with their doctor. Dubard, Garrett, and Gizlice (2006) observed that fewer than 10 percent of Latina/o participants identified all heart attack symptoms and fewer than 20 percent identified all stroke symptoms. Latina/os are also likely to hold incorrect beliefs regarding diabetes. For instance, they may believe their diabetes complications are the result of insulin therapy instead of prolonged hyperglycemia. In addition, compared to non-Latina/os, they are more likely to hold myths about insulin therapy, such that insulin therapy indicates that the disease progressed. They also perceive that insulin injections will be extremely painful and cause long-term complications, such as blindness (Campos 2007).

Personal Barriers to Healthcare

Latina/os are more likely to work in low wage occupations that provide limited socioeconomic mobility and insurance benefits. If health coverage is available from employers, it is not easily affordable (American Cancer Society 2009) or inadequate (Valdez et al. 2011). The purchase of health insurance also poses economic hardships, as health insurance is viewed in terms of costs and benefits rather than risks and benefits (Martinez and Carter-Pokras 2006). Unfortunately, the lack of insurance creates a decreased likelihood of having a primary care provider, preventive services, referrals, early detection, and adequate treatment (Betancourt, Carrillo, Green, and Maina 2004).

Research also suggests that while Latina/os have lower rates of preventive care, they have higher rates of emergency department visits for routine care and mental health services (Vega et al. 2009, Vélez et al. 2008). For instance, 53 percent of Latina/os use emergency rooms and outpatient departments as sources of medical care (Betancourt et al. 2004). However, the delays in preventive care are also attributed to economic constraints and the lack of health insurance. Martinez and Carter-Pokras (2006) found that Latinas postpone their own health care visits until they require emergency room services and rely upon home remedies due to the lack of health insurance. However, their children's health is their top priority and they actively seek preventive services for them despite their limited economic resources.

Other personal barriers include linguistic factors, such as limited English proficiency. Latina/os with limited English proficiency are more likely to experience difficulties scheduling a medical appointment and interacting with medical staff. The lack of written information in Spanish, as well as poorly translated materials, also creates difficulties completing and understanding medical documents. Limited English proficiency also makes it difficult to maintain drug compliance, as Latina/os do not always understand their medical condition. Moreover, they report difficulties reading drug labels, understanding their medications, and report that the side effects of their medication were inadequately explained by their health provider (Wallace et al. 2009).

Among Spanish-speaking Latina/o patients, language is one of the most important factors that influence the patient-physician encounter and quality of care. The lack of language concordance also contributes to decreased communication and patient satisfaction (Betancourt et al., 2004). Linguistic barriers with primary care providers are also common among primarily Spanish-speaking Latina/os, as the majority of healthcare providers are non-Spanish speaking (Buki and Selem 2009, Campos 2007; Valdez et al. 2011). It is estimated that only 5 percent of medical providers are Spanish-speaking (Campos 2007). In addition, not all medical facilities provide trained or qualified interpreters. While medical facilities may provide interpreters, Latina/os with limited English proficiency prefer to work with a Spanish-speaking health provider to avoid difficulties communicating with their provider. When Latina/os are unable to fully express themselves, they risk receiving incomplete information regarding their health (Shelton et al. 2011) and a lack of preventive services. Similarly, they face greater risk for misdiagnosis, poor compliance, medical errors, and poor outcomes (Betancourt et al. 2004, NCLR 2010).

Organizational and Structural Barriers to Healthcare among Latina/os

Betancourt and colleagues (2004) suggest that Latina/os are more likely to receive medical care in community-based clinics, hospital outpatient departments, emergency rooms, and other safety-net settings. Consequently, they receive health services in settings that often fail to provide continuity of care, utilize dated medical record systems, maintain limited after-hours services, and frequently depend upon residents and fellows as primary providers. Unfortunately, the U.S. healthcare system is inherently complex, underfunded, and bureaucratic. Furthermore, organizational barriers also make it difficult for Latina/os to receive preventive screening and referrals to medical specialists, diagnostic screenings, and medical interventions (Betancourt et al. 2004).

Institutional barriers, such as organizational and structural practices also contribute to health disparities among Latina/os. The lack of transportation and limited mobility make it difficult to travel to health facilities, particularly facilities that require significant travel (Betancourt et al 2004, Salazar 1996). The high clinical demands that are placed upon health providers often lead to shorter patient visits and limit the amount of time spent with patients. Long waiting periods and crowded medical facilities are also realities for most patients and contribute to high dissatisfaction (Betancourt et al. 2004). Limited hours of operation and the timing of visits also create hardships, particularly for Latina/os who work during traditional office hours (Martinez and Carter-Pokras 2006). A doctor's visit may amplify their economic burden, as they might not be able to leave their place of employment for their medical needs, due to the lack of leave benefits (Valdez et al., 2011) or inflexible work schedules.

Among Latina/o immigrants, the poor quality of health services often due to long wait periods, limited hours of operation, lack of Spanish-speaking bilingual and bicultural services, and fear of deportation contribute to the distrust of the health care system and providers (NCLR, 2010; Song et al., 2012). Distrust of the medical establishment may also extend into the area of medical research (Shelton et al., 2011). There is ample research suggesting that discrimination also contributes to the distrust of the medical establishment and perceptions of inferior medical services (Shariff-Marco, Klassen, and Bowie, 2010; Shelton et al., 2011). For instance, research suggests that Latina/os are less likely to receive certain procedures and surgeries such as coronary artery bypass graft, angioplasty, and kidney transplant based upon provider bias (Betancourt et al., 2004). In addition, perceptions of poor medical care due to racism also adversely impact health delivery and outcomes. In an examination of racial bias,

Latina/os reported that their doctor did not listen to them or actively involve them in the decision-making of their treatment. They also reported that the medical staff judged them unfairly or treated them with disrespect because they were Latina/o (Johnson, Saha, Arbelaez, Beach, and Cooper, 2004).

Culturally Tailored Health Promotion Programs for Latina/os

It is particularly important to avoid making stereotypes of Latina/os, and remember that there are both within-group and between-group variations among Latina/os. For instance, Cubans may not hold the same cultural values and health beliefs as Mexican Americans. Moreover, due to factors such as acculturation, immigration, generation, and education, certain Latina/os may share health-related practices similar to European Americans when compared to other Latina/os (Betancourt and Flynn, 2009). However, the empirical literature suggests that Latina/os expect to receive information during their health visits but often fail to receive this needed information and largely rely upon their social networks and word-of-mouth to obtain health information (Martinez and Carter-Pokras, 2006). Unfortunately, the information that they receive from their social networks is not always accurate. Latina/os also obtain health information from media sources, such as television, radio, and printed sources, such as magazines and the newspaper (Olson, Sabogal, and Perez 2008). The lack of English proficiency, limited or inaccurate health knowledge, and limited health access proves challenging.

There is an immediate need for health care providers to increase their understanding of the diversity that exists among Latina/os, as Latina/os are a heterogeneous group. One method to improve the patient-provider relationship is to practice culturally competent care by respecting the cultural values of Latina/os. A bilingual and culturally responsive staff is also critical. In particular, cultural values such as *simpatia, personalismo, respeto,* and *familismo* appear to impact the medical encounter (Buki and Selem 2009, Campos 2007, Huff and Kline 2008). Cumulatively, these values emphasize formal friendliness, respect, and recognition of the family's importance. When these values are absent within the clinical encounter, they serve as barriers to treatment because providers are perceived as uncaring, which results in noncompliance, delayed treatment, and potential conflict (Campos 2007).

In addition to the integration of Latina/o cultural values within medical encounters, the literature suggests that these values are important within health promotion programs. Linguistically simple and visually appealing materials that are culturally relevant are also regarded as credible (Buki et al. 2009) among Latina/os. Efficacious strategies for promoting health education with Latina/os include the use of *promotoras,* bilingual print materials, mass media, technology, and English as a Second Language venues. However, due to space limitations, a brief overview of these strategies is provided below.

Use of *Promotoras de Salud*

There is a significant amount of literature suggesting that community health advisors, also known as *promotoras de salud* or *promotoras,* are beneficial in improving the health, knowledge, and behaviors of Latina/os. Their success is often attributed to their roles as community advocates, role models, health advisors, and providers of social support (Larkey 2006, Keane, Nielsen and Dower 2004). An appealing aspect of promotoras is their ability to increase access to care and provide preventive services. However, the success of *promotora* programs lies in the fact that promotoras are trusted individuals, as they are members of their social networks and thus model cultural values in health care (Elder et al. 2009, Keane et al. 2004).

Promotora programs are provided within various facilities and also focus upon various individuals within Latina/o families. In their review of the literature regarding promotoras with Latina/os, Rhodes and colleagues (2007) identified the following eleven intervention areas: cancer prevention and screening, prenatal health, general health promotion and disease prevention, cardiovascular disease prevention, HIV, access to health care services, diabetes, eye safety, environmental health, and asthma management. However, despite successful outcomes, *promotora* programs are not without limitations. Most *promotoras* within these studies are females and few interventions specifically focus upon Latina/o men. Similarly, a significant portion of these studies focus upon Mexican Americans in the Southwestern regions of the United States. Methodological challenges are also noted due the diversity within methodologies, as not all programs include control or comparison groups (Rhodes et al. 2007). Lastly, *promotora* programs require a significant amount of time to recruit, train, and sustain *promotoras* (Elder et al. 2009).

Use of Print Materials

As identified by the literature, print materials are effective in changing health-related knowledge and behaviors. Communication research regarding Latina/os suggests that they tend to prefer written materials and hands-on demonstrations by well-informed experts. These materials are perceived as highly credible when they are culturally relevant and emphasize the family

(Buki et al. 2009). They are also efficacious when they include visually appealing pictures and illustrations and convey linguistically simple messages. In addition, pictorial messages and testimonials, such as *telenovelas* (Spanish soap operas) are also appealing to Latina/os (Buki et al. 2009, Elder et al. 2005), as illustrated within the *Secretos de la Buena Vida* (Secrets of the Good Life) program.

Secretos de la Buena Vida was a 12 week randomized controlled trial that targeted the diets of Latina/os from San Diego through a tailored communication approach (Elder et al. 2005). The three conditions included a *promotora* and tailored print materials (treatment group), tailored print materials only (tailored), and off-the shelf print materials (control). The content of the tailored print materials included culturally relevant behavioral strategies and tips, a lifestyle column addressing common concerns among Latinas, and a *novela* (story) that depicted a family who dealt with nutrition-related challenges, colorful pictures, and other personalized information. Results indicated that the *promotora* condition successfully attained lower levels of total fat grams and energy intake, total saturated fat, total carbohydrates, glucose, and fructose at immediate post-intervention. However, at one-year follow-up, these changes did not persist and additional changes were observed within the tailored mailed condition.

Use of Mass Media

Latina/os consume most types of media but appear to utilize radio and television at higher rates. The use of radio and television for health promotion has proven effective with Latina/os. For instance, in an effort to improve diabetes care among Latina/o Medicare beneficiaries, *Viva La Vida* (Live Life), was developed (Olson et al. 2008). In addition to improving diabetes care, the program was developed to reduce annual glycosylated hemoglobin (A1C) testing disparities between White/European American and Latina/o Medicare beneficiaries within four Southern California counties. *Viva La Vida* utilized a multifaceted approach to target health care providers and beneficiaries through bilingual, low literacy and well-illustrated health education materials and tools, community and provider partnerships, and the mass media. For instance, in addition to free bilingual materials on their websites, partner organizations also distributed program materials to their health providers and Latina/o constituents that included colorful graphics and materials with messages for individuals with low literacy and limited knowledge regarding diabetes.

A physician-patient prompt card helped to facilitate communication and record important test results. Evidence-based materials for quality improvement and cultural competency were also distributed to providers. To reinforce these messages, the mass media was also utilized, such as public service announcements for radio and television, live interviews, and the placement of ads and articles within bilingual and Spanish community newspapers. Program messages were also placed in physician trade magazines. Program results suggested that A1C testing between White/European American and Latina/o beneficiaries decreased considerably during the 18 months of program interventions, from 7.1 to 3.0 percent.

Video interventions with Latina/os are effective at changing health-related knowledge, attitudes, and behaviors (Elder et al. 2009), particularly as Latina/os view more television than the general U.S. population and are more likely to utilize information from these television sources (Wilkin et al. 2007). The *telenovela* (Spanish soap opera) is a popular form of entertainment among Spanish-speaking Latina/os. Thus, Wilkin and associates (2007) examined the efficacy of a *telenovela* in providing breast cancer information to Spanish-speaking viewers within the United States. Health professionals consulted on a breast cancer storyline that was featured within a Spanish-language telenovela, *Ladrón de Corazones,* and evaluated its impact upon viewers' knowledge and behavioral intentions. Calls placed to 1-800-4-CANCER significantly increased when a PSA was featured with the phone number during the telenovela. Secondly, a nationwide telephone survey indicated viewers gained specific knowledge from viewing the story, and men who viewed the telenovela were significantly more likely to recommend that women obtain mammograms.

Use of Technology

Given the increased use of social marketing technologies, multimedia technology is a promising venue for providing accurate health information. In particular, health information kiosks, ATM-style terminals with touch screens are promising when working with Latina/os. Kiosks are effective since they do not require technological expertise to navigate and are also flexible in disseminating information. They also assist researchers with data collection because they record confidential patient health information, such as weight and blood pressure. In addition, kiosks are considered economical in providing important health information to underserved communities, such as Latina/os. Matthews and colleagues (2009) investigated the use of electronic, web-enabled touch-screen information kiosks to provide culturally and linguistically appropriate diabetes information to Latina/os in Northeastern Georgia. Two kiosk models provided bilingual, read-aloud diabetes education and local resource information regarding health care. Data indicated that users found the kiosks and their functions helpful and easy to use. However, participants preferred to use the kiosks when supported by a human resource, such as a *promotora* to provide additional encouragement because they felt this type of technology was initially intimidating.

Use of English as a Second Language (ESL) Venue

The use of an English as a Second Language (ESL) setting is a beneficial method for reaching a population that does not traditionally receive public health messages, due to activities that compete for their time. In a creative format, Elder and colleagues (2000) addressed the issue of language literacy and health promotion with Latina/o immigrants through their *Language for Your Health* program, by integrating health messages within English as a second language (ESL) courses in San Diego, CA. The goal of the *Language for Your Health* program was to create changes in students' nutrition-related knowledge, attitudes, behaviors, and physiological measures. The intervention group received nutrition/heart health education that was integrated into ESL classes, while the control group received the same quality of education in the area of stress management. Post-test data indicated that Latina/os successfully reduced their HDL ratio, systolic blood pressure, fat reduction, and nutritional knowledge. Interestingly, these differences disappeared at follow-up, suggesting that the control group also indicated positive health changes.

Recommendations for Public Policy

An increased focus regarding chronic disease prevention and control is essential. The aforementioned programs and others, are warranted to engage Latina/o communities in addressing environmental, policy, and behavioral changes (NCLR 2010). These changes can occur through partnerships with community-based organizations and collaboration with *promotoras*. The ability to link prevention and treatment programs with a policy agenda will also help increase opportunities for long-term funding and the integration of community-based practices into broader use in society (Betancourt et al. 2004, NCLR 2010). Moreover, this political agenda will help decrease health disparities among Latina/os. Because *promotoras* also have the potential to create social change (Keane et al. 2004), community-based partnerships are needed to work with *promotoras* to reduce linguistic and economic barriers. Large scale efforts are needed to address the lack of access to health insurance among Latina/os. Despite the current U.S. economic crisis and political climate, the issue of healthcare remains controversial. This controversy is further amplified by unprecedented budget cuts (Betancourt et al. 2004). However, policy makers should work to make health insurance more affordable and identify ways to decrease the numbers of uninsured Latina/os. Efforts to increase affordability and access to healthcare should not solely rest upon Latina/os. In addition, increased education is needed regarding current social service programs so that Latina/os may meet eligibility criteria, such as health benefits (Bentancourt et al 2004, Daniels 2010).

Given the low ratio of Spanish-speaking and Latina/o health professionals, there is a significant need to develop a significant cadre of bilingual health professionals (NCLR 2010). Colleges and universities should focus upon recruiting greater numbers of Latina/os into health care professions. In addition, increased governmental funding is needed to provide scholarships and grants for education and training as healthcare professionals (Daniels 2010). The paucity of Spanish-speaking health providers necessitates that academic institutions integrate cultural competencies throughout their curriculum. Similarly, health care settings must provide their staff with regular cultural competency training. In addition, these organizations must focus upon eliminating other barriers within their infrastructure that contribute to health care disparities (Daniels 2010, Valdez et al. 2011).

Collaboration is also needed between physicians and mental health providers due to the co-occurrence of physical illnesses and psychological disorders. For instance, it is not uncommon for depression or anxiety to co-occur with chronic diseases and cancer. In addition, depression may manifest itself through depressive symptoms. However, due to the stigma associated with mental illness among Latina/os, they are more likely to seek care within primary health settings. Because Latina/os tend to postpone their delivery of care, they often present with acute psychological and medical conditions in emergency rooms. Thus, collaborative arrangements are needed to ensure consultation, coordination, and co-delivery of care (Valdez et al. 2011). In addition, policy and research efforts are needed to integrate physical and mental health care and interdisciplinary research and practice.

Recommendations for Future Research

Because clinical trials are considered the "gold standard" of evidence regarding the efficacy of disease prevention, early detection, and treatment interventions, it is important to include Latina/os within clinical trials to ensure their applicability. Unfortunately, little is known about Latina/o clinical trial participation, as they are absent from clinical trials. In one of the first studies to examine awareness of cancer clinical trials, and willingness to participate, Wallington and colleagues (2012) observed that participants from Central, South, and North America were largely unfamiliar (52 percent) with clinical trials but once explained, 65 percent indicated a willingness to participate. Findings also suggest that informational channels, such as the internet and Spanish-language telephone call centers are effective in conveying clinical trial information. While this study is informative, additional studies are needed to identify ways to increase their participation within clinical trials. However, given the need for preventive services among Latina/os, their participation in clinical trials is vital to ensure generalizability of results and benefits from the advances within such research.

There is an increased need to develop large scale epidemiological studies that include diverse groups of Latina/os from different regions, such as the current SOL Study. Sponsored by the National Heart, Lung, and Blood Institute (NHLBI) and the National Institutes of Health (NIH), the *Hispanic Community Health Study (HCHS)/ Study of Latinas/os (SOL)*, is the largest study ever conducted regarding the health of Latina/os within the U.S (Sorlie et al. 2010). This national study is a multi-center epidemiologic study that includes 16,000 adults between the ages of 18 to 74. As an epidemiologic study, SOL focuses upon Latina/os to determine the role of acculturation within the prevalence and development of disease, and to identify risk factors that play a protective or harmful role within Latina/os. Thus, researchers and practitioners should familiarize themselves with the various findings of this large study and integrate them within their work (for additional information visit http://www.cscc.unc.edu/hchs/).

Conclusions

The need to eliminate health disparities among Latina/os and other underserved populations is paramount and requires continuous attention and effort. Unfortunately, Latina/os face a myriad of barriers to health promotion and disease prevention. While there are no easy solutions to eliminate these disparities, multifaceted approaches are needed, including programming, outreach, and research initiatives. However, increased advocacy and policy initiatives are also needed to improve the overall well-being of Latina/os and to empower the Latina/o community.

References

American Cancer Society. 2009. *Cancer Facts and Figures for Hispanics/Latinos 2009–2011*. Atlanta, GA: American Cancer Society.

Austin, L. T., M. McNally, and D. E. Stewart. 2002. "Breast and Cervical Cancer Screening in Hispanic Women. A Literature Review Using the Health Belief Model." *Women's Health Issues 12:* 122–128.

Betancourt, J. R., J. E. Carrillo, A. R. Green, and A. Maina. 2004. "Barriers to Health Promotion and Disease Prevention in the Latino Population." *Clinical Cornerstone 6:* 16–29.

Betancourt, J. R., and Flynn. 2009. "The Psychology of Health. Physical Health and the Role of Culture and Behavior." In *Handbook of U.S. Latino psychology. Developmental and Community-Based Perspectives,* edited by F. A. Villarruel, G. Carlo, J. A. Grau, M. Azmitia, N. J. Cabrera, and T. J. Chahin, 347–361. Thousand Oaks, CA: Sage.

Borrell, L. N., and N. D. Crawford. 2009. "All-Cause Mortality among Hispanics in the United States: Exploring Heterogeneity by Nativity Status, Country of Origin, and Race in the National Health Interview Survey-Linked Mortality Files." *Annals of Epidemiology 19:* 336–343.

Buki, L. P., S. I. Salazar, and V. O. Pitton. 2009. "Design Eelements for the Development of Cancer Education Print Materials for a Latina/o Audience." *Health Promotion Practice 4:* 564–572.

Buki, L. P. and M. Selem. 2009. "Cancer Screening and Survivorship in Latino Populations. A Primer for Psychologists." In *Handbook of U.S. Latino Psychology. Developmental and Community-Based Perspectives,* edited by F. A. Villarruel, G. Carlo, J. A. Grau, M. Azmitia, N. J. Cabrera, and T. J. Chahin, 363–378. Thousand Oaks, CA: Sage.

Campos, C. 2007. "Addressing Cultural Barriers to the Successful Use of Insulin in Hispanics with Type II Diabetes." *Southern Medical Journal* 100: 812–820.

Centers for Disease Control and Prevention. 2010. *Cultural Insights: Communicating with Hispanics/Latinos.* Office of the Associate Director for Communication. Washington DC.

Christian, A. H., W. Rosamond, A. R. White, and L. Mosca. 2007. "Nine-Year Trends and Racial and Ethnic Disparities in Women's Awareness of Heart Disease and Stroke: An American Heart Association National Study." *Journal of Women's Health 16:* 68–81.

Chong, N. 2002. *The Latino Patient: A Cultural Guide for the Health Care Providers.* Boston, MA: Intercultural Press.

Daniels, M. 2010. "Strategies for Targeting Health Care Disparities among Hispanics." *Family and Community Health 33:* 329–342.

Delgado-Romero, E. A., N. Galvan, M. R. N. Hunter, and V. Torres. 2008. "Latino/Latina Americans." In *Culturally Alert Counseling: A Comprehensive Introduction,* edited by G. McAulifee, 323–352. Thousand Oaks, CA: Sage.

Diaz, J. A., R. Goldman, N. Arellano, J. Borkan, and C. B. Eaton. 2011. "Brief Report: Exploration of Colorectal Cancer Risk Perceptions among Latinos." *Journal of Immigrant Minority Health 13:* 188–192.

DuBard, A. C., J. Garrett, and Z. Gizlice. 2006. "Effect of Language on Heart Attack and Stroke Awareness among U.S. Hispanics." *American Journal of Preventive Medicine 30:* 189–196.

Elder, J. P., J. I. Candelaria, S. I. Woodruff, M. H. Criqui, G. A. Talavera, and J. W. Rupp. 2000. "Results of Language for Health: Cardiovascular Disease Nutrition Education for Latino English-as-a-Second-Language Students." *Health Education and Behavior 27:* 50–63.

Elder, J. P., G. X. Ayala, N. R. Campbell, D. Slymen, E. T. Lopez-Madurga, M. Engelberg, and B. Baquero. 2005. "Interpersonal and Print Nutrition Communication for a Spanish-Dominant Latino Population." *Secretos de la Buena Vida. Health Psychology* 24: 49–57.

Elder, J. P., G. X. Ayala, D. Parra-Medina, and G. A. Talavera. 2009. "Health Communication in the Latino Community: Issues and Approaches." *Annual Review of Public Health* 30: 227–251.

Falicov, C. J. 1995. *Latino Families in Therapy. A Guide to Multicultural Practices.* New York, NY: The Guilford Press.

Fernández-Esquer, M. E., P. Espinoza, A. G. Ramirez, and A. L. McAlister. 2003. "Repeated Pap Smear Screening among Mexican American Women." *Health Education Research: Theory and Practice* 18: 477–487.

Galarraga, J. "Hispanic-American Culture and Health." Retrieved August 12, 2011, from http://www.cwru.edu/med/epidbio/mphp439/Hispanic_Healthcare.pdf

Gallardo, M. 2012. "Therapists as Cultural Architects and Systemic Advocates. Latina/o Skills Identification Stage Model." *Culturally Adaptive Counseling Skills. Demonstrations of Evidence-Based Practices,* edited by M. E. Gallardo, C. A. Yeh, J. E. Trimble, and T. A. Parham, 77–112. Thousand Oaks, CA: Sage.

Gans, K.M., G. J. Burkholder, D. I. Upegui, P. M. Risica, T. M. Lasater, and R. Fortunet. 2002. "Comparison of Baseline Fat-related Eating Behaviors of Puerto Rican, Dominican, Columbian, and Guatemalans who Joined a Cholesterol Education Project." *Journal of Nutrition Education and Behavior* 34: 202–210.

Giachello, A. L. 1996. "Latino women." In *Race, Gender, and Health,* edited by M. Bayne-Smith, 121–171. Thousand Oaks, CA: Sage.

Goldman, R. E., J. A. Diaz, and I. Kim. 2009. "Perspectives of Colorectal Cancer Risk and Screening among Dominicans and Puerto Ricans: Stigma and Misperceptions." *Qualitative Health Research* 19: 1559–1568.

Huff, R. M., and M. V. Kline. 2008. "Tips for Working with Hispanic/Latino Population Groups." In *Health Promotion in Multicultural Populations. A Handbook for Practitioners and Students,* edited by M. V. Kine and R. M. Huff, 278–283. Thousand Oaks, CA: Sage.

Johnson, R. L., S. Saha, J. J. Arbelaez, M. C., Beach, and L. A. Cooper. 2004. "Racial and Ethnic Differences in Patient Perceptions of Bias and Cultural Competence in Health Care." *Journal of General Internal Medicine* 19: 101–110.

Keane, D., C. Nielsen, and C. Dower. 2004. *Community Health Workers and Promotores in California.* UCSF Center for Health Professions. San Francisco, CA.

Larkey, L. 2006. "*Las Mujeres Saludables* Reaching Latinas for Breast, Cervical, and Colorectal Cancer Prevention and Screening." *Journal of Community Health* 31: 69–77.

Lopez, A. G., and E. Carrillo. 2001. *The Latino Psychiatric Patient: Assessment and Treatment.* Washington, DC: American Psychiatric Publishing, Inc.

Martinez, I. L., and O. Carter-Pokras. 2006. "Assessing Health Concerns and Barriers in a Heterogeneous Latino Community." *Journal of Health Care for the Poor and Underserved* 17: 899–909.

Matthews, P. H., C. Darbisi, L. Sandmann, R. Galen, and D. Rubin. 2009. "Disseminating Health Information and Diabetes Care for Latinos via Electronic Information Kiosks." *Journal of Immigrant Minority Health 11*: 520–526.

Miniño, A. M., S. L. Murphy, J. Xu, and K. D. Kochanek. 2011. "Deaths: Final Data for 2008." In *National Vital Statistics Reports, Vol 59* (10). Hyattsville, MD: National Center for Health Statistics.

Motel, S. 2012. *Statistical Portrait of Hispanics in the United States, 2010.* Washington DC: Pew Hispanic Center.

National Council of La Raza. 2010. *Heart Health in the Latino Community.* Washington, DC: NCLR.

Olson, R., F. Sabogal, and A. Perez. 2008. "*Viva La Vida:* Helping Latino Medicare Beneficiaries with Diabetes Live Their Lives to the Fullest." *American Journal of Public Health 98*: 205–208.

Organista, K. C. 2007. *Solving Latino Psychosocial and Health Problems: Theory, Practice, and Populations.* Hoboken, NJ: John Wiley and Sons, Inc.

Ortiz, F. A., K. G. Davis, and B.W. McNeill. 2008. "Curanderismo: Religious and Spiritual Worldviews and Indigenous Healing Traditions." In *Latina/o Healing Practices. Mestizo and Indigenous Perspectives,* edited by B.W. McNeill and J. M. Cervantes, 271–302. New York, NY: Routledge.

Penn, N. E., J. Kramer, J. Skinner, R. J. Velasquez, B.W.K. Yee, L. M. Arellano, and J. P. Williams. 2000. "Health Practices and Health-Care Systems among Cultural Groups." In *Handbook of Gender, Culture, and Health,* edited by R. M. Eisler and M. Hersen, 105–138. Mahwah, NJ: Lawrence Erlbaum Associates.

Pew Hispanic Center. "Country of Origin Profiles." Retrieved October 4, 2012, from http://www.pewhispanic.org.

Poss, J. and M. A. Jezewski. 2002. "Mexican Americans' Explanatory Model of Type II Diabetes." *Western Journal of Nursing Research 24*: 840–858.

Ramirez, A. G., L. Suarez, L. Lufman, C. Barroso, and P. Chalela. 2000. "Hispanic Women's Breast and Cervical Cancer Knowledge, Attitudes, and Screening Behaviors." *American Journal of Health Promotion 14*: 292–300.

Rhodes, S. D., K. L. Foley, C. S. Zometa, and F. R. Bloom. 2007. "Lay Health Advisor Interventions among Hispanics/Latinos. A Qualitative Systematic Review." *American Journal of Preventive Medicine 33*: 418–427.

Ruiz, P. 1994. "Cuban Americans: Migration, Acculturation, and Mental Health." In *Theoretical and Conceptual Issues in Hispanic Mental Health,* edited by R. G. Malgady, O. Rodriguez, F. L. Malabar, 70–89. Krieger Publishing.

Salazar, M. K. 1996. "Hispanic Women's Beliefs about Breast Cancer and Mammography." *Cancer Nursing 19*: 437–446.

Santiago-Rivera, A. L., P. Arredondo, and M. Gallardo-Cooper. 2002. *Counseling Latinas/os and la Familia: A Practical Guide.* Thousand Oaks, CA: Sage.

Santos, S. J., Hurtado-Ortiz, M. T., and Sneed, C. D. 2009. "Illness Beliefs regarding the Causes of Diabetes among Latino College Students." *Hispanic Journal of Behavioral Sciences 31*: 395–412.

Shariff-Marco, S., A. C. Klassen, and J. V. Bowie. 2010. "Racial/Ethnic Differences in Self-Reported Racism and Its Association with Cancer-Related Health Behaviors." *American Journal of Public Health 100*: 364–374.

Shelton, R. C., R. E. Goldman, K. M. Emmons, G. Sorensen, and J. D. Allen. 2011. "An Investigation into the Social Context of Low-Income, Urban Black and Latina Women: Implications for Adherence to Recommended Health Behaviors." *Health Education and Behavior 38*: 471–481.

Song, E., J. S. Leichliter, F. R. Bloom, A.T. Vissman, M. C. O'Brien, and S. D. Rhodes. 2012. "The Use of Prescription Medications Obtained from Non-Medical Sources among Immigrant Latinos in the Rural Southeastern U.S." *Journal of Health Care for the Poor and Underserved 23*: 678–693.

Sorlie, P. D., L. M. Avilés-Santa, S. Wassertheil-Smoller, R. C. Kaplan, M. L. Daviglus, A. L. Giachello, G. Heiss. 2010. "Design and Implementation of the Hispanic Community Health Study/Study of Latinos." *Annals of Epidemiology 20*: 629–641.

Spector, R.E. 2009. *Cultural Diversity in Health and Illness* (7th ed.). Upper Saddle River, NJ: Pearson.

U.S. Census Bureau. "Overview of Race and Hispanic Origin, 2010." Retrieved November 11, 2011, from http://www.census.gov/prod/cen2010/briefs/c2010br -02.pdf

U.S. Department of Health and Human Services (USDHHS). 2000. *Healthy People 2010: Understanding and Improving Health and Objectives for Health* (2nd ed.). Washington, DC: U.S. Government Printing Office.

Valdez, C. R., M. J. Dvorscek, S. L. Budge, and S. Esmond. 2011. "Provider Perspective about Latino Patients: Determinants of Care and Implications for Treatment." *The Counseling Psychologist 39*: 497–526.

Vega, A., M. A. Rodriguez, and E. Gruskin. 2009. "Health Disparities in the Latino Population." *Epidemiologic Reviews 31*: 22–112.

Vélez, L. F., P. Chalela, and A. G. Ramirez. 2008. "Hispanic/Latino Health and Disease." In *Health Promotion in Multicultural Populations. A Handbook for Practitioners and Students*, edited by M. V. Kine and R. M. Huff, 187–222. Thousand Oaks, CA: Sage.

Viladrich, A. 2010. "Botánicas in America's Backyard: Uncovering the World of Latino Healers' Herb-Healing Practices in New York City." In *Health Care*, edited by I. Stavans, 86–108. Santa Barbara, CA: Greenwood.

Wallace, L. S., J. E. DeVoe, J. D. Heintzman, and G. E. Fryer. 2009. "Language Preference and Perceptions of Healthcare Providers' Communication and Autonomy Making Behaviors among Hispanics." *Journal of Immigrant Minority Health 11*: 453–459.

Wallington, S. F., G. Luta, A. Noone, L. Caicedo., M. Lopez-Class, V. Sheppard, C. Spencer, and J. Mandelblatt. 2012. "Assessing the Awareness of and Willingness to Participate in Cancer Clinical Rrials among Immigrant Latinos." *Journal of Community Health 37*: 335–343.

Wilkin, H. A., T. W. Valente, S. Murphy, M. J. Cody, G. Huang, and V. Beck. 2007. "Does Entertainment-Education Work with Latinos in the United States? Identification with the Effects of a Telenovela Breast Cancer Storyline." *Journal of Health Communication* 12: 455–469.

Yang, W., F. Qeadan, and J. Smith-Gagen. 2009. "The Hispanic Epidemiological Paradox in the Fastest-Growing State in the United States." *Hispanic Health Care International* 7: 130–140.

CHAPTER FIVE

Acculturation and Health

Sabrina Crawford and Kavita Avula

As rates of international migration have reached unprecedented levels in the United States, acculturation has become a well-recognized and increasingly worthwhile area of study. The current massive wave of immigration is larger than those that took place in the 19th and early 20th centuries and is not showing any signs of slowing (Schwartz, Unger, Zamboanga and Szapocznik 2010). This trend is also reflected in Western Europe and Canada. Additionally, Australia is also experiencing one of the largest immigrant influxes in recent history. In the most recent, post-1960s wave, migrants originated primarily from Latin America, Asia, Africa, the Caribbean, and the Middle East. The regions from which these migrants hail have societies that operate based on collectivism or a focus on the well-being of the group, family, clan or religion. These migrants settled mostly in North America, Western Europe, and Oceania, areas that are more centered on individualism that incorporates a focus on the needs of the individual person over the group. Inevitably, immigrants will be confronted with gaps in cultural values between their own society and the one receiving them.

The sizeable flow of migrants worldwide has stimulated more scholarly interest in acculturation and with the rates of immigration ever-increasing, it is becoming especially relevant to understand the impact of these trans-regional migrations and the process by which individuals and groups recover from sociocultural contextual change. In this chapter, we provide an overview of immigration, measuring acculturation and acculturation theory, acculturative stress, group dynamics, health disparities and trends, stressors, and barriers to health services on the largest immigration groups to the United States, including those from Africa, Asia, and Latin America.

An Overview of Immigration

Africans

A key component affecting the process of acculturation has to do with whether or not the migration is voluntary (Aponte and Barnes 1995). The earliest immigration of Africans to the Western Hemisphere was an involuntary one and occurred during transatlantic slavery, during which Africans were forcibly removed from their homelands to be slaves. The first African slaves arrived in the 1600s with the largest influx of forced African immigrants arriving between 1700 and 1840; they represented half a million of the 10–12 million Africans who were enlisted as slaves and taken elsewhere (Venters and Gany 2011). Those brought during this time period came mainly from West Africa, including the areas between present-day Senegal and the eastern region of Benin. After slavery was abolished, there was a sharp decline in African immigration to the United States that lasted through the 1950s. The quotas set at this time permitted less than 2,000 African immigrants annually, the lowest quota when compared with those of groups coming from other regions. In 1965, the Hart-Cellar Immigration Act, part of the civil rights movement, overhauled immigration laws by establishing criteria for admission such as professional skills and family ties. The Refugee Act of 1980 granted permanent residence after one year, and the Immigration Reform and Control Act of 1986 legalized the status of 31,000 Africans residing in the United States at that time. The Diversity Visa Lottery offered visas to Africans from underrepresented countries and established the Temporary Protected Status program, which gave refugee status to those from natural disaster zones and conflict-affected areas such as Liberia, Somalia, Sierra Leone, Sudan, and Burundi (Venters and Gany 2011).

The forced nature of early immigration and the history of oppression of African Americans in the United States cannot be separated from our understanding of acculturation of Africans and African Americans today. The oppression that the group as a whole suffered for decades in the form of physical violence, loss of human rights, and dehumanization has had far-reaching impacts that are relevant today. African Americans continue to experience limited opportunities and barriers as evidenced by their levels of health, education, occupations, and poverty (Aponte and Barnes 1995). Historically, African American families have been characterized by high birth rates among single African American women and a predominance of mother-only households, high rates of unemployment among African American men, a decline in the number of married couples with small children, and an increase in the proportion of children being raised in single-parent households (Wilson et al.

1995). Additionally, African American families have been subjected more frequently to violent crime, in particular, assault and homicide targeting males which makes them more vulnerable to economic, social, and psychological stress.

There are approximately one million African immigrants currently residing in the United States, with over half having immigrated between 1990 and 2000 (Venters and Gany 2011). Most recently, immigrants from Africa have come from West Africa (35 percent), East Africa (26 percent), North Africa (20 percent), South Africa (7 percent), and Central Africa (3 percent). They tend to be unemployed, in poverty, and less often from Anglophone countries than from non-English speaking areas. Between 1990 and 2000, the number of immigrants rose by 166 percent (Venters and Gany 2011). In recent years, a large concentration of African immigrants has settled in Washington D.C., New York City, Minneapolis-St. Paul, and Atlanta.

Latinos

Currently, Latinos comprise 15 percent of the U.S. population and represent the largest and fastest-growing ethnic minority group in the country. It is estimated that by the year 2050, the percentage of Latinos in the United States will rise to 25 percent (Valencia-Garcia et al. 2012). A heterogeneous group, Latinos originate from 43 Spanish-speaking countries, with the majority (67 percent) hailing from Mexico. Puerto Ricans make up the nation's second largest immigrant group of Latino origin at 9.2 percent, followed by Cubans (3.7 percent), Salvadorans (3.6 percent), Dominicans (3.0 percent), Guatemalans (2.2 percent), Colombians (1.9 percent), Hondurans (1.4 percent), Ecuadorians (1.3 percent), and Peruvians (1.2 percent), according to the U.S. Census Bureau, 2010.

A variety of general terms are used to refer to members of this group including Latino, Hispanic, Central and South American (Comas-Diaz 2006). Although these groups share a history of being colonized by the Spanish, each subgroup has its own unique cultural identity and challenges. Mexicans and Mexican-Americans have had to contend with job discrimination, immigration restrictions, more legal pressures, school segregation, and electoral disenfranchisement (Aponte and Barnes 2005). Although Puerto Ricans have also experienced job discrimination, they have the distinct legal and practical advantage of being citizens and being afforded easily accessible transportation back to their place of birth. The Cuban experience, in contrast, has been more politically linked with services including the Cuban Refugee Program being in place to facilitate migration and integration (Aponte and Barnes 1995). Dominicans tend to be subjected to more overt racism as a consequence of their African phenotype and many South

Americans vacillate between detachment and belonging (Comas-Diaz 2006). Some Latinos choose to politically identify by referring to themselves as Chicanos, Ricans, or Boricuas while others identify according to their national origins and describe themselves as Mexican Americans, Colombians, Cuban Americans, Peruvians or Venezuelans.

Latino immigrants face numerous social and economic barriers including poverty, low education levels, housing in poor neighborhoods, language challenges, lack of or insufficient health care, isolation, discrimination, and segregation. In the early 1990s, the proportion of mother-only households among Latino families increased by 10 percent while the proportion of dual-parent households decreased by 6 percent, a trend heightened by high birth and poverty rates among Latino groups (Wilson et al. 1995). Of all the racial groups in the United States, Latinos are the least likely to be insured and the least likely to use preventive health care services (Comas-Diaz 2006).

Asians and Pacific Islanders

The Asian American and Pacific Islander (AAPI) group, constituting 5 percent of the population, or over 12 million people, is another rapidly growing minority in the United States (Esperat et al. 2004, Valencia-Garcia et al. 2012). The Asian contingent hails from Asia and Southeast Asia with the largest representation of people from China, the Philippines, Japan, Korea, and the Pacific Islands. Not all of the individuals included in the designation AAPI are considered immigrants since some who carry the designation reside in the Pacific Rim, where they are native to Polynesia, Micronesia, and Melanesia. Within AAPI, there are over 60 different ethnic groups that speak over 100 different languages (Esperat el al. 2004). When it comes to societal generalizations, this group has had to contend with the "model minority" label that arose due to their touted high-achieving capacities in the socioeconomic and academic spheres. While some members of this group may indeed perform above average, the label is inappropriate and misleading as it does not capture the vast diversity that exists within the AAPI group. The stereotype may also create the tendency to dismiss and overlook the actual needs of the group. In terms of family trends, marriage rates are higher and divorce rates are lower among Asian Americans when compared to other ethnic minorities in the United States (Wilson et al. 1995). The cultural socialization process of various Asian groups tend to be more supportive of traditional sex roles than mainstream American culture and families that uphold misogynistic values can display a devaluation of girls and women by denying them the opportunities afforded to boys and males (Koo et al. 2012).

While much of the literature focuses on inter-racial and inter-ethnic differences, the authors wish to underscore the idea that intra-racial and intra-ethnic differences are paramount. Each immigrant group has a multitude of vastly distinct subgroups represented within each characterized by different beliefs, customs, and values. It is impossible and beyond the scope of this chapter to capture these distinctions and nuances. While this chapter will summarize acculturation trends by group, it is with the intent of providing an overview and a knowledge base from which to work. In providing treatment to a member of any of these groups, the individual's own narrative should always guide the health provider's understanding of the client, *not* the generalizations that are associated with each group.

Acculturation

Broadly defined, acculturation refers to the multidimensional process of adaptations that occur when a group of people migrate to a new culture and make contact with culturally dissimilar people, groups, and social influences. Acculturation is the degree to which individuals adapt to a whole new way of life by learning about and adopting the attitudes, values, customs, beliefs, and behaviors of another culture, typically the dominant culture of the receiving country (Abraido-Lanza et al. 2006, Castillo and Carver 2009, Esperat et al. 2004). Most often, acculturation is studied in individuals living in regions other than where they were born; for example, immigrants, refugees, asylum seekers, international students, and seasonal farm workers (Schwartz et al. 2010). Acculturation research tends to focus on immigrants, refugees, and asylum seekers permanently settled in their new homeland.

Early acculturation theorists depicted acculturation as a one-dimensional process in which preservation and retention of the heritage culture and acquisition of the receiving culture were conceptualized as opposing ends of a single continuum (Aponte and Barnes 1995, Schwartz et al. 2010). This unilinear perspective was based on the idea that an individual would identify with *either* their culture of heritage *or* the receiving culture. Biculturalism was pinpointed as the midpoint between the two cultures (Castillo and Carver 2009). The major flaw in this model was the assumption that acquiring the receiving culture's values, beliefs, and practices was contingent on letting go of those from the heritage culture.

Enculturation refers to the process of selectively retaining elements of one's heritage culture while selectively acquiring some elements of the receiving culture (Schwartz et al. 2010). Historically, acculturation and enculturation have been mistakenly thought to be mutually exclusive (Castillo and Carver 2009, Reynold et al. 2011).

Measuring Acculturation

Since the early 1980s, cross-cultural psychologists have established the notion that taking on the beliefs, values, and practices of the receiving country does not necessitate discarding native beliefs, values, and practices. There have been two influential models that emerged to conceptualize and measure the extent and nature of acculturation: the biculturalism model and the ethnic identity model. The biculturalism model, also known as the multiculturalism model, was created in the context of immigration and cultural competence. This model focuses on acquisition of cultural skills and knowledge necessary to function in the new environment. The question of identity is not as pressing for recent immigrants because their primary task is to negotiate and survive the demands of a new environment.

Alternatively, the ethnic identity model, also referred to as cultural identification model, or racial identity model, was created in the context of racial and ethnic minority experience and emphasizes the consequences of oppression. For American born members of racial ethnic minority groups, language and knowledge are not a major concern; rather, oppression and marginalization hinder the establishment of a positive sense of one's cultural identity. The identity models hold that the best resolution of acculturative conflicts is contingent upon the establishment of a positive sense of identity as a members of one's own cultural group while retaining competence in the society at large (Birman 1984).

One of the most well-known models of biculturalism, Berry's bilinear model holds that acculturation and enculturation are two discrete entities; acculturation is seen as the level of identification and affiliation with the receiving culture and enculturation is seen as the level of identification and affiliation with the native culture (Schwartz et al. 2010). Proponents of the bilinear model contend that an individual can be bicultural without losing his or her core cultural identity; that is, they can maintain an affiliation to the native culture while also adapting to the receiving country's culture - these are no longer thought of as mutually exclusive. In the bilinear model, individuals confront two primary issues: whether or not the heritage culture continues to be of value and should be retained and whether or not the receiving culture is of value and therefore something be sought out instead of avoided (Castillo and Carver 2009).

Berry studied the intersection of these two dimensions and theorized that there are four acculturation categories: assimilation, separation, integration and marginalization. The first, *assimilation,* absorbs the receiving culture and discards the heritage culture. Individuals in this group have high levels of acculturation and low levels of enculturation. *Separation* rejects the receiving culture and holds onto the heritage culture. *Integration,* also referred to as biculturalism, entails proficiency in the receiving culture while simultaneously retaining proficiency in the heritage culture at the same time (Castillo and Carver 2009, Kim and Omizo 2006). *Marginalization* rejects both the heritage and receiving cultures.

Classifying people according to different ethnic identity stages or acculturation categories has been criticized when applied rigidly as this type of classification can suggest that individuals have immutable characteristics; rather, the stages should be viewed as fluid as opposed to linear. It should also be noted that it is common for individuals to move through stages out of order and more than once depending on where they are in their lives and the interplay of intrapersonal and interpersonal dynamics, self-concept, and situational factors (Aponte and Barnes 1995).

Berry's bilinear model of acculturation has been criticized for its lack of empirical rigor. The model rests on the assumption that all four categories exist and are equally valid. The two-by-two acculturation matrix classifies individuals as high or low on receiving culture acquisition and heritage culture retention (Schwartz et al. 2010). A priori values such as sample median are used to classify individuals as high or low which results in equal numbers of individuals in each category. The problem is that the cut-off point between classifications of "high" and "low" is arbitrary and will inevitably differ across samples, hindering comparisons between studies. Furthermore, the validity of marginalization as an accurate construct has been brought into question. The chances that a person will develop a cultural self that does not include his or her heritage or the receiving culture seems highly unlikely. Rather, this category may capture a smaller number of individuals who reject or feel rejected by both cultures. The scales that have attempted to measure marginalization have poor reliability and validity compared with the scales for the other categories. Research has started to respond to these criticisms and some degree of validity has been documented. The studies found that the acculturation categories are not as well-differentiated within Berry's model with three of the four categories - integration, separation, and assimilation. Even though further research is necessary to establish greater empirical rigor, Berry's is a leading model on acculturation.

Recent research suggests that Berry's integration category is indeed the most favorable, in particular, among young immigrants (Schwartz et al. 2010). The degree of actual or perceived similarity between receiving and heritage culture influences the degree of ease versus difficulty in integrating the two. When ethnicity is held constant, those coming from English-speaking countries, or who are otherwise proficient in English, tend to experience less stress and resistance in the United States than those who are not as adept at the English language. For example, among Black Caribbean immigrants, Jamaicans might experience less discrimination and acculturative stress than Haitians due to common language (Schwartz et al. 2010).

LaFromboise, Coleman, and Gerton (1993) developed a theoretical model of bicultural competence that includes six dimensions:

> (a) Knowledge of Cultural Beliefs and Values—the degree to which a person is aware of and knowledgeable about the history, institutions, rituals, and everyday practices of a given culture; (b) Positive Attitudes Toward Both Groups—the degree to which a person regards both cultural groups positively; (c) Bicultural Efficacy—the belief that a person can function effectively within two cultural groups without compromising one's cultural identity; (d) Communication Ability—the person's ability to communicate verbally or nonverbally in both cultural groups; (e) Role Repertoire—the range of culturally appropriate behaviors or roles a person possesses or is willing to learn/ perform; and (f) Social Groundedness—the degree to which a person has established social networks in both cultural groups. (David, Okazaki, and Saw 2009).

These authors' beliefs are consistent with other researchers who theorize that a strong bicultural identity results in improved physical and psychological health.

Another acculturation model—The Concordance Model of Acculturation (CMA)—differs from Berry's model in that it focuses on the receiving culture's influence on the immigrant's transition (Piontkowski, Rohmann, and Florack 2002) and describes the dominant group's influence on the acculturation process. However, the CMA does agree with Berry's model in that it also positively correlates the size of the cultural differences between the cultures with greater difficulty adapting and, moreover, asserts that significant discrepancies may threaten minority group identity. As a result, the CMA predicts that mismatch in acculturation attitudes could lead to intergroup conflict and impact psychological well-being (Castillo et al. 2007).

Other acculturation and ethnic identity measures that can provide information on current levels of acculturation and ethnic identity include the Development Inventory of Black Consciousness, the Hispanic Acculturation Scale, the Ethnic Identity Questionnaire, the Rosebud Personal Opinion Survey for Native Americans, and the Suinn-Lew Asian Self Identity Acculturation Scale (Aponte and Barnes 1995).

Acculturative Stress

Acculturative stress refers to the difficulties and stressors that arise during the acculturative process, such as language differences, perceived cultural incompatibilities, and cultural self-consciousness. Acculturative stress studies have tended to focus on stress due to the differences between heritage culture and dominant culture group behaviors, such as limited knowledge of the English language and American customs (Hovey 2000; Lee, Koeske, and Sales 2004). Scholars have speculated that acculturative stress can also be experienced when an individual faces criticism from family, such as the inability to speak the heritage culture's language or perceived inactivity in practicing cultural customs. Thus, the expectation to maintain the heritage culture group's norms may be related to acculturative stress (Castillo et al. 2007).

As individuals adapt to a new physical and cultural environment, sources of stress include the acquisition of new language skills, development of competitive work skills, and comprehension of new social and behavioral norms, social isolation, and possible racism. High stress levels are experienced as individuals negotiate how to maintain cultural ties, values, traditions, economic challenges, and oppression when it comes to employment.

In the dominant literature on acculturation, language preference and proficiency are key considerations when it comes to the social integration of immigrants and are widely used in the development of tools to measure acculturation (Esperat et al. 2004). Research shows that a shared language is part of the fabric of national identity and migrants who do not speak English may be deemed a threat to unity by the majority. For example, a white, English-speaking Canadian individual will probably have much less difficulty in acculturating to the United States when compared to an indigenous migrant from Latin America. The Canadian's transition will be buffered not only by shared language but also by shared values and belief systems as well as the ability of white migrants to more readily blend into the American mainstream. Level of language proficiency impacts entry into the labor force and basic functioning and establishment of a support system. Poor English can interfere with ability to find and obtain medical services, obtain employment, and navigate public transportation. Acculturation measures also include acceptance of new culture, preferences for food, and friends.

Length of time since migration may also impact how stress affects immigrant mental health. One theory asserts acculturative stress should be more prevalent in recent immigrants, and greater vulnerability to stress (acculturative and general) may exist because of compromised social networks. A competing theory asserts that recent immigrants often exhibit healthier outcomes than their counterparts who have been in the United States longer (McDonald and Kennedy 2005, Stephen et al. 1994). For instance, Finch and Vega (2003) found that immigrants residing in the United States longer than 10 years reported poorer health than those in the United States fewer than 10 years. Given competing hypotheses, it is important to continue examining how migration time affects mental health (Kiang et al. 2010).

Group Dynamics

Many acculturation models examine the bi-dimensional relationship regarding cultural acquisition versus cultural retention. For acculturating individuals, an emphasis on "our practices, values, and identifications" can be reflective of an "in-group orientation" whereas, an emphasis on the dominant culture's orientation of "their practices, values, and orientations" is reflective of an "out-group orientation" (Roysircar-Sodowsky and Maestas 2000).

According to social identity theory, belonging to a social group (i.e. an ethnic group) provides members with a sense of social identity that directs appropriate behaviors for an individual's membership (Tajfel 1991). Group dynamics research suggests that in-group members who are perceived as threatening to the distinctiveness of a group may be marginalized by those same members of the group. The literature suggests that friends, members of the ethnic group, and family members can enforce heritage culture group norms. Social identity theory asserts that groups maintain their identity by the distinctive behaviors of their members. When an acculturating individual displays behaviors or attitudes that differ from the group's norms, the group may respond to the threat with social isolation of the individual.

When in-group versus out-group dynamics result in an unequal distribution of power and the subjugation of the minority group to the dominant group, this system of subordination is referred to as racism (Derman-Sparks and Phillips, 1997). An institutionalized system of power, racism comprises an interplay of economic, political, social and cultural beliefs and values that systematically results in thwarted privileges, resources, and power for the minority group in favor of the dominant group. It is important to note that the lack of intentionality in a situation does not change the consequences for people of color, a term used to refer not to actual skin color but rather immigrant or ethnic minority status. The level of severity of prejudice and discrimination resulting from racism experienced by immigrant groups unequivocally impacts one's sense of self worth and sense of belonging to the culture at large (Derman-Sparks and Phillips 1997).

Intra-group marginalization focuses on the heritage culture group's reaction to the individual (Castillo et al. 2007), and is defined as the interpersonal distancing that occurs when an acculturating individual is believed to exhibit behaviors, values, and beliefs that are outside the native culture's group norms. This, when exacerbated by the receiving culture's negative stereotypes and attitudes, can lead to the extreme yet common phenomenon of internalized racism, or self-directed aggression and devaluation around one's race.

Internalized racism, or racism directed at one's own ethnic group, occurs when members of marginalized cultural groups unknowingly internalize negative attitudes held by society and this can have a deleterious effect, in particular, on psychological health. Internalized racism can be defined as the conscious and/or unconscious incorporation and acceptance of negative stereotypes of the dominant culture by persons of color. Of importance is the racial context in the immigrants' country of origin and the extent to which American society mirrors or departs from this previous reality. Internalized racism can lead to complicated acculturation in which the individual takes on negative attitudes towards their own ethnic group and, consequently, toward themselves and can have a significant impact on sense of self-worth.

Adaptation can be complicated by internalized racism that can result in "hazing" or "ostracizing," causing individuals to feel rejected by their cultural group or from the majority culture or by both. On the basis of social identity theory, according to Nesdale and colleagues (2005), the importance of social identification is highlighted, particularly in the context of inter-group interactions. This theory also makes a distinction between bias (e.g., a preference for one's group) and prejudice (e.g., derogation of out-groups). This phenomenon is profound with the Native American populations, who although not immigrants per se, have had to contend with centuries of trauma that have had a significant impact on Native American health. The large-scale actions that deliberately threatened the physical integrity of the indigenous people have resulted in widespread intergenerational stress, post-traumatic stress, anger, depression, suicidal ideology, unresolved grief, alcoholism, and survivor's guilt. The loss of territory and environmental devastation created major barriers to health and resilience in that the Native people could no longer access their traditional foods and medicines. These losses occurred in conjunction with the psychological suffering that results from historical trauma, defined as the "cumulative emotional and psychological wounding from massive group trauma experiences" (Weaver and Congress 2010, 215). The forced loss of traditional practices and culture is a major contributor to health disparities that plague the Native American population today.

The Impact of Acculturation on the Family

Historically, the "normal" family referred to one with a nuclear structure derived from immediate family membership with all else labeled abnormal. Immigration in conjunction with changing demographic patterns has broadened the traditional definition of the family with the greatest impact on minority and immigrant groups (Wilson et al. 1995). The extended family that goes beyond the nuclear family unit to include a greater range of relatives takes on special meaning for many ethnic minority groups. This larger group plays a primary role in the establishment of family members' values, beliefs and behaviors. For ethnic minority families these relatives and non-blood relatives create a cohesive force that informs social interaction, transmits values, influences lifestyle trends such as economic cooperation and childcare responsibilities (Wilson et al. 1995).

Although the family and community can create a support structure for immigrants, this does not preclude the impact of discrimination. In a study that comprised six focus groups with 30 immigrants from Cambodia, Eastern Europe, Iran, Iraq, Africa, and Vietnam, all six groups reported having experienced discrimination since arriving in the United States (Saecho et al. 2011). Children may be ridiculed at school for being different, and adults may experience being shunned at work or in social situations due to having an accent or being from a culture that has a strong negative stereotype in the United States.

Immigrant children can demonstrate resiliency in light of acculturative pressures. Rapid behavioral acculturation in immigrant youth may be associated with gains in overall functioning. Immigrant children tend to adopt roles of responsibility, often having to act as cultural brokers and translators for their parents, and some researchers contend that these demands and responsibilities may actually enhance rather than compromise functioning (Fugligni et al. 2002). This interpretation is consistent with findings that language brokering is associated with positive social and academic outcomes among Latino adolescents (Buriel et al. 1998). Fuligni and colleagues (1998, 2002) have described how minority youth are able to artfully balance their cultural obligations to their immigrant families with the demands of being an adolescent in U.S. society with few psychological costs and notable benefits to emotional and academic functioning. Despite the benefits highlighted in the literature regarding gains of heightened responsibility for some children, others may suffer from its impact.

Some research indicates that when immigrant parents allow children to make their own choices concerning their cultural identity, their children will be more likely to internalize the culture of origin and will experience greater well-being in different aspects of their lives (Farver et al. 2002). Families in which both parents are first-generation immigrants typically experience elevated stress as their second-generation children develop. Second-generation immigrants must simultaneously explore two (or more) potentially conflicting cultures to become comfortable in their identities.

Second-generation immigrants report more daily hassles, in-group conflict, and lowered self-esteem; they also receive more frequent diagnoses of internalizing disorders than either first-generation immigrants or American-born peers of the same age and socioeconomic status (Lay and Safdar 2003; Farver et al. 2002). One reason for these differences in wellbeing may be that, unlike first-generation immigrants, second-generation individuals do not necessarily have sustained, direct experiences with their native culture from which to draw meaning in times of stress (Schwartz and Montgomery 2002).

As a way to mediate acculturative stress, immigrants can display a stronger tolerance for ambiguity, change and contradictions regarding how they see themselves as being a part of their culture. As a result, these individuals tend to be more tolerant of self-inconsistencies. The concept described is known as "dialectical self-views." Spencer-Rodgers and colleagues (2004) highlight the tendency of people from Eastern cultures and traditions to be more likely to have dialectical self-views than those from Western cultures. This stems from deeply rooted Eastern religious and philosophical traditions that promote acceptance of contradiction and change.

Key Health Issues

Research on cross-cultural health has uncovered what is now referred to as the *healthy immigrant effect,* a term that arose from the finding that immigrants tend to arrive in the United States in better health than their counterparts who were born in the United States (Acevedo-Garcia et al. 2010, Antecol and Bedard 2006, Newbold 2005; Cho et al. 2004, Jasso et al. 2004; McDonald and Kennedy 2004, 2005). Studies have revealed a higher life expectancy for immigrants to the United States compared with native-born individuals. Specifically, immigrants have better perinatal and adult health, and lower disability and mortality rates than non-immigrants born in the United States (Singh and Miller 2004).

Immigrants tend to smoke less, consume less alcohol and fewer illicit drugs, and are less likely to be overweight than Americans. However, the positive health outcomes that are associated with increased immigrant health disappear over time and tend to eventually reflect the health outcomes of the individual's racial and ethnic groups in the United States (Hamilton and Hummer 2011). Hamilton and Hummer (2011) surmise that a possible contributing factor to the erosion of immigrant health associated with time in the United States is exposure to racism and discrimination as well as other negative social, economic, and environmental factors that have detrimental effects on health.

African immigrants self-report their own health to be better than African Americans, followed by West Indian blacks, then European-born blacks (Read et al. 2005). The longer African immigrants reside in the United States, and the more acculturated immigrants become, the more they take on the characteristics of the population around them. Among African immigrants, rates of obesity, smoking and hyperlipidemia increase with length of time in the United States (Koya and Egede 2007). Although African-born immigrants are less likely to smoke or to be obese when compared to African-Americans, increased acculturation and language ability are positively associated with smoking and obesity (Bennet et al. 2008). It appears that the more an individual adapts to American culture, the more his or her behaviors, and eventually health, reflect that of those that are lifelong residents of the receiving culture.

Read et al (2005), introduced "the racial context of origin hypothesis," which contends that Black immigrants who faced racism and discrimination in their countries of origin similar to that faced by Blacks born in the United States will mirror the health outcomes of Blacks born in the United States. Read and Emerson's research found that the healthiest groups of Black immigrants migrated from Africa or South America, regions in which the white population is significantly less than the black population. The next healthiest group comes from the West Indies which has a racially diverse population. Lastly, Black immigrants from Europe, a region in which the Black population is significantly less than the white population, report the worst health (Hamilton and Hummer 2011).

Noteworthy Health Trends

Higher levels of acculturation that result from increased adaptation were not linked to increased health risk behaviors; rather, the disavowal of one's heritage culture was more problematic (Schwartz et al. 2010, Abraído-Lanza et al. 2006). Retaining at least one element of the heritage culture was found to be protective against health risk behaviors for all of the racial/ethnic groups. The immigrant paradox—the positive association of acculturation with risky health practices—can be largely attributed to the loss of the heritage culture, not the acquisition of the new one (Schwartz et al. 2010).

Reckless alcohol use was linked with Black, East Asian, and South Asian participants; illegal drug use was linked to Black, Hispanic, and East Asian participants; unsafe sexual practices were linked to Hispanic and East Asian participants; and impaired driving was linked to white and black participants.

White immigrants showed the least amount of health risks related to acculturation. Researchers cited the phenotypic and cultural similarities of white immigrants to white Americans as key factors that facilitated being looked upon more favorably than negatively. In contrast, dark-skinned immigrants with foreign accents were perceived as "other" and consequently viewed negatively. Furthermore, white immigrants with foreign accents including British, French and Australian individuals were perceived as interesting rather than different (Steiner, 2009).

For Latino and Asian groups, the centrality of collectivistic values was protective against health risks across racial/ethnic groups (Ramirez et al., 2004; Le et al., 2009; Le and Kato, 2006). Specifically, factors such as interdependence, fear of embarrassment, and maintaining a respectable image for self and family inoculated these groups from health risk behaviors (Nagayama Hall, Teten, and Sue, 2003). Self-focused or pleasure-seeking behaviors tended to be be associated with negative long-term consequences resulting from family tensions and dissent.

Stressors and Barriers to Using Health Services

Cultural factors intrinsic to each immigrant group directly impact help-seeking behaviors. National epidemiological studies show that 17.9 percent of the general U.S. population use mental health services while far fewer ethnic minorities make use of these services. For example, only 8.6 percent of Asian American adults seek mental health assistance (Nguyen 2011). Unfortunately, reaching out for psychological support is highly stigmatized in many cultures.

A significant factor that places immigrants at risk for poor management of mental health symptoms is the pattern of health care use among their heritage culture population. While recent immigrants tend to utilize clinics and emergency rooms for medical care, they are often more reticent to seek mental health services because of stigma and cultural shame associated with having a mental illness (Kandula et al. 2004, Snowden 2003). While it is positive that recent immigrants are able and willing to seek care in emergency rooms and clinic settings, utilization of treatments in these settings can make it difficult to create effective therapeutic relationships as there is limited opportunity for continuity of care. This population may also have difficulty accessing specialty services such as mental health assessment and treatment due to their immigration status (documented vs. undocumented), lack of insurance, and frustration with long wait times to see a mental health care provider. Wang and colleagues (2005) reviewed data from the National Comorbidity Survey Replication of more than

9,000 respondents and found that when treatment is not immediately accessed upon the initial onset of psychiatric symptoms, it can take up to six to eight years for immigrants to receive treatment for mood disorders.

Both the stigma attached to mental health as well as the lack of awareness about mental health services are major barriers to seeking treatment (Saechao et al. 2011). Some immigrants may have lived in a region in which access to mental health services was limited or unavailable, compounded by the stereotype that only very disturbed individuals need such services. Consequently, immigrants have opted to see a medical doctor, which is seen as more acceptable according to societal standards. This may be why immigrants tend to frame their psychological distress in terms of somatic complaints; however, this can result in a focus on reducing physical distress while overlooking emotional distress which is actually the primary problem. Thus, it becomes important that physicians assess for psychological causes, in particular, when no known biological precipitant is found.

Asian Americans seek professional assistance for psychological concerns at a significantly lower rate than white Americans (Nguyen 2011). Among some Asian American families, the use of mental health services is seen as shameful, and professionals are often consulted as a last resort. For mental illness, AAPIs have often opted to go to primary care and general practitioners, in addition to Chinese herbalists and acupuncturists, rather than a mental health professional. Studies have shown that Asian Americans report communication difficulties with physicians, finding language to be a barrier in some cases, and tend to use referrals from others they may know and community-based programs over formal health care. They may also attempt to handle their problems on their own or seek help from their support network before seeking formal services (Esperat et al. 2004). Japanese-American participants in one study rated family, friends, self-help and support groups as significantly more useful than white American participants. Additional barriers to accessing services include stigma, deficits regarding culturally relevant interventions, language barriers resulting from insufficient bilingual providers, finances, lack of information, and geographic proximity.

A study on Vietnamese refugees and dementia found that obtaining services from formal sources was only considered when symptoms of dementia were severe. Korean immigrants experiencing high levels of distress did not consider their symptoms severe enough to seek help outside of the family (Esperat et al., 2004). In contrast, Chinese immigrants and U.S.-born Chinese were more likely to seek formal services when family conflict levels were high.

Atkinson and Gim (1989) found that more highly acculturated Asian American students were more likely to recognize a personal need for professional psychological services and be open to discussing problems with a psychologist and tolerant of the stigma associated with psychological help in comparison to their white American counterparts. Increased levels of acculturation among Chinese-American adults was positively correlated with utilizing mental health services (Nguyen 2011).

Much of the research that focuses on between-group differences recommends a directive approach in counseling with Asian Americans. However, as contemporary psychodynamic psychologists, we challenge this overly simplified perspective and contend that a non-directive, insight-oriented approach is not only effective but indicated for many. We hold that the most important aspect in an effective cross-cultural encounter is, as consistently reflected in the research, the quality of the therapeutic relationship. In the cross-cultural encounter, while sensitivity and awareness are instrumental, it remains essential that the therapeutic process develops in a comfortable environment. This therapeutic environment should allow for the individual to feel safe to disclose.

The relationship between acculturation and depression is complex with higher levels of acculturation associated with elevated depressive symptoms and higher stress levels. However, these relationships are significantly impacted by the presence of both socioeconomic status and social support (Trinh et al. 2009). A screening for depression in Los Angeles showed significant concern around stigma and lower likelihood to seek treatment among African immigrants. Similarly, in a study of Ethiopian immigrants in Toronto, low levels of utilization of services were found within this community despite high levels of need.

The prevalence of mental health issues among African immigrants varies tremendously throughout the research. One study revealed lower rates of depression, alcohol and drug use than other immigrant and native-born groups among low-income women in Los Angeles. The literature also highlights that Africans may tend to somaticize their mental health issues and describe physical symptoms instead of emotional ones. In an investigation of somatic pain in Senegalese immigrants in New York, participants reported a grouping of abdominal and back pains they referred to as *Toy* as part of a manifestation of "heartache."

European mental health professionals who have worked with African immigrants that have experienced distinct stressors from dangerous sea voyages have referred to their symptom picture as *Chronic and Multiple Stress Syndrome*. These experts have differentiated "Chronic and Multiple Stress Syndrome" from post-traumatic stress disorder and adjustment disorders.

"Chronic and Multiple Stress Syndrome" refers to the "atypical presentation of depressive symptoms, dissociative symptoms, or somatoform symptoms that escalate during a dangerous voyage and continue to worsen as an immigrant encounters new difficulties upon arrival" (Carta et al. 2005).

Somali immigrants can demonstrate a propensity to report that they are healthier and less symptomatic regarding their psychological distress. These individuals may feel more comfortable reporting somatic symptoms including headaches, heart palpitations, and tiredness than directly expressing psychological discomfort. As a result, challenging and alleviating symptoms, especially more severe symptoms, can be difficult to treat when not considering cultural or religious attitudes. For example, for Somalis there can be externalization of agency that comes from the stance that their problematic circumstance is God's will. There may also be a tendency to minimize suicidal thoughts because this is considered a sin. Consequently, traditional medicine may be considered the optimal treatment because for this group, supernatural forces may hold more value than Western medicine, science, and technology (Scuglik et al. 2007).

Scuglik and colleagues (2007) describe varying somatization and conversion reactions among Somali immigrants that include spirit possession and suffering caused by the "evil eye." Individuals can be perceived as being "cursed" or "possessed by Satan" as punishment when mental health issues are present. As is often the case with immigrant clients that are from countries that have experienced political and societal instability, individuals in roles of authority can be seen as untrustworthy. The authors suggest a way to build rapport with Somali clients is to focus on the physical symptoms and how they are impacting the family. In the spirit of transparency, it will likely be more effective to thoroughly explain and provide rational options when making recommendations.

Traditional practices of African immigrants and the ways in which they adapt to a new society remain unknown in the literature. "What is known is that: they seldom seek help; they are ambitious and dedicated people; they are also naturally shy and show a great respect for elders and authorities. This sometimes becomes problematic because such respect often gets misinterpreted by the host society" (Behnia 1993).

In many African societies, the use of rituals can be employed when a member of a tribe is in conflict with the spirit world and ancestral principles. This conflict between the individual and spiritual world can cause emotional and psychological turmoil. The turmoil can manifest in symptoms of anxiety or any other noticeable change in behavior. Outside of Africa, the behavioral reaction may not be identified as significant or problematic. However, for those embedded in the culture, it is a delicate process that does require effective intervention (Chaboud 1998). To resolve the conflict, elders of the community or tribe are called upon to engage in a collective sacred ritual (Sullivan 1989, 288) to rid the individual from the afflictions brought about by others in the community or ancestral world.

The level to which acculturation impacts the use of traditional health practices versus more Western healing methods is an area for continued research. Specifically factors around cultural practices, religion, and dietary factors, were found to impact traditional health practices. However, the utilization of these practices are not only impacted by the aforementioned factors, but also by legal implications and policy trends. For example, in a survey of 500 Ghanaians residing in Canada, 75 percent reported they continued to hold positive beliefs towards traditional healing practices (Venters and Gany 2011).

When Western practitioners work with a member of a distinct cultural group, "cultural brokers" have been helpful in facilitating communication between populations and other providers to create a useful system leading to effective treatment. These individuals can help immigrants to be amenable to services by discussing treatment in a cultural context consistent with the heritage country's belief systems. Bilingual and bicultural services are becoming a standard of care, especially in providing services to racially and ethnically diverse groups (Esperat et al. 2004).

Special Considerations: Pre-Migration Stress

Among new immigrants to the United States are refugees and asylum seekers. In 2008, the U.S. Committee for Refugees and Immigrants resettled about 60,200 refugees from other countries and granted asylum to 20,500 individuals (Saechao et al. 2011).

Research has shown that the circumstances under which cultural groups have migrated to the Unites States significantly impact mental health (Saechao et al. 2011). Persons forced to leave their countries as a result of war, persecution, and human rights abuses face a major disadvantage as they attempt to adjust to living in a new country. Pre-migration risk factors for emotional distress include previous torture or traumatic experiences such as exposure to political violence and the conditions of loss, lower education, fewer social contacts, no occupation, and pain. Resettled refugees in western countries are about ten times more likely to have post-traumatic stress disorder (PTSD) than an age-matched sample in the country of resettlement. Post-migration circumstances, such as inadequate English language skills, low socioeconomic status, and lower understanding of new cultural expectations, further impede healthy adjustment and adaptation (Saecho et al. 2012).

African asylum seekers are identified as being a vulnerable group (Steel et al. 2006). Statistics from a 2005 study of mental health problems among asylum seekers detained in the United States found that 77 percent were from Africa and of these, 86 percent had clinically significant symptoms of depression, 77 percent had anxiety, and 50 percent were found to have post-traumatic stress disorder. It is hypothesized that these high rates of mental health symptoms may be attributed to both prior traumatization and ongoing detention.

In Conclusion

A predominant criticism of the acculturation literature is its tendency towards a "one size fits all" approach. The need for a more nuanced approach that more accurately captures the complexity and many variations among immigrants and their experiences is substantial. When examining data found in the literature, it is challenging to capture the variety that does exist within each cultural group.

The process through which acculturation takes place is a journey comprised of one's past and present experiences. Personal characteristics, cultural contexts, and societal membership provide a schema to capture how socioeconomic status, geographical location, and language abilities impact acculturation. These distinct factors must be understood and respected to facilitate effective assessment and treatment when working with individuals not belonging to the dominant culture. Furthermore, by leveraging one's perceived strengths, including self-affirmation skills, effective coping strategies, and a positive sense of self, including ones ethnic identity, can be used as tools for service providers to collaboratively work with immigrant clients. The salient ways that immigrants feel either comfortable and empowered, or limited, in their ability to express their identity is also an important treatment consideration (Tsai et al. 2000). Through the facilitation of a strong therapeutic alliance, one that reflects the specific cultural experiences of the client, service providers can enhance their ability to effectively work with their clients. Furthermore, also making space to acknowledge within–cultural group differences will continue to highlight the gaps and promote a more comprehensive approach to examining the relationship between acculturation and health. Smith and colleagues (2011) assert that by highlighting within-group differences, it will minimize the data on acculturation and health to be used improperly.

Finally, the discrepancy between low levels of accessing mental health services and high levels of psychological need must be addressed. Greater interaction is warranted between the mental health providers and immigrant communities to counter the perceived lack of services, lack of information, language barriers, and perceptions about cost (Saechao et al. 2012.). This can be achieved via enhanced public education and more targeted outreach by mental health service providers to new immigrant communities in different languages. Until mental health service providers forge stronger relationships with resettlement and clinical agencies that new immigrants access, years may pass before immigrants even know about the option to receive psychological care.

With the rate of the immigrant population predicted to show exponential increases over the next 20 years, it behooves our behavioral health system developers to understand health trends among and within these groups in order to effectively plan for the future and develop culturally sound and competent services that can meet the needs of a changing population (Nguyen 2011).

References

Abraído-Lanza, A. F., A. N. Armbrister, K. R. Flórez, and A. N. Aguirre. 2006. "Toward a Theory-Driven Model of Acculturation in Public Health Research." *American Journal of Public Health* 96(8): 1342–1346. doi:10.2105/AJPH.2005.064980

Acevedo-Garcia, D., L. M. Bates, T. L. Osypuk, and N. McArdle. 2010. "The Effect of Immigrant Generation and Duration on Self-rated Health among US adults 2003–2007." *Social science & medicine* 71(6): 1161–1172.

Antecol, H., and Bedard, K. 2006. "Unhealthy Assimilation: Why do Immigrants Converge to American Health Status Levels?" *Demography,* 43(2): 337–360.

Aponte, J., and J. Barnes. 1995. "Impact of Acculturation and Moderator Variables on the Intervention and Treatment of Ethnic Groups." *Psychological Interventions and Cultural Diversity,* ed. by J. F. Aponte and J. Wohl, 19–39. Needham Heights, MA: Allyn and Bacon.

Atkinson, D. R., and R. H. Gim. 1989. Asian-American cultural identity and attitudes toward mental health services. *Journal of Counseling Psychology* 36(2): 209.

Behnia, B. 2007. "An Exploratory Study of Befriending Programs with Refugees: The Perspective of Volunteer Organizations." *Journal of Immigrant & Refugee Studies,* 5(3): 1–19.

Bennet, G. G., K.Y. Wolin, C. A. Okechukwu, and K. M. Emmons. 2008. "Nativity and Cigarette Smoking among Lower Income Blacks: Results from the Healthy Directions Study." *Journal of Immigrant and Minority Health* 10(4): 305–311.

Bennet, G. G., K. Y. Wolin, S. Askew, R. Fletcher, and K. M. Emmons. 2007. "Immigration and Obesity among Lower Income Blacks." *Obesity* 1515(6): 13911–13914. doi:10.1038/oby.2007.166.

Berry, J. W. 1980. "Acculturation as Varieties of Adaptation." *Acculturation: Theory, Models and Some New Findings,* 9–25.

Birman, D. 1984. "Biculturalism and Ethnic Identity: An Integrated Model." *Society for the Psychological Study of Ethnic Minority Issues* 8(1): 9–11.

Buriel, R., W. Perez, L. Terri, D. V. Chavez, and V. R. Moran. 1998. "The Relationship of Language Brokering to Academic Performance, Biculturalism, and Self-efficacy among Latino Adolescents." *Hispanic Journal of Behavioral Sciences* 20(3): 283–297.

Carta, M. G., M. Bernal, M. C. Hardoy, and J. M. Haro-Abad. 2005. "Report on the Mental Health in Europe Working Group. Migration and Mental Health in Europe (the State of the Mental Health in Europe Working Group; Appendix 1)." *Clinical Practice and Epidemiology in Mental Health* 1(13). doi.10.1186/1745 -0179-1-13.

Castillo, L. G., and K. A. Caver. 2009. "Expanding the Concept of Acculturation in Mexican American Rehabilitation Psychology Research and Practice." *Rehabilitation Psychology* 54(4): 351–362. doi:10.1037/a0017801

Castillo, L. G., C. Conoley, D. Brossart, and A. Quiros. 2007. "Construction and Validation of the Intragroup Marginalization Inventory." *Cultural Diversity and Ethnic Minority Psychology* 13(3): 232–240.

Chaboud, E. 1998. *The African Immigrants Use of Traditional Healing Practices as Part of Their Process of Re-settlement into Canada.* University of British Columbia, Canada.

Cho, Y., W. P. Frisbie, R. A. Hummer, and R. G. Rogers. 2004. "Nativity, Duration of Residence, and the Health of Hispanic Adults in the United States." *International Migration Review* 38(1): 184–211.

Comas-Diaz, L. 2006. "Latino Healing: The Integration of Ethni Psychology into Psychotherapy." *Psychotherapy: Theory, Research, Practice, Training, 43*(4): 436.

David, E., S. Okazaki, and A. Saw. 2009. "Bicultural Self-Efficacy among College Students: Initial Scale Development and Mental Health Correlates." *Journal of Counseling Psychology* 56(2): 211–226.

Derman-Sparks, L. and C. B. Phillips. 1997. *The Dynamics of Racism. Teaching/ Learning Anti-Racism: A Developmental Approach.* New York: Teachers College Press, 9–21.

Esperat, M., J. Inouye, E. Gonzalez, D. Owen, and D. Feng. 2004. "Health Disparities among Asian Americans and Pacific Islanders." *Annual Review of Nursing Researcha* 22: 135–159.

Farver, J., S. Narang, and B. Bhada. 2002. "East Meets West: Ethnic Identity, Acculturation, and Conflict in Asian Indian Families." *Journal of Family Psychology* 16(3): 338–350.

Finch, B. K., and Vega, W. A. 2003. "Acculturation Stress, Social Support, and Self-rated Health among Latinos in California." *Journal of immigrant health* 5(3): 109–117.

Fuligni, A. J. 2001. "A Comparative Longitudinal Approach to Acculturation among Children from Immigrant Families." *Harvard Educational Review* 71(3): 566–578.

Fuligni, A. J., T. Yip, and V. Tseng. 2002. "The Impact of Family Obligation on the Daily Activities and Psychological Wellbeing of Chinese American Adolescents." *Child Development* 73(1): 302–314.

Hall, G. C. N., A. L. Teten, and S. Sue. 2003. "The Cultural Context of Sexual Aggression." *Annals of the New York Academy of Sciences* 989(1): 131–143.

Hamilton, T. and R. Hummer. 2011. "Immigration and the Health of United States Black Adults: Does Country of Origin Matter?" *Social Science and Medicine* 73: 1551–1560.

Hovey, J. D. 2000. "Acculturative Stress, Depression, and Suicidal Ideation among Central American Immigrants." *Suicide and Life-Threatening Behavior* 30(2): 125–139.

Hyman, D. J., K. Ogbonnaya, V. N. Pavlik, W. S. Poston, and K. Ho. 2003. "Lower Hypertension Prevalence in First-Generation African Immigrants Compared to U.S. Born African Americans." *Ethnicity and Disease* 13(3): 316–323.

Jasso, G., D. S. Massey, M. R. Rosenzweig, and J. P. Smith. 2004. "Immigrant Health: Selectivity and Acculturation." *Critical Perspectives on Racial and Ethnic Differences in Health in Late Life,* 227–266.

Kandula, N., M. Kersey, and N. Lurie. 2004. "Assuring the Health of Immigrants: What the Leading Health Indicators Tell Us." *Annual Review of Public Health* 25: 357–376.

Kiang, L., J. Grzywacz, A. Marín, Arcury, A. Thomas, and S. Quandt. 2010. Mental Health in Immigrants from Nontraditional Receiving Sites." *Cultural Diversity and Ethnic Minority Psychology* 16(3): 386–394.

Kim, B. S., and M. M. Omizo. 2006. "Behavioral Acculturation and Enculturation and Psychological Functioning among Asian American College Students." *Cultural Diversity and Ethnic Minority Psychology* 12(2): 245.

Koo, K. H., S. A. Kari, K. P. Lindgren, and W. H. George. 2012. "Misogyny, Acculturation, and Ethnic Identity: Relation to Rape-Supportive Attitudes in Asian American College Men." *Archives of Sexual Behavior* 41(4): 1005–1014.

Koya, D. L. and L. E. Egede. 2007. "Association between the Length of Residence and Cardiovascular Disease Risk Factors among an Ethnically Diverse Group of United States Immigrants." *Journal of General Internal Medicine* 22(6): 841–846. doi:10.1007/s11606-007-0163-y.

LaFromboise, T., H. L. Coleman, and J. Gerton. 1993. "Psychological Impact of Biculturalism: Evidence and Theory." *Psychological bulletin* 114(3): 395.

Lay, C. H., and S. F. Safdar. 2003. "Daily Hassles and Distress among College Students in Relation to Immigrant and Minority Status." *Current Psychology* 22(1): 3–22.

Le, T. N., and T. Kato. 2006. "The Role of Peer, Parent, and Culture in Risky Sexual Behavior for Cambodian and Lao/Mien Adolescents." *Journal of Adolescent Health* 38(3): 288–296.

Lee, J. S., G. F. Koeske, and E. Sales. 2004. "Social Support Buffering of Acculturative Stress: A Study of Mental Health Symptoms among Korean International Students." *International Journal of Intercultural Relations* 28(5): 399–414.

McDonald, J. T., and S. Kennedy. 2004. "Insights into the 'Healthy Immigrant Effect': Health Status and Health Service Use of Immigrants to Canada." *Social Science & Medicine* 59(8): 1613–1627.

Nesdale, D., A. Maass, K. Durkin, and J. Griffiths. 2005. "Group Norms, Threat, and Children's Racial Prejudice." *Child Development* 76(3): 652–663.

Newbold, K. 2005. "Self-rated Health within the Canadian Immigrant Population: Risk and the Healthy Immigrant Effect." *Social science & medicine* 60(6): 1359–1370.

Nguyen, D. 2011. "Acculturation and Perceived Mental Health Need among Older Asian Immigrants." *Journal of Behavioral Health Services and Research* 38(4): 526–533. doi:10.1007/s11414-011-9245-z

Piontkowski, U., A. Rohmann, and A. Florack. 2002. "Concordance of Acculturation Attitudes and Perceived Threat." *Group Processes & Intergroup Relations* 5(3): 221–232.

Ramírez, M., M. E. Ford, A. L. Stewart, and J. Teresi. 2005. "Measurement Issues in Health Disparities Research." *Health Services Research* 40(5p2): 1640–1657.

Read, J. G., M. O. Emerson, and A. Tarlov. 2005. "Implications of Black Immigrant Health for United States Racial Disparities in Health." *Journal of Immigrant Health* 7(3): 205–212. doi:10.1007/s10903-005-3677-6.

Reynolds, A. L., S. M. Sodano, T. R. Ecklund, and W. Guyker. 2012. "Dimensions of Acculturation in Native American College Students." *Measurement and Evaluation in Counseling and Development* 45(2): 101–112.

Roysircar-Sodowsky, G., and M. Maestas. 2000. "Acculturation, Ethnic Identity, and Acculturative Stress: Evidence and Measurement." In *Handbook of Cross Cultural and Multicultural Personality Assessment,* edited by R. H. Dana, 131–172. Mahwah, NJ: Lawrence Erlbaum.

Ryan, T., and M. Willcox. 2011. "Collaboration with Traditional Health Practitioners in the Provision of Skin Care for all in Africa." *International Journal of Dermatology* 50: 564–570.

Saechao, F., S. Sharrock, D. Reicherter, J. Livingston, A. Aylward, J. Whisnant, and S. Kohli. 2011. "Stressors and Barriers to Using Mental Health Services among Diverse Groups of First-Generation Immigrants to the United States." *Community Mental Health Journal* 48(1): 98–106. doi:10.1007/s10597-011-9419-4

Schwartz, S. J. and M. J. Montgomery. 2002. "Similarities or Differences in Identity Development? The Impact of Acculturation and Gender on Identity Process and Outcome." *Journal of Youth and Adolescence* 31: 359–372.

Schwartz, S. J., J. B. Unger, B. L. Zamboanga, and J. Szapocznik. 2010. "Rethinking the Concept of Acculturation: Implications for Theory and Research." *American Psychologist* 65(4): 237–251.

Scuglik, D., R. Alarcon, A. Lapeyre, M. Williams, and K. Logan. 2007. "When the Poetry No Longer Rhymes: Mental Health Issues among Somali Immigrants in the USA." *Transcultural Psychiatry* 44(4): 581–595. doi:10.1177/1363461507083899

Singh, G., B. Miller. 2004. "Health, Life Expectancy, and Mortality Patterns among Populations in the United States." *Canadian Journal of Public Health* 95(3): 14–21.

Smith, T., M. Rodríguez, and G. Bernal. 2011. "Adapting Psychotherapy to the Individual Patient." *Journal of Clinical Psychology* 67(2): 166–175. doi: 10.1002/jclp.20757

Sodi, T., P. Mudhovozi, T. Mashamba, M. Radzilani-Makatu, J. Takalani, and J. Mabunda. 2011. "Indigenous Healing Practices in Limpopo Province of South Africa: a Qualitative Study." *International Journal of Health Promotion and Education* 49(3): 101–110.

Spencer-Rodgers, J., K. Peng, L. Wang, and Y. Hou. 2004. "Dialectical Self-esteem and East-West Differences in Psychological Well-being." *Personality and Social Psychology Bulletin* 30(11): 1416–1432.

Steel, Z., D. Silove, R. Brooks, S. Momartin, B. Alzuhairi, and I. Suslijik. 2006. "Impact of Immigration Detention and Temporary Protection on the Mental Health of Refugees." *British Journal of Psychiatry* 188: 58–64. doi:10, 1192/bjp. bj.104.007864.

Stephen, E. H., K. Foote, G. E. Hendershot, and C. A. Schoenborn. Advance Data. 1994. "Health of the Foreign-Born Population." *Advance Data from Vital and Health Statistics 241:* 1–10.

Tajfel, H., C. Flament, M. G. Billig, and R. P. Bundy. 1971. "Social Categorization and Intergroup Behaviour." *European Journal of Social Psychology 1:* 149–178.

Trinh, N., Y. C. Rho, F. G. Lu, and M. Sanders, eds. 2009. *Handbook of Mental Health and Acculturation in Asian American families.* New York: Humana Press.

Tsai, J. L., Y. Ying, and P. A. Lee. 2000. "The Meaning of 'Being Chinese' and 'Being American': Variation among Chinese American Young Adults." *Journal of Cross-Cultural Psychology 31:* 302–322.

Valencia-Garcia, D, J. M. Simoni, M. Alegria, and T. Takeuchi. 2012. "Social Capital, Acculturation, Mental Health, and Perceived Access to Services among Mexican American Women." *Journal of Consulting and Clinical Psychology 80* (2): 177–185.

Venters, H. and F. Gany. 2011. "African Immigrant Health." *Journal of Immigrant and Minority Health 13:* 333–344.

Wang, S., and Lo, L. 2005. "Chinese Immigrants in Canada: Their Changing Composition and Economic Performance." *International Migration* 43(3): 35–71.

Wilson, M. N., D. G. Phillip, L. P. Kohn, and J. A. Curry-El. 1995. "Cultural Relativistic Approach toward Ethnic Minorities in Family Therapy." In *Psychological Interventions and Cultural Diversity,* edited by J. F. Aponte and J. Wohl, 92–108. Needham Heights, MA: Allyn and Bacon.

Zacharias, S. 2006. "Mexican Curanderismo as Ethnopsychotherapy: A Qualitative Study of Treatment Practices, Effectiveness, and Mechanisms of Change." *International Journal of Disability, Development, and Education* 53(4): 381–400.

CHAPTER SIX

Yoga, Meditation, and Other Alternative Methods for Wellness: Prevalence and Use in the United States

Sonia Suchday, Lauren Hagemann, Yvette Fruchter, and Miriam Frankel

Historically Western medicine and Eastern medicine have differed in their approach to health and disease. Western medicine derived from the medical model, and focuses on distinguishing between disease and wellness. Eastern approaches emphasize a holistic approach to treatment where illness is considered a function of disequilibrium (Tsuei 1978). However, globalization has led to an amalgamation of cultures and practices among Eastern and Western cultures related to health and healing. In the West, the treatment of acute illness and chronic disease are no longer limited to the medical model. Within the past decade, the use of Complementary and Alternative Medicine (or CAM) in the United States has continued to increase at a steady rate (Nahin et al. 2009). Deriving from traditional Eastern medicine roots, these CAM techniques focus on a combination of physical postures and mental exercises coupled with breathing techniques to achieve a harmonious integration of mind, body, and soul. The most popular therapies in the United States are yoga, meditation, and breathing exercises (Wardle, Lui, and Adams 2012).

This chapter will provide an overview of Eastern approaches to wellness, vis-à-vis yoga, meditation, and other methods of alternative medicine. A specific focus on use and development in the Western world in addition to user characteristics will also be explored, as many of Eastern practices appeal to specific populations for vastly different reasons whether for health as used in conjunction with or in place of conventional medical treatment (NCAM 2012), emotional or recreational purposes. Understanding how ancient approaches to wellness can be accommodated efficiently in a modern world is a fruitful piece of knowledge that will help preserve the physical and psychological well being of American society.

Use of CAM, Yoga, and Meditation in the United States

The use of CAM, specifically yoga and meditation, continues to grow in popularity throughout the United States (Wardle et al. 2012). According to various nationally representative samples, the percentage of adults who use CAM practices, products, and therapies dramatically increased between 1990 and 2002, citing that one-third of the adults in the United States reported using at least some form of CAM (Barnes et al. 2004). A substantive increase was also noted between 2002 and 2007 (Pagan and Pauly 2005, Su and Li 2011). By 2007, four out of ten adults in the United States reported some modality of CAM use (Barnes et al. 2008).

Recent estimates of yoga and meditation use indicate approximately 15 million individuals in the United States practice yoga and about 10 million report the practice of meditation ("Yoga in America Study," 2008, Ospina et al. 2008, Saper et al. 2004). Growing consumer interest in mind-body therapy techniques is demonstrated by statistically significant increases in NHIS respondents' use of yoga and meditation: from 5.1 percent to 6.1 percent and from 7.6 to 9.4 percent, respectively (Barnes et al. 2008). This increased prevalence in the United States demonstrates the growing influence of yoga and meditation in Western populations.

User Characteristics

Characteristics of CAM users, as per recent literature include women, middle-aged adults with higher education or income, alcohol users, those living in the South or West, those with chronic conditions resulting in functional limitations, and those who have been hospitalized in the last year (Barnes et al. 2008, Ryder et al. 2008, Saper et al. 2004). National surveys have indicated yoga users to be predominantly white, female, college educated, urban dwellers with a mean age of 39.5 years (Birdee et al. 2008, Saper et al. 2004). Additionally yoga users compared to non-yoga users were less likely to smoke cigarettes but more likely to drink alcohol (Birdee et al. 2008). Yoga users were also more likely to have a better health status, and be of average weight (Birdee et al. 2008).

Gender. Numerous studies, including the nationally representative samples of the NHIS, have demonstrated women as more likely than men to use CAM practices and therapies (Barnes et al. 2008, Clayton 2005, Fouladbakhsh 2007, Fouladbakhsh and Stommel 2008, Ryder et al. 2008). In fact, women are approximately twice as likely to engage in CAM practices such as yoga, meditation, and guided imagery than men (Birdee et al. 2008, Fouladbakhsh and Stommel 2008). It is hypothesized that women's penchant for using active CAM techniques such as yoga and meditation is due to women being generally more active and engaged in self-care rituals and practices (Fouladbakhsh and Stommel 2010).

Racial Disparities

Estimates based on surveys of nationally representative U.S. samples indicate CAM utilization varies with regards to race and ethnicity (Barnes et al. 2004, Graham et al. 2005, Keith et al. 2005, Kronenberg et al. 2006, Su and Li 2011). Non-Hispanic whites have been cited to have the highest CAM use as compared to ethnic minorities. Additionally, the reasons for engaging in complementary and alternative medication appear to differ with regards to race and ethnicity. Surveys examining reasons for CAM use among U.S. women found Mexican-American women were most likely to use CAM both due to the cost of conventional medication and because they grew up with family members who engaged in these practices (Chao et al. 2006, Graham et al. 2005). African American women were most likely to use CAM as a result of exposure to these practices in the media. Non-Hispanic white women were most likely to report using CAM because of personal beliefs and philosophy.

With respect to yoga and meditation specifically, Non-Hispanic whites were significantly more likely to engage in these practices as compared to African Americans, Mexican Americans, and Chinese Americans. Non-Hispanic white CAM users remained more likely than Mexican American and African American users to engage in yoga and meditation in the last year even after accounting for socioeconomic factors.

The growth of yoga and meditation use and all other CAM therapies is unevenly distributed across racial and ethnic groups in the United States. A comparative analysis of data from 2002 and 2007 NHIS studies revealed CAM growth, including yoga and relaxation techniques, for non-Hispanic whites and Asian Americans was significantly greater as compared to African Americans and Hispanics (Su and Li 2011). It appears the gap between

Caucasians and racial minorities with regards to use of complementary and alternative medicine is therefore widening.

Notably, Hispanics have demonstrated the lowest rate of CAM use, including yoga and meditation, as compared to other ethnicities. They also demonstrated a general lack of growth in their utilization of CAM between 2002 and 2007 (Su and Li 2011). Within the Hispanic population, Mexican-born adults in the United States have shown the lowest rate of CAM use as compared to Puerto Rican, Mexican American, Dominican, and Central or South American adults (Barnes et al. 2008). Su and Li (2011) suggested the low use of CAM techniques stems from Hispanic immigrants' lack of knowledge and exposure to these practices. Additionally, many Hispanic immigrants practice *Curanderismo* (see chapter 10, this volume), a holistic system of folk medicine that is commonly practiced in Latin America (Su and Li 2011). Therefore, they may be less inclined to practice or engage in other unfamiliar forms of CAM therapies.

Analyses from a CAM supplement to the 2002 National Health Interview Survey found that the level of acculturation, measured by length of stay in the United States and language of interview, is strongly associated with CAM use. Specifically, the greater the acculturation of immigrants (via their time in the United States and their proficiency of English), the more likely they are to use CAM therapies, gradually approaching the level of CAM use by native-born Americans (Su, Li, and Pagan 2008). Thus, acculturation appears to be a central factor in the disparity of CAM use between immigrants and U.S.-born Americans with regards to CAM use.

Socioeconomic Factors

With regards to socioeconomic status, use of CAM is inconclusive. While studies have demonstrated adults with higher income are more likely to utilize complementary and alternative medicine, including yoga and meditation (Barnes et al. 2008), two national surveys examining prevalence of yoga use found no significant relationship between income and yoga use (Birdee et al. 2008, Saper et al. 2004). Regardless of the relationship between income and CAM use, research indicates people are more likely to use CAM for health care when financial obstacles disturb access to standard medical care (Su and Li 2011). National survey data from 2002 and 2007 confirm adults in the United States are inclined to use CAM when medical needs are unmet or conventional care is delayed because of cost (Barnes et al. 2008). Further, findings from a study examining CAM growth between 2002 and 2007 indicate that rising prices of standard medical treatment and the resulting decreased access to medical care is contributing to the increasing prevalence in CAM use (Su and Li 2011). Type of insurance also may play a role in CAM use: adults with private insurance are more likely than those with public health insurance or uninsured adults to use biologically-based therapies, body-based therapies, and mind-body therapies. Adults with public insurance have demonstrated to be less inclined to use CAM as compared to uninsured adults or adults with private health insurance (Barnes et al. 2008).

A recent cross-sectional study of women in the United States highlights the importance of accounting for socioeconomic factors when examining CAM use among racial and ethnic groups (Kronenberg et al. 2006). Without accounting for socioeconomic factors, overall CAM use among Caucasians was higher than minorities. When CAM use was adjusted for socioeconomic factors, there was no difference of CAM use by Caucasians and Mexican Americans. However, socioeconomic factors did not account for differences in utilization of CAM between whites and African Americans. Interestingly, Kronenberg et al. (2006) also found that racial minorities were the highest users of culturally relevant CAM practices, including herbal medicine among Mexican Americans and acupuncture among Chinese Americans.

Health Status

While some studies have found CAM use is associated with worse self-rated health, secondary analyses of the 2007 NHIS survey illuminated a remarkable paradox: CAM users reported more chronic illnesses but were also more likely to report their health as excellent and as better than the prior year (Keith et al. 2005; Wolsko et al. 2000). Researchers speculated high self-rated health might be the product of participants' optimism and positive feelings regarding their CAM use (Nguyen et al. 2010). However, randomized controlled studies are needed to establish whether CAM therapies and mind-body medicine in particular lead to better health status and improvement in addition to a better understanding of the impact of self rated health.

Medical Conditions

Despite the positive association between CAM utilization and number of medical conditions and doctor's visits over a twelve months period, approximately 20 percent of adults without health conditions and 25 percent of adults without any doctor visits also practiced CAM in general (Barnes et al. 2008). Leading a lifestyle that incorporates yoga and relaxation techniques in particular can have long term benefits of preventing and ameliorating illness (Yang 2007). People often use CAM to improve their health as well as mitigate symptoms of chronic or terminal illnesses. Research indicates most individuals use CAM in addition to conventional care rather than as a substitute (Astin 1998, Eisenberg et al. 1998). According to 2007 NHIS survey data, the top five health problems reported by U.S. adults as reasons for CAM use were back pain, neck pain, anxiety, arthritis, and joint pain (Wells et al. 2011). According to a recent study, approximately one-third of patients with Acute Coronary Syndrome practice some form of mind-body medicine (Leung et al. 2008). Additionally, CAM is widely used with cancer patients, as it is estimated at least 39 percent of United States individuals diagnosed with cancer at some point in their lifetime have used CAM (Fouladbakhsh and Stommel 2008). A recent survey found those with cancer were more likely to use low-cost practices such as meditation as compared to higher cost practices such as yoga, which requires expenses for class attendance and purchase of materials (Fouladbakhsh and Stommel 2010). Specific examination of 2002 NHIS yoga consumers indicates yoga users are more likely to have mental health conditions, musculoskeletal conditions, severe sprains and asthma (Birdee et al. 2008). Additionally, yoga appears to be most commonly used to treat musculoskeletal and mental health conditions. Interestingly, hypertension and chronic obstructive lung disease has been associated with less yoga use, and based on this finding, researchers suggested that yoga users may be a particular group of people less likely to have hypertension (Birdee et al. 2008).

Defining Yoga and Meditation

Yoga

Yoga, a set of ancient teachings and exercises, produces inner peace and wellbeing by tapping into the physical, emotional, and mental aspects of a person (Ross and Thomas 2010). Diverse physical and psychological pathways bring about such effects. Yoga is defined as Buddhi which means the joining of Prakriti (nature) and Purusha (spirit) (DeMichelis 2004). The more classical methods of yoga include an ethical, disciplined lifestyle, physical postures, breathing control, and meditation. Effective practice of yoga results in the achievement of the highest potential, leading to an enduring life of happiness and health (Eggleston 2009).

The most commonly practiced forms of yoga in the West include Hatha, Iyengar, Sudarshan Kriya, and Meditative yoga; each type stresses a different construct of relaxation (Cabral, Meyer, and Ames 2011). Hatha yoga, the most popular form of yoga in Western society, emphasizes the progression through a series of physical postures or poses (Asanas). Iyengar yoga, a derivative of Hatha yoga, is a low impact practice that utilizes props and other aids such as foam blocks and straps, to help with performing a set series of poses. It also entails holding poses for a longer period of time (Field 2011). This form of yoga is recommended in populations stricken with physical limitations and other disabilities, for example, those recovering from surgery or other injuries (Duncan 2008). Sudarshan Kriya yoga is a practice that stresses slow and modulated breathing, allowing for oxygenated blood to flow freely to all parts of the body, increasing parasympathetic drive and homeostasis of various hormones including cortisol (Brown and Gerbarg 2009).

Meditation

Although traditionally meditation was conceptualized as a component of yoga practice, it is frequently utilized as an independent practice in the West. Meditation entails training the mind to concentrate and focus. This focus is achieved by repetition of a word, focus on a scene, or watching your breath. Practice of meditation leads to the relaxation response, which is a set of physical changes that include increased blood flow to the brain and release of muscle tension (Cabral et al. 2011). There are many forms of meditation practiced in Western society, the most popular being Transcendental Meditation (TM) and various forms of Mindfulness Meditation (Horowitz 2010). Transcendental meditation aims to prevent distracting thoughts by way of a mantra (word, sound, or symbol). The notion of TM is that repetition of the mantra will prevent other cognitive activity such as racing thoughts and excess worry from occurring, yielding superlative focus and attention on the meditative exercise. Individuals engaged in TM are instructed to remain passive and if distracting thoughts come to mind are encouraged to notice them but quickly return to the mantra at hand (Manocha 2000). Mindfulness based meditative practices involve features such as enhanced awareness and attention to sensations occurring within the body such as thoughts and emotions. It also requires refraining from reacting to internal stimuli by staying present focused and non-judgmental (Baer 2003). Unlike TM, mindfulness meditation is not mantra based; instead it encourages an individual to wholly accept a stimulus as it unfolds, without attempts to change or avoid it.

Methods of mindfulness meditation include mindfulness based stress reduction or MBSR, which combines mindfulness meditation techniques, gentle yoga, and psychoeducation. Specifically, psychoeducation for mindfulness meditation includes education on how techniques can impact various pathways that, when implemented appropriately, can effectively treat and/or influence various psychological and physical disorders (Olivo et al. 2009). This form of meditation practice has been associated with a decrease in anxiety, depression, and fatigue (Carlson and Garland 2005, Carlson et al. 2004). Various techniques of this method of meditation include guided imagery, body scans, deep breathing and Zen meditation. Mindfulness meditation is also utilized in clinical modalities such as dialectical behavior therapy (Linehan 1993, Ospina et al. 2008).

Meditation: Pranayama or Breathing Exercises

A key element of yoga and meditation deserves special mention—Pranayama. This is one of the eight components of yoga described in traditional Indian texts and is comprised of a combination of specialized breathing techniques and patterns that include deep breathing into the abdomen, holding the breath at different points in the breathing cycle, breathing through one or both nostrils and the mouth alternately, and breathing against airway resistance (Brown and Gerbarg 2009). Pranayama has gained recent attention in the West through the efforts of organizations such as the Art of Living, which conduct training sessions on pranayama.

The value of combining meditation and pranayama is hypothesized to be in their ability to create altered states of consciousness, a state of calm, parasympathetic activation, and neuroendocrine activity that decreases the stress response (Brown and Gerbarg 2005, 2009). Depending on the teachers and settings, pranayama is used along with other yoga and meditation techniques. Even when no specific mention is made of pranayama, breath regulation is a key element of yoga and meditation. Recent evidence points to the importance of pranayama in the treatment of depression, anxiety, post-traumatic stress disorders, increasing longevity, and medical conditions (Brown and Gerbarg 2005, 2009). It is considered a powerful stress management technique that may be used by itself or in conjunction with yoga and meditation. All three are thought to be synergistic in their benefits to health and wellbeing.

History of Yoga and Meditation

Eastern Perspectives

Yoga and meditation are commonly used practices that originated in India between 5000 BC and 3000 BC (DeMichelis 2004). Yoga and meditation overlap in their philosophy and practice to emphasize the mind-body-spirit connection. Foundational and historic texts such as the *Yoga Sutras of*

Patañjali detail the ancient yogic teaching, postures and ethnics and provide clarity regarding the practice of yoga and meditation (Feuerstein 1998).

Traditional yoga and meditation practices are a way of life and a means to sustain optimal well-being; they are not viewed as two separate entities. A lifestyle of yoga and meditation includes a series of regimented commitments that range from strict dietary rules to time dedicated to various yogic, meditative and breathing exercises during the day, especially the morning hours. The core of yoga has traditionally been described as having eight aspects or "limbs" that holistically bring completeness to an individual. These eight "limbs" of yoga include Yama, the ethical or moral principles such as non-harm; Niyama, purification and cleansing; Asanas, physical postures; Pranayama, breath; Pratyahara, withdrawal of the senses; Dharana, concentration; Dhyana, meditation; and Samadhi, awareness of the self or the achievement of ecstasy (Ross and Thomas 2010). Faithful engagement in these components or "limbs" is believed to be a pathway to connect with a higher being and essential for the attainment of a superior conscious state (Desikachar 2003).

Western Perspectives

Unlike Eastern cultures where yoga and meditation are a way of life, Western culture views yoga and meditation as therapies. Specifically in Western cultures, yoga and meditation are utilized as supplemental or alternative therapies to Western medicine. Practice of yoga and meditation in Western cultures can be traced back to the late 19th century as a result of the British occupation of the Indian peninsula (DeMichelis 2004). However, these practices did not make it into mainstream American society until the late 1960s, following the Vietnam War and Civil Rights movement, in an era renowned for its evolution of alternative worldviews and free and forward thinking.

While there has always been a distinct focus on spiritual healing through the practice of yoga and meditation in the east, the popularity of yoga and meditation practice grew, not for their spiritual context, but more so for their espoused physical and health benefits (Reder 2001). For example, dissimilar to traditional practice and the focus on the eight components mentioned above, Westernized practice tends to stress only Asana (postures) and Pranayama (breath). The Western world places emphasis on the secondary gains of yoga (e.g., flexibility, strength, and balance), while the primary spiritual objectives of the practice emphasized in the east appear to be less relevant. An online survey of yoga and meditation showed that despite participation and interest in yoga, less than half of the sample engaged in meditation and/or breathing exercises, suggesting poor adherence to the more spiritual facets of the practice (Yogasite 2006). Participants who engaged in yoga were more concerned with having certain physical and lifestyle characteristics, including a more toned and lean physique, and the acquisition of a lifestyle viewed as more peaceful.

Yoga and Meditation: Physiological and Psychological Impact

The effects of yoga and meditation may be through a direct impact on physiological and biological systems or indirect through their impact on affective states, including stress, anger, depression, and anxiety. Research has also examined the positive effect of these practices on chronic disease risk factors such as obesity, elevated blood pressure, elevated blood glucose, and cholesterol (Yang 2007).

Recent data has shown that the physiological mechanisms responsible for the effects of yoga and meditation include parasympathetic activation and the neuroendocrine management of the stress response (Brown and Gerbarg 2009; Kuntsevich, Bushell, and Theise, 2010). A recent review of physiologic and biological systemic mechanisms underlying the effects of yoga and meditation on health and disease (Kuntsevich et al. 2010) includes immune system responses (hormones, neurotransmitters, growth factors, cytokines, chemokines, adipokines) the central and peripheral nervous system, macrophage and lymphocyte activity, and electromagnetic activity.

Psychological pathways associated with chronic illnesses, such as cardiovascular disease and diabetes, include depression, anger/hostility, anxiety and stress. Stress, anxiety, and depression pathways to illness include disturbed mood and activation of the hypothalamic-pituitary-adrenal axis, which are associated with negative health outcomes (Anisman and Merali 2003). Yoga, meditation, and pranayama with their mind-body focus are appealing stress management strategies and research has demonstrated their ability to positively impact chronic illness outcomes (Rozanski et al. 2005).

Yoga has also demonstrated efficacy for weight loss, reducing chronic pain, improving outcomes of coronary heart disease and diabetes, decreasing stress, and improving psychiatric diagnoses including depression, anxiety, posttraumatic stress disorder, and schizophrenia (Bijlani et al. 2005, Kristal et al. 2005, Morone and Greco 2007, Smith et al. 2007; Culos-Reed, Carlson Daroux, and Hately-Aldous, 2006; Suchday et al. 2012; Cabral, Meyer, and Ames 2011).

Another means by which yoga can influence health includes the alleviation of the body's natural stress response. By using inward focus, one is said to hold the power to redirect attention away from external triggers of stress and re-regulate them into a more peaceful state. This relaxation response is further enhanced through breathing exercises and other techniques, which help modulate physiological stimuli associated with increased sympathetic activation (Hayes 2010). Due to yoga's meditative component, there is an emphasis on heightened bodily awareness, which allows practitioners to increase awareness of their anxiety and physiological responses (Javnbakht et al. 2009). This attunement to physiological and psychological responses leads to a plethora of positive side effects, such as enhanced concentration and performance speed, beyond what is typically seen in traditional exercise (Manjunath and Telles 2001). This use of increased mindfulness is hypothesized to lead to better management of health issues.

Recent research shows the benefit of stress mitigation as an important mechanism by which yoga positively influences wellness. Evidence comparing the level of salivary cortisol, a factor associated with stress, between Hatha yoga and African dance participants demonstrated the calming impact Hatha yoga practice had on lowering cortisol levels (West, et al. 2004). These aforementioned benefits have also been proven useful in early breast cancer patients. A study including a yoga program in tangent with adjuvant radiotherapy found significant declines in anxiety, depression, perceived stress, and salivary cortisol when compared to controls (Vadiraja et al. 2009). Yoga and meditation have also been found to decrease music performance anxiety, general anxiety, tension, depression, and anger in professional musicians (Khalsa et al. 2009). These studies provide evidence of the range of benefits that yoga can have on improving practitioners' wellness, health, and mindfulness.

A systematic review of meditation's efficacy for the treatment of medical and psychological illnesses found meditation has beneficial effects for epilepsy, premenstrual syndrome symptoms, menopausal symptoms, mood and anxiety disorders, autoimmune illness, and emotional disturbance in neoplastic disease (Arias 2006). Specific forms of meditation, such as the use of MBSR, improved mood, decrease perceived stress, and influenced positive immunological changes such as decreased production of interferon and increased production of anti-inflammatory cytokine in a sample consisting of breast cancer patients (Carlson et al. 2003). Additional studies observing healthy controls found those who completed an eight week meditation program before receiving influenza vaccination demonstrated better antibody responses compared to a weight-list control group, decreased trait anxiety, and increased positive affect (Davidson et al. 2003). The practice of TM lowers the indicators of psychosocial stress such as anger, hostility, and depression (Barnes 2012). This form of meditation also mitigates psychosocial stress and anxiety in addition to lowering the rates of smoking and alcohol abuse (Rainforth et al. 2007). Other studies have found that forms of meditation are more effective than somatic relaxation at enhancing positive mood and reducing distractive thoughts and were also more effective in reducing ruminative thoughts and behaviors compared to a control condition (Jain et al. 2007).

Additional Benefits of Yoga and Meditation

Not only are there notable physical and psychological benefits to regular yoga and meditation, there are more practical and fiscal benefits to their use. The high rate of CAM utilization is associated with considerable out-of-pocket payments by U.S. adults for practitioner visits, products, and other relevant materials. Data analysis of the 2007 NHIS study demonstrates while the amount spent on CAM was only 1.5 percent of total health care expenditure; it comprised a sizeable amount of out-of-pocket health care costs (Nahin et al. 2009). In 2007, adults in the United States paid 33.9 billion dollars out of pocket on CAM visits, products, classes and materials. Close to two-thirds of these total costs were related to self-care therapies including natural products, homeopathic products, and yoga. Specifically, adults spent 4.1 billion dollars out of pocket on yoga, tai chi, or quigong classes, approximately 12 percent of total out-of-pocket costs. With regards to relaxation techniques, individuals spent 0.2 billion dollars total on relaxation techniques, which is approximately 0.6 percent of total out-of-pocket costs (Nahin et al. 2009). The high level of expenditure points to the high value placed on complementary and alternative therapies. One possible reason for the increasing popularity and sometimes even greater demand of yoga and meditation may be the integration of these therapies into regular healthcare. Healthcare consumers are taking control of these types of services and are educating themselves on a variety of CAM practices to use in lieu of Westernized medicine. This is especially relevant in the face of rising health care costs, negative medication side effects and poor treatment results from conventional care.

Medication Side Effects

Components of CAM therapies are used to complement conventional care (Astin 1998, Eisenberg et al. 1998), and are prescribed by healthcare providers in an effort to go beyond treating the physical and biochemical manifestations of illness. One way in which CAM serves complementary to other health care modalities is via its impact on replacing prescription medication use. Negative side effects of conventional medications may prevent patient adherence to treatment, especially in children and adolescents. In a sample of adolescents with asthma, negative response to medications was identified as a key factor in adolescents' lack of adherence to treatment. Some adolescents even reported using CAM, specifically relaxation and prayer, instead of their prescribed asthma medication (Cotton, Luberto, Yi, and Tsevat 2011).

Cost of Healthcare and Use

The high cost of healthcare coverage and conventional care has led people to seek these alternative therapies for medical and psychological ailments. When adults and children are concerned with the cost of conventional care, they delay treatment and are more likely turn to CAM providers for help (Barnes et al. 2008). To offset health care expenses, employers and insurance companies have begun responding to the growing demand for these services in substitute of or along with conventional medical treatment. In some states, legislation ensures that employers offer certain alternative services to employees, such as massage therapy and chiropractors. Furthermore, there are new insurance plans that cover CAM expenses or affinity programs where members receive discounts to visit CAM providers in their coverage network. Employers and insurance companies alike are motivated to provide coverage for these practices for various reasons. Firstly, because of its preventative benefits and efficacy with improving overall wellness. Secondly, research posits that such alternative practices hold the potential to improve work performance and efficiency. For example a study comparing yoga therapies with traditional exercise in areas of focus and concentration found that yoga significantly decreased the time needed to perform certain concentration tasks (Manjunath and Telles 2001).

The use of CAM is not limited to the medical population; people seek CAM, like yoga and meditation for stress reduction, to improve health and enhance quality of life. Various CAM modalities have been proven to be useful alternatives to pharmaceutical interventions or more invasive approaches to treatment (Chapman and Bredin 2010). In addition, Western culture has also adopted the practice of yoga and meditation as a means of stress management, recreation and exercise.

Yoga and Meditation Use for Stress Management

The leading cause of death in the United States is predominately related to chronic diseases, which tend to develop over the lifespan (Center for Disease Control 2004). These conditions, including heart disease, cancer and diabetes, are exacerbated by our day-to-day exposure to stress. With stress related illness on the rise, the availability of and access to stress reduction strategies is crucial to sustaining optimal, long term well being. Research posits that individuals are drawn to yoga as a mechanism to control stress (Van der Klink et al. 2001). In a review of the most useful stress-reducing interventions in work settings, research posits that relaxation techniques such as yoga and meditation are found to be some of the most useful modalities in alleviating stress (Van der Klink et al. 2001). Such improvements can be specifically explained by the various mechanisms and pathways that these practices can alter such as cognitive, sensory, affective, and biological processes (Newberg and Iversen 2003).

The utility of yoga, meditation and other CAM practices as stress management tools is currently widely researched. One study found that certain forms of yoga acted as effective stress management programs when incorporated into cognitive behavioral therapy (Granath et al. 2006). Results showed that both standard cognitive behavioral therapy (CBT) and yoga programs resulted in a statistically significant reduction in scores on many stress related subjective and physiological variables. Importantly, it is useful to be cognizant of the therapeutic effectiveness of a more mind-body based treatment modality among individuals who are less inclined to pursue more traditional methods of therapy. Such individuals may find yoga and meditation a less stigmatizing and more acceptable avenue to explore when requiring assistance with stress related issues (Milligan 2011).

Utilization of yoga as a stress management tool appears to have both immediate and long term effects. In research conducted by Gupta (2006) and replicated by Sharma (2008), the short term impact of a brief yoga intervention was found to be beneficial at reducing anxiety scores in both healthy and diseased participants (e.g., those diagnosed with hypertension, obesity). Engaging in a simple series of asanas (postures) and pranayama (breathing) exercises, combined with other stress management strategies, has the ability to influence anxiety scores and improve quality of life in a brief period of time. Likewise, longitudinal studies addressing yoga participants across several years, report similar findings, indicating that longer term yoga exposure can also impact mental health, thus reducing levels of anxiety, anger and fatigue (Yoshihara et al. 2011).

Meditation alone has also been shown to be a useful stress management technique. Research has shown that brief meditation interventions, as short as eight weeks, can yield improvements in perceived stress, overall mood, depression, sleep, memory and blood pressure in groups of community dwelling adults diagnosed with cognitive impairment and their caregivers (Innes et al. 2012). Although there are many forms of meditation practices, research has demonstrated the type of meditation does not seem to impact improvement outcomes. For example, in a study comparing the effectiveness of two meditation types (mindfulness and transcendental meditation), it was found that there appear to be no difference in outcome in relation to the form of meditation engaged in (Schoormans 2011).

Other Psychological Benefits of Yoga and Meditation

Not only do yoga, meditation and other CAM practices enhance one's spiritual and physical well being, these activities are also viewed as an avenue to enhance opportunities for recreation and socialization. The benefits of maintaining regular recreational and social activities are plentiful. Such benefits include the acquisition of a sense of meaning and purpose in life in addition to better overall and self-rated health, strengthened immune system functioning and improved mortality (Cohen, Gottlieb, and Underwood 2004). Similarly those who reportedly engage in a regular yoga practice endorse a significant social connection that can lead to a wide range of positive outcomes including various health benefits, improved self esteem, self efficacy and self awareness.

Yoga is an active form of recreation. Individuals engaged in a local practice experience an increased sense of acceptance both personally and within society, oftentimes inspiring those to give back to their communities (Stelzer 2009). Additionally, yoga and meditative practices performed regularly in a group setting can lead to bonding, yielding new interpersonal relationships and friendships and social opportunities, thereby improving mental health by decreasing feelings of depression and isolation (Stelzer 2009).

Mind-body therapies are no longer bound to the constraints of a yoga studio. Due to the minimalist and simplistic requirements to engage in a yoga and/or meditation practice, there has been a steady rise in the integration of such activities into various settings (Stelzer 2009). For example, many schools, churches, and other public establishments are incorporating mind-body therapies into their congregations with the goal to not only maintain wellness but also promote a sense of community. Additionally, various classes which are specific to age, gender, and physical condition, such as pre-natal yoga and classes or individuals recovering from surgery or medical conditions, have been proven to enhance the therapeutic experience while providing a sense of acceptance, connectedness, and belonging amongst its participants (Chapman and Bredin 2010).

Yoga and Meditation Use for Exercise

With the increasing popularity of CAM to improve wellness and quality of life, people are incorporating yoga and meditation into their daily exercise regimens. In a national survey exploring the prevalence and patterns of yoga use in the United States, of the 3.8 percent of respondents who confirmed practicing yoga in the previous year, 64 percent validated use for wellness purposes while 48 percent engaged for health reasons (Saper et al. 2004).

It is noted that yoga has over 200 variations of poses and sequences (Ripoll and Mahowald 2002). Due to the multitude of postures and variations available in the practice of yoga, people are able to accommodate their exercise regimen accordingly and adapt their practice to whatever physical or medical ailment as needed. For example, different types of yoga provide varying forms of physical exercise, ranging from the gentle and meditative to more vigorous and exhaustive forms like Ashtanga or power yoga. Additionally, yoga exercises can be used to target specific areas requiring strengthening or improvement, such as upper and lower body muscle strength, endurance, balance, and flexibility, cardiovascular functioning, and weight loss (Bhutkar et al. 2011, Chen et al. 2006).

Yoga and meditation have been found to be equal or superior to traditional methods of exercise (Ross and Thomas 2010). These practices have proven to be effective for both healthy and diseased populations, and are particularly effective in relieving symptoms associated with diabetes, kidney disease and chronic pain disorders and improving blood pressure and blood glucose levels. Research has noted that yoga exercise is significantly more effective at reducing pain related disability and improving flexibility compared to a physical exercise regimen that excludes yoga and meditation (Tekur et al. 2008). Literature on the topic of yoga and meditation as a method of exercise defends the notion that the practices can serve as a supplement or substitute for other exercises in patient populations that benefit from exercise, and many individuals may find yoga a less intense but equally effective workout (Ripoll and Mahowald 2002).

Users should be cognizant when performing yoga and meditation practices as risks do exist. Novices to yoga postures may overexert and strain muscles or cause physical injury. Therefore, prescribers of such alternative healing as well as consumers themselves should be mindful of personal limitations and maneuver their practice with patience and awareness.

Future Directions

In order for yoga and meditation to maintain their growing popularity in the United States, it is essential these practices evolve in accordance with the changing American demographic. Recent estimates indicate there are an estimated 11.5 million unauthorized immigrants living in the United States as of January 2011 (Hoefer, Rytina, and Baker 2012). According to a May

2012 U.S. Census Bureau report, racial minorities, including Hispanics, Asians, and African Americans, comprised the majority of American births for the 12-month period ending in July 2011. This milestone in American history leads to an interesting paradox: the United States continues to grow in diversity while the majority of CAM consumers remain well-educated Caucasian women (Barnes et al. 2008, Su and Li 2011). Innovative and personalized methods of yoga and meditation dissemination are recommended to close the gap for CAM use between whites and minorities as well as between men and women.

Racial health-care disparities in America are well documented and caused by many factors, including socioeconomic and environmental conditions (Peek et al. 2012, Smedley, Stith, and Nelson 2002). Therefore, the racial imbalance of CAM use is not unusual or unexpected. It has been hypothesized immigrants and racial minorities are less likely to use yoga and meditation due to economic disadvantage, rendering them less able to afford paying for materials and classes, coupled with lack of exposure to these practices (Su and Li 2011). Notably, there are actually a variety of options and resources for underprivileged individuals looking to start or maintain the practice of yoga and meditation. While many studio classes are costly, free or low cost classes are becoming increasingly more available. Further, there are many free video tutorials for yoga and meditation on websites such as www.myfreeyoga.com, www.doyogawithme.com, and www.freemeditation.org. One lesser-used option yoga studios may wish to consider is incorporating a "work-service" program, which would allow individuals to participate in classes in exchange for working at the studio.

The larger issue appears to be educating individuals who are not exposed to yoga and meditation or are not aware of the benefits of this practice. Opening yoga studios with low-cost options within the geographic location of immigrant and minority communities may improve awareness and accessibility among these populations. Additionally, in order for yoga and meditation to reach a wider audience, it is essential for these practices to be integrated into a variety of environments, including health-care settings, community centers, churches, schools, and the workplace. Incorporation of CAM into these other settings increases the convenience of practice and makes it more likely people will add such activities to their daily routine. Further, people are more likely to try these novel techniques in a setting that is familiar and comfortable to them. Individuals are also more likely to obtain accurate and important information on yoga and meditation through these avenues.

In addition to decreasing the racial imbalance, another future goal of researchers and consumers alike should be to decrease the gender gap widely exhibited in Western societies. As stated above, women are more likely to engage in health care services and generally more active with self-care, which may result in their greater likelihood of using yoga and meditation. Engaging men in these CAM practices may be accomplished by encouraging them to become more involved with their health-care and self-maintenance. Research has also indicated yoga improves men's sexual functioning, which may be another incentive for men to practice yoga (Dhikav et al. 2010). Future studies may wish to examine why men are less prone to use these techniques and whether men are aware of the health benefits of yoga and meditation. Additionally, it is important for doctors and other health-care practitioners to remain informed about the health benefits of CAM for men and to provide this information to their patients.

Concluding Thoughts

Yoga and meditation are ancient forms of alternative medicine. Despite the evolution of these practices, they continue to prove effective for both physical and mental health ailments as they target specific pathways to enhance and improve wellness. The practice of yoga and meditation has evolved with changing times. From its early beginnings during the Vietnam era as a spiritual endeavor, to its more recent evolution as a health care essential and recreational activity, the benefits of yoga and meditation have been widely claimed. What remains elusive in Western society is the practice of yoga and meditation as a lifestyle as it is practiced in Eastern cultures rather than a means to an end (e.g., health care, recreation, etc.). Although popularity is widespread, the literature suggests that middle-aged women, those with higher socioeconomic status and higher education, are more likely to use such practices. Yoga and meditation are also used frequently in populations suffering from acute and chronic physical and mental health conditions.

Tough economic times have also influenced people to discover and implement alternative treatment modalities within their lifestyles to better manage their health without the supports of traditional medicine. For example, CAM practices are commonplace for those who are uninsured or underinsured as well in populations that are unable to afford prescription medications (Su and Li 2011) or for those leery of the side effects of certain prescribed medications. Employers are also including incentives for alternative medicine usage in their staff, so as to prevent spikes of absenteeism and to improve work efficacy and performance.

Yoga and meditation is no longer strictly a spiritual and physical experience confined to the studio walls. Society now regards these practices as functional activities that are used to combat stress, improve socialization and sense of community. Various communal establishments are incorporating yoga, meditation, and other methods of relaxation not only to improve wellness, but to foster interpersonal bonds. The widespread functional use of yoga and meditation has increased curiosity and popularity of these therapies in Western culture.

References

Anisman, H., and Z. Merali. 2003. "Cytokines, Stress, and Depressive Illness: Brain-Immune Interaction." *Annals of Medicine 35*: 2–11.

Arias, A. J., K. Steinberg, A. Banga, and R. L. Trestman. 2006. "Systemic Review of the Efficacy of Meditation Techniques as Treatment for Medical Illness." *The Journal of Alternative and Complementary Medicine 12*(8): 817–832.

Astin, J.A. 1998. "Why Patients Use Alternative Medicine: Results of a National Study." *The Journal of American Medical Association 19*: 1548–1553.

Baer, R. 2003. "Mindfulness Training as a Clinical Intervention: A Conceptual and Empirical Review." *Clinical Psychology: Science and Practice 10*(2): 125–143.

Barnes, P. M., B. Bloom, and R. L. Nahin. 2008. "Complementary and Alternative Medicine Use among Adults and Children: United States, 2007." *National Health Statistics Reports 12*: 1–24.

Barnes, P. M., E. Powell-Griner, K. McFann, and R. L. Nahin. 2004. "Complementary and Alternative Medicine Use among Adults: United States, 2002." *Advance Data from Vital and Health Statistics,* no 343. Hyattsville, MD: National Center for Health Statistics.

Barnes, V. A. and D. W. Orme-Johnson. 2012. "Prevention and Treatment of Cardiovascular Disease in Adolescents and Adults through the Transcendental Meditation® Program: A Research Review Update." *Current hypertension reviews 8*(3): 227.

Bhutkar, M.V., P. M. Bhutkar, G. B. Taware, and A. D. Surdi. 2011. "How Effective is Sun Salutation in Improving Muscle Strength, General Body Endurance, and Body Composition?" *Asian Journal of Sports Medicine 2*(4): 259–266.

Bijlani, R. L., R. P. Vempati, R. K. Yadav, R. B. Ray, V. Gupta, R. Sharma, S. C. Mahapatra. 2005. "A Brief but Comprehensive Lifestyle Education Program Based on Yoga Reduces Risk Factors for Cardiovascular Disease and Diabetes Mellitus." *The Journal of Alternative and Complementary Medicine 11*(2): 267–274.

Birdee, S. G., A. T. Legedza, R. B. Saper, S. M. Bertisch, D. M. Eisenberg, and R. S. Phillips. 2008. "Characteristics of Yoga Users: Results of a National Survey." *The Journal of General Internal Medicine 23*(10): 1653–1658.

Bloom, B., and R. L. Nahin. 2008. "Complementary and Alternative Medicine Use among Adults and Children: United States, 2007." *National Health Statistics Reports,* no 12. Hyattsville, MD: National Center for Health Statistics.

Brown, R. P. and P. L. Gerbarg. 2005. "Sudarshan Krita and Yogic Breathing in the Treatment of Stress, Depression and Anxiety. Part I – Neurophysiologic Model." *The Journal of Complementary and Alternative Medicine 11*(1): 189–201.

Brown, R. P. and P. L. Gerbarg. 2009. "Yoga Breathing, Meditation, and Longevity." *Longevity, Regeneration, and Optimal Health: Annals of the N.Y. Academy of Sciences* 1172: 54–62.

Burke, A., and A. Gonzalez. 2011. "Growing Interest in Meditation in the United States." *Biofeedback* 39(2): 49–50.

Cabral, P., H. B. Meyer, and D. Ames. 2011. "Effectiveness of Yoga Therapy as a Complementary Treatment for Major Psychiatric Disorders: A Meta-Analysis." *Primary Care Companion for CNS Disorders* 13 (4). doi: 10.4088/PCC.10r01068.

Carlson, L. E. and S. Garland. 2005. "Mindfulness-Based Stress Reduction (MBSR) on Sleep Quality in Cancer Patients." *International Journal of Behavioral Medicine* 12(4): 278–285.

Carlson, L. E., M. Speca, K. D. Patel, and E. Goodey. 2003. "Mindfulness-Based Stress Reduction in Relation to Quality of Life, Mood, Symptoms of Stress, and Immune Parameters in Breast and Prostate Cancer Outpatients." *Psychosomatic medicine* 65(4): 571–581.

Carlson, L. E., M. Speca, K. Patel, and E. Goodey. 2004. "Mindfulness-Based Stress Reduction in Relation to Quality of Life, Mood, Symptoms of Stress and Levels of Cortisol, Dehydroepiandrosterone Sulfate (DHEAS) and Melatonin in Breast and Prostate Cancer Outpatients." *Psychoneuroendocrinology* 29: 448–474.

Chao, M.T., C. Wade, F. Kronenberg, D. Kalmuss, and L. F. Cushman. 2006. "Women's Reasons for Complementary and Alternative Medicine Use: Racial/ Ethnic Differences." *Journal of Complementary and Alternative Medicine* 12(8): 719–720.

Chapman, E. L. and S. S. D. Bredin. 2010. "Why Yoga? An Introduction to the Philosophy, Practice and the Role of Yoga in Health Promotion and Disease Prevention." *Health and Fitness Journal of Canada* 3(2): 13–21.

Chen, K., A. Hassett, F. Hou, J. Staller, and A. Lichtbroun. 2006. "A Pilot Study of External Qigong Therapy for Patients with Fibromyalgia." *The Journal of Alternative and Complementary Medicine* 12(9): 851–856.

Clayton, A. H. 2005. "Complementary and Alternative Medicine." *Primary Psychiatry* 12(8): 20–201.

Cohen, S., B. H. Gottlieb, and L. G. Underwood. 2004. "Social Relationships and Health." *American Psychologist* 59(8): 676–684.

Cotton, S., C. M. Luberto, M. S. Yi, and J. Tsevat. 2011. "Complementary and Alternative Medicine Behaviors and Beliefs in Urban Adolescents with Asthma." *The Journal of Asthma* 48(5): 531–538.

Culos-Reed, S. N., L. E. Carlson, L. M. Daroux, and S. Hately-Aldous. 2006. "A Pilot Study of Yoga for Breast Cancer Survivors: Physical and Psychological Benefits." *Psychooncology* 15(10): 891–897.

Davidson, K.W., M. Goldstein, R. M. Kaplan, et al. 2003. "Evidence Based Behavioral Medicine: What Is It and How Do We Achieve It?" *Annals of Behavioral Medicine* 26: 161–171.

De Michelis, E. 2004. *A History of Modern Yoga: Patanjali and Western Esotericism.* London and New York: Continuum.

Desikachar, T. K. V. 2003. *Reflections on Yoga Sutras of Patañjali.* Chennai, India: Krishnamacharya Yoga Mandiram.

Dhikav, V., G. Karmarkar, M. Verma, R. Gupta, S. Gupta, D. Mittal, and K. Anand. 2010. "Yoga in Male Sexual Functioning: A Non-Comparative Pilot Study." *Journal of Sexual Medicine* 7: 3460–3466.

Duncan, M. D., A. Leis, and J. W. Taylor-Brown. 2008. "Impact and Outcomes of an Iyengar Yoga Program in a Cancer Center." *Integrative Oncology* 15(2): S72-S78.

Duraiswamy, G., J. Thirthalli, H. R. Nagendra, and B. N. Gangadhar. 2007. "Yoga Therapy as an Add-On Treatment in the Management of Patients with Schizophrenia: A Randomized Controlled Trial." *Acta Psychiatr Scand* 10: 226–232.

Eggleston, B. 2009. "Psychosocial Determinants of Attending Yoga Classes: An Application of the Theory of Planned Behavior." Doctoral dissertation, Indiana University. *ProQuest* 48–01 (UMI No: 3344775).

Eisenberg, D. M., R. B. Davis, S. L. Ettner, S. Appel, S. Wilkey, M. Van Rompay, et al. 1998. "Trends in Alternative Medicine Use in the United States, 1990–97: Results of a Follow-up National Survey." *The Journal of American Medical Association* 280(18): 1569–1575.

Feuerstein, G. 1998. *The Yoga Tradition: Its History, Literature, Philosophy, and Practice.* Prescott, Arizona: Hohm Press.

Field, T. 2011. "Yoga Clinical Research Review." *Complementary Therapies in Clinical Practice* 17(1): 1–18.

Fouladbakhsh, J. M. and M. Stommel. 2008. "Comparative Analysis of CAM Use in the U.S. Cancer and Non-Cancer Populations." *Journal of Complementary and Integrative Medicine* 5(1): 19–29.

Fouladbakhsh and M. Stommel. 2010. "Gender, Symptom Experience, and Use of Complementary and Alternative Medicine Practices among Cancer Survivors in the U.S. Cancer Population." *Oncology Nurse Forum* 37(1): E7–15.

Fouladbakhsh, J. M., and M. Stommel. 2007. "Using the Behavioral Model for Complementary and Alternative Medicine: The CAM Healthcare Model." *Journal of Complementary and Integrative Medicine* 4(1).

Graham, R. E., A. C. Ahn, R. B. Davis, B. B. O'Connor, D. M. Eisenberg, and R. S. Phillips. 2005. *The Journal of the National Medical Association* 97(5): 535–545.

Granath, J., S. Ingvarsson, U. von Thiele, and U. Lundberg. 2006. "Stress Management: Randomized Study of Cognitive Behavioural Therapy and Yoga." *Cognitive Behaviour Therapy* 35(1): 3–10.

Gupta, N., S. Khera, R. P. Vempati, R. Sharma, and R. L. Bijlani. 2006. "Effect of Yoga Based Lifestyle Intervention on State and Trait Anxiety." *Indian Journal of Physiology and Pharmacology* 50: 41–47.

Hayes, M and S. Chase. 2010. "Prescribing Yoga." *Primary Care: Clinics in Office Practice* 37: 31–47.

Hoefer, M. N. Rytina, and B. Baker. 2012. *Estimates of Unauthorized Population Residing in the United States: January 2011.* Fact Sheet. Office of Immigration Statistics, Department of Homeland Security, Washington, DC.

Horowitz, S. 2010. "Health Benefits of Meditation: What the Newest Research Shows." *Alternative and Complementary Therapies* 16(4): 223–228.

Innes, K. E., T. K. Selfe, C. J. Brown, K. M. Rose, and A. Thompson-Heisterman. 2012. "The Effects of Meditation on Perceived Stress and Related Indices of Psychological Status and Sympathetic Activation in Persons with Alzheimer's Disease and Their Caregivers: A Pilot Study." *Evidence-Based Complementary and Alternative Medicine.* doi:10.1155/2012/927509.

Jain, S., S. L. Shapiro, S. Swanick, S. C. Roesch, P. J. Mills, I. Bell, and G. E. Schwartz. 2007. "A Randomized Controlled Trial of Mindfulness Meditation Versus Relaxation Training: Effects on Distress, Positive Stress of Mind, Rumination, and Distraction." *Annals of Behavioral Medicine* 33(1): 11–21.

Javnbakht, M., R. Hejazi Kenari, and M. Ghasemi. 2009. "Effects of Yoga on Depression and Anxiety of Women." *Complementary Therapies in Clinical Practice* 15: 102–104.

Jayadevappa, R., J. C. Johnson, B. S. Bloom, S. Nidich, S. Desai, S. Chhatre, R. Schneider. 2007. "Effectiveness of Transcendental Meditation on Functional Capacity and Quality of Life of African Americans with Congestive Heart Failure: A Randomized Control Study. *Ethnic Disparities* 17(1): 72–77.

Keith, V. M., J. J. Kronenfeld, P. A. Rivers, and S. Liang. 2005. "Assessing the Effects of Race and Ethnicity on Complementary and Alternative Medicine Therapies in the USA." *Ethnicity and Health* 10(1): 19–32.

Khalsa, S., S. Shorter, S. Cope, et al. 2009. "Yoga Ameliorates Performance Anxiety and Mood Disturbance in Young Professional Musicians." *Applied Psychophysiology Biofeedback* 34(4): 279–289.

Kristal, A. R., A. J. Littman, D. Benitez, and E. White. 2005. "Yoga Practice is Associated with Attenuated Weight Gain in Healthy, Middle-Aged Men and Women." *Alternative Therapies in Health Medicine* 11: 28–33.

Kronenberg, F., L. F. Cushman, C. M. Wade, D. Kalmuss, and M. T. Chao. 2006. "Race/Ethnicity and Women's Use of Complementary Alternative Medicine in the United States." *The American Journal of Public Health* (97) 7: 1236–1242.

Kuntsevich, V., W. C. Bushell, and N. D. Theise. 2010. "Mechanisms of Yogic Practices in Health, Aging, and Disease." *Mount Sinai Journal of Medicine* 77: 559–569.

Lee, J. H., M. S. Goldstein, R. Brown, and R. Ballard-Barbash. 2010. "How Does Acculturation Affect the Use of Complementary and Alternative Medicine Providers among Mexican and Asian Americans?" *The Journal of Immigrant Minority Health* 12: 302–309.

Leung, Y. W., H. Tamim, D. E. Stewart, H. M. Arthur, and S. L. Grace. 2008. "The Prevalence and Correlates of Mind-Body Therapy Practices in Patients with Acute Coronary Syndrome." *Complementary Therapies in Medicine* 16: 254–261.

Linehan, M. M. 1993. *Cognitive-Behavioral Treatment of Borderline Personality Disorder.* New York: Guilford Press.

Macy, D. 2013. "Yoga in America" market study. *Yoga Journal.* http://www. yogajournal.com/advertise/press_ releases/10.

Manjunath, N. K., and S. Telles. 2001. "Improved Performance in the Tower of London Test Following Yoga." *Indian Journal of Physiology and Pharmacology 45*: 351–354.

Manocha, R. 2000. "Why Meditation?" *Australian Family Physician* 29(12): 1135–1138.

Milligan, C. K. 2011. "Yoga for Stress Management Program as a Complementary Alternative Counseling Resource in a University Counseling Center." *Journal of College Counseling* 9(2): 181–187.

Morone, N. E., and C. M. Greco. 2007. "Mind-Body Interventions for Chronic Pain in Older Adults: A Structured Review." *Pain Medicine 8*: 359–375.

Nahin, R. L., P. M. Barnes, B. J. Stussman, and B. Bloom. 2009. "Cost of Complementary and Alternative Medicine and Frequency of Visits to CAM Practitioners: United States, 2007." *National Health Statistics Report 18*: 1–15.

National Institutes of Health. 2004. "Expanding Horizons of Health Care National Center for Complementary and Alternative Medicine Strategic Plan 2005–2009." National Institutes of Health: Author.

NCAM 2012. http://nccam.nih.gov/health/whatiscam

Newberg, A. B. and J. Iversen. 2003. "The Neural Basis of the Complex Mental Task of Meditation: Neurotransmitter and Neurochemical Considerations." *Medical Hypothesis* 61(2): 282–291.

Nguyen, L. T., R. B. Davis, T. J. Kaptchuk, and R. S. Phillips. 2010. "Use of Complementary and Alternative Medicine and Self-Rated Health Status: Results from a National Survey." *The Journal of General Internal Medicine* 26(4): 399–404.

Nguyen, L. T., R. B. Davis, T. J. Kaptchuk, and R. S. Phillips. 2011. "Use of Mind-Body Medicine and Improved Self-Rated Health: Results from a National Survey." *The International Journal of Person-Centered Medicine* 1(3): 514–521.

Olivo, E. L., B. Dodson-Lavelle, A. Wren, Y. Fang, and M. C. Oz. 2009. "Feasibility and Effectiveness of a Brief Meditation-Based Stress Management and Intervention for Patients Diagnosed with or at Risk for Coronary Heart Disease: A Pilot Study." *Psychology, Health, and Medicine* 14(5): 513–523.

Ospina, M. B., K. Bond, M. Karkhaneh, N. Buscemi, D. M. Dryden, V. Barnes, L. E. Carlson. J. A. Dusek, and D. Shannahoff-Khalsa. 2008. "Clinical Trials of Meditation Practices in Healthcare: Characteristics and Quality." *The Journal of Complementary and Alternative Medicine* 14(10): 1199–1213.

Pagan, J. A. and M. V. Pauly. 2005. "Access to Conventional Medical Care and the Use of Complementary and Alternative Medicine." *Health Affairs* 24(1): 255–262.

Peek, M. E., S. C. Wilson, J. Bussey-Jones, M. Lypson, L. Cordasco, E. A. Jacobs, C. Bright, and A. F. Brown. 2012. "A study of National Physician Organizations' Efforts to Reduce Racial and Ethnic Health Disparities in the United States." *Academic Medicine* 87: 694–700.

Pelletier, K. R. and J. A. Astin. 2002. "Integration and Reimbursement of Complementary and Alternative Medicine by Managed Care and Insurance Providers: 2000 Update and Cohort Analysis." *Alternative Therapies in Health and Medicine* 8(1): 38–44.

Rainforth, M. V., R. H. Schneider, S. I. Nidich, C. Gaylord-King, J. W. Salerno, and J. W. Anderson. 2007. "Stress Reduction Programs in Patients with Elevated Blood Pressure: A Systematic Review and Meta-Analysis." *Current Hypertension Reports* 9(6): 520–528.

Ray, U. S., S. Mukhopadhyaya, S. S. Purkayastha, V. Asnani, O. S. Tomer, R. Prashad, et al. 2001. "Effect of Yogic Exercises on Physical and Mental Health of Young Fellowship Course Trainees." *Indian Journal of Physiology and Pharmacology* 45: 37–53.

Reder, A. 2001. "Reconcilable Differences: Yoga and Religion." *Yoga Journal* March/April: 78–85.

Ripoll, E. and D. Mahowald. 2002. "Hatha Yoga Therapy Management of Urologic Disorders." *World Journal of Urology* 20: 306–309.

Ross, A. and S. Thomas. 2010. "The Health Benefits of Yoga and Exercise: A Review of Comparison Studies." *The Journal of Alternative and Complementary Medicine* 16(1): 3–12.

Rozanski, A., J. A. Blumenthal, K. W. Davidson, P. G. Saab, and L. Kubzansky. 2005. "The Epidemiology, Pathophysiology, and Management of Psychosocial Risk Factors in Cardiac Practice: The Emerging Field of Behavioral Cardiology." *Journal of the American College of Cardiology* 45(5): 637–651.

Ryder, P.T., B. Wolpert, D. Orwig, O. Carer-Pokras, and S. A. Black. 2008. "Complementary and Alternative Medicine Use among Older Urban African Americans: Individual and Neighborhood Associations." *The Journal of the American Medical Association* 100(10): 1186–1192.

Saper, R, D. Eisenberg, R. Davis. L. Culpepper, and R. Phillips. 2004. "Prevalence and Patterns of Adult Yoga Use in the United States: Results of a National Survey." *Altern. Ther. Health Med.* 10: 44–48.

Schneider, R. H. 2007. "Effectiveness of Transcendental Meditation on Functional Capacity and Quality of Life of African Americans with Congestive Heart Failure: A Randomized Control Study." *Ethnic Disparities* 17(1): 72–77.

Schoormans, D. and I. Nyklicek. 2011. "Mindfulness and Psychologic Wellbeing: Are they Related to Type of Meditation Technique Practiced?" *The Journal of Alternative and Complementary Medicine* 17(7): 629–634.

Scott, L. 2008. "Yoga off the Mat: How Far and to Whom Do the Benefits Extend" The University of Texas School of Public Health. Health Promotion and Behavioral Sciences Management: ProQuest.

Sharma, R., N. Gupta, and R. L. Bijlani. 2008. "Effect of Yoga Based Lifestyle Intervention on Subjective Wellbeing." *Indian Journal of Physiology and Pharmacology* 52(2): 123–131.

Smedley, B., A. Stith, and A. Nelson. 2002. *Unequal Treatment: Confronting Racial and Ethnic Disparities in Health Care.* Washington, DC: National Academies Press.

Smith, C., H. Hancock, J. Blake–Mortimer, and K. Eckert. 2007. "A Randomized Comparative Trial of Yoga and Relaxation to Reduce Stress and Anxiety." *Complementary Therapies in Medicine* 15: 77–83.

Stelzer, S. 2009. "New Yoga Studio Encourages Positive Impact on Community through Communication and Leadership." *ProQuest* 48–01. (UMI No. 1468978).

Su, D. J., and L. Li. 2011. "Trends in the Use of Complementary and Alternative Medicine in the United States: 2002–2007." *Journal of Health Care for the Poor and Underserved* 22: 296–310.

Su, D. J.,L. Li, and J. A. Pagan. 2008. "Acculturation and the Use of Complementary and Alternative Medicine." *Social Science and Medicine* 66: 439–453.

Suchday, S., M. Dziok, M. Katzenstein, E. Kaplan, and M. Kahan. 2012. "The Effects of Meditation and Yoga on Cardiovascular Disease." In *Stress Proof of the Heart: Behavioral Interventions for Cardiac Patients,* edited by E. A. Dornelas, 223–248. New York, NY: Springer.

Tacon, A. M., J. McComb, Y. Caldera, and P. Randolph. 2003. "Mindfulness Meditation, Anxiety Reduction, and Heart Disease: a Pilot Study." *Family and Community Health* 26(1): 25–33.

Tekur, P., C. Singphow, H. R. Nagendra, and N. Raghuram. 2008. "Effect of Short-Term Intensive Yoga Program on Pain, Functional Disability, and Spinal Flexibility in Chronic Low Back Pain: A Randomized Control Study." *The Journal of Alternative and Complementary Medicine* 14(6): 637–644.

Tsuei, J. J. 1978. "Eastern and Western Approaches to Medicine." *Western Journal of Medicine* 128(6): 551–557.

U.S. Census Bureau. 2012. "Most Children Younger than Age 1 Are Minorities, Census Bureau Reports." http://www.census.gov/newsroom/releases/archives/population/cb12–90.html

U.S. Department of Health and Human Services. 2004. The Health Consequences of Smoking: A Report of the Surgeon General. *Atlanta, GA: U.S. Department of Health and Human Services, Centers for Disease Control and Prevention, National Center for Chronic Disease Prevention and Health Promotion, Office on Smoking and Health,* 62.

Vadiraja, H., R. Raghavendra, R. Nagarathna, et al. 2009. "Effects of a Yoga Program on Cortisol Rhythm and Mood States in Early Breast Cancer Patients Undergoing Adjuvant Radiotherapy: A Randomized Controlled Trial." *Integrative Cancer Therapy* 8(1): 37–46.

Van der Klink, J. L., R. B. Blonk, A. H, Schene, and F. H. van Dijk. 2001. "The Benefits of Interventions for Work-Related Stress." *American Journal of Public Health* 91: 270–276.

Wardle, J., C. Lui, and J. Adams. 2012. "Complementary and Alternative Medicine in Rural Communities: Current Research and Future Directions." *The Journal of Rural Health* 28: 101–112.

Wells, R. E., S. M. Bertisch, C. Buettner, R. S. Phillips, and E. P. McCarthy. 2011. "Complementary and Alternative Medicine Use among Adults with Migraines/Severe Headaches." *Headache* 51: 1087–1097.

West, J., C. Otte, K. Geher, J. Johnson, and D. C. Mohr. 2004. "Effects of Hatha Yoga and African Dance on Perceived Stress, Affect, and Salivary Cortisol." *Annals of Behavioral Medicine* 28(2): 114–118.

Wolsko, P., L. Ware, J. Kutner, C. Lin, G. Albertson, L. Cyran, L. Schilling, and R. J. Anderson. 2000. "Alternative/Complementary Medicine: Wider Usage than Generally Appreciated." *Journal of Alternative and Complementary Medicine* 6(4): 321–6.

Yang, K. 2007. "A Review of Yoga Programs for Four Leading Risk Factors of Chronic Diseases." *Evidence-Based Complementary and Alternative Medicine* 4(4): 487–491.

Yogasite 2006. "Yoga Now: Results of an Online Survey by Yogasite." www.yogasite .com/surveyreport.html on June. 26, 2012.

Yoshihara, K., T. Hiramoto, N. Sudo, and C. Kubo. 2008. "Profile of Mood States and Stress Related Biochemical Indices in Long-Term Yoga Practitioners." *Biopsychosocial Medicine* 5(6). doi: 10.1186/1751-0759-5-6

CHAPTER SEVEN

Ayurveda: An Alternative in the United States

*Sonia Suchday, Natasha P. Ramanayake,
Amina Benkhoukha, Anthony F. Santoro,
Carlos Marquez, and Gen Nakao*

Globalization has led to a changing picture of health and wellness; increased interaction and porous borders have created a situation where diseases spread rapidly between communities and countries, creating a demand for health and wellness services. As diverse communities converge to urban areas across the world, they bring their traditional practices of health and wellness. These traditional practices coexist with mainstream practices and systems of health care. These rapid changes in demand from a diverse population for health care, requires a change in health care systems and practices to better serve the health of diverse individuals and communities.

This chapter offers a brief introduction to the core principles, philosophies, and basic treatment approaches of Ayurveda, prevalence rates of Ayurveda in the United States, ways in which it differs from conventional U.S. health and healthcare practices, and, finally, available scientific research investigating the various treatments associated with Ayurveda, discussed in terms of the appropriateness and translation to Western methodologies.

History and Definition of Ayurveda

Ayurveda is an ancient, traditional paradigm of medicine and health care. Originating from the Vedic civilization of ancient India, Ayurveda has been actively practiced for 5,000 years, making it one of the oldest known systems of medicine (Mukherjee et al. 2012, Patwardhan 2010, Ramchandani et al. 2012, Sharma et al. 2007, Sharma, Triguna, and Chopra 1991). Ayurveda practices are still prominent in present day India, representing a large proportion of the readily available health care in most rural areas. Rather than being considered antiquated or obsolete, Ayurveda is practiced in conjunction with existing systems of allopathic medicine and is highly regarded for its time-tested efficacy. There was a decline in the prevalence of Ayurveda during the colonial rule; however, independence from colonial rule saw the revival of Ayurvedic practices (Sharma et al. 2007). Global interest in this medical tradition has steadily increased throughout the last few decades (Islam 2010, 2012, Mamtani and Mamtani 2005, Manohar 2012, Sharma et al. 2007). Beyond Indian borders, Ayurveda practices, conceptualizations, and ideologies are becoming increasingly more apparent in Western countries, such as the United States (Mamtani and Mamtani 2005, Manohar 2012).

In the United States, Ayurvedic medicine has been grouped under complementary and alternative medicine, better known as CAM (National Center for Complementary and Alternative Medicine [NCCAM] 2009) along with other approaches, including acupuncture, homeopathy, and traditional healers such as shamans (Barnes, Bloom, and Nahin 2008). These practices grouped under CAM include treatment modalities, which may be biologically-based, or mind-body therapies and practices like Ayurveda or Homeopathy that represent a complex system of medicine (Varker et al. 2012).

Ayurveda and other alternative therapies have gained increasing popularity since the 1960s and 1970s in the United States and other western cultures and are associated with disillusionment with the mainstream culture, a fascination for eastern thought, a movement to commune with nature, holistic medicine, and New Age culture (Park et al. 2012).

Philosophy and Theory of Ayurveda

The term *Ayurveda,* comes from the Sanskrit roots *ayus* and *veda;* literally translated, *Ayus* refers to lifespan of anything living (including a cell) and Veda means knowledge (Hankey 2001). Based on this translation, Ayurveda is the accumulation of knowledge on health and wellness, managing disease or illness, and promotion of harmony between one's mind, body, spirit, and natural systems or environment (Mamtani and Mamtani 2005, Sharma et al. 2007, Sharma et al. 1991).

Ayurveda is an integrative and holistic approach to optimal health, which may be achieved through addressing a multitude of indivisible dimensions of the human condition: the body, mind and spirit (Ramchandani et al. 2012, Patwardhan 2010). These indivisible aspects are reflected in the Ayurvedic term for health, which is *swastha; swastha* is the combination of *swa*, translated as *self*, and *astha*, meaning *established*. The interpretation of this term is that the self can be realized through a harmonious balance between mind, body, and spirit (Sharma et al. 2007a). This harmony or equilibrium can be achieved through an appropriate lifestyle and the practice of appropriate nutrition and cleansing practices, meditation and yoga, massage, etc. In the translation to therapeutic practice, emphasis on wholeness is manifest in Ayurvedic practices which are geared towards treating the individual rather than the presenting symptomology (Mamtani and Mamtani, 2005).

There are two paradigms or ideologies incorporated in the practice of Ayurveda: *Charaka* and the *Sushruta* (Manohar 2012). Based on the teachings of a famous Indian physician, Atreya, the *Charaka* dates back to around 300 B.C. and is the first text to advance medical practices from superstition and sorcery. It defines the *self* as the perpetual amalgam of mind, body, spirit, and senses. According to the *Charaka*, an individual's health is not predetermined, but influenced by his or her lifestyle. Based on this approach there is an emphasis on integrated practices of illness prevention over aggressive treatment of disease. The *Sushruta*, ascribed to a 6th century B.C. physician of the same name, is a descriptive text outlining over 1,100 illnesses, invasive procedures and surgical instruments. Ayurveda, as practiced today, is the product of the *Charaka's* holistic scope and preventive orientation and the *Sushruta's* structured coding and meticulous practices (Ramchandani et al. 2012).

Ayurveda names five core elements—*fire, water, earth, air,* and *ether*, or space—that make up life and the universe, referred to as *panchamahabhutas*. However, these elements are not emphasized in a physical or material sense. Instead, Ayurveda speaks of the unique essences, or natural forces, and properties of these five elements. For example, fire represents light and heat while water represents the cohesive strength of matter. The *panchamahabhutas* elements comprise the three basic tenets that regulate physiology and health called *doshas* or humors: *Vata, Pitta,* and *Kapha* (Islam 2012, Mamtani and Mamtani 2005, Mukherjee et al, 2012). Each *dosha* relates to specific aspects of movement. *Vata* (space) presides over physiological functions that relate to motion and mobility, including the movement of blood through veins. *Pitta* (fire and water) presides over the processes of transformation, including those related to metabolism and digestion. *Kapha* (earth and water) presides over bodily form and muscle fluidity. Contrary to Charaka, *doshas* possess a genetic component called *prakrit*, which represents an individual's unique proportion of *vata, pitta,* and *kapha* that they are born with. However, lifestyle influences can disrupt the balanced doshas and such disproportion is referred to as *vikriti*. Moreover, the three *doshas* are viewed as universal tenets of nature, existing in animals, plants, minerals, seasons, and planets. This allows conceptualizing the human being as innately and naturally existing in connection to the universe and nature (Sharma et al. 2007).

Prevalence of Ayurveda in the United States

Despite increasing technological sophistication in understanding illness and health, and in prevention, treatment, and cure of disease, many challenges remain in the United States. Prevalence of chronic disease is increasing and obesity has reached pandemic proportions. The healthcare system has been inadequate in preventing or controlling the spread of chronic disease and rising costs have made it inaccessible to a large number of people (Sharma et al. 2007). In addition to increased prevalence of chronic disease, the challenge of preventing and managing multiple risk factors that lead to these disorders and the inadequacy of conventional allopathic medicine in targeting these conditions have led people to seek alternatives to the predominant system of healthcare in the United States.

Ayurvedic medicine, as mentioned earlier, is one of many modalities grouped under complementary and alternative medicine, or CAM (NCCAM, 2009). Although Ayurveda is considered a complex system of medicine, simpler treatment modalities and mind-body practices such as acupuncture are also considered as falling under the CAM umbrella (Barnes et al. 2008, Varker et al. 2012). In general, people in the United States use CAM therapies to supplement rather than replace conventional medicine, and this medical pluralism in the United States has important implications for individual patient care and for the health care system as a whole (Eisenberg et al. 1993, Nemer 2010). An important point about CAM use in the United States including Ayurveda is that individuals may use some component of the treatment rather than utilizing all aspects of it. According to the 2007 National Health Interview Survey (NHIS) (Barnes et al. 2008), almost four out of 10 adults used CAM therapy in the last twelve months, with the most commonly used therapies being non-vitamin, non-mineral, natural products (17.7 percent) and deep breathing exercises (12.7 percent).

From this national survey, it was also found that approximately one in nine children (11.8 percent) used CAM therapy in the past 12 months. Accordingly, children whose parents used CAM were almost five times as likely (23.9 percent) to use CAM as children whose parents did not use CAM (5.1 percent). Although detailed rate or method of use is not reported, in 2002 approximately 154,000 adult people had used Ayurvedic medicine in the United States Comparatively, more than 200,000 adult people in the United States reported specifically using Ayurvedic medicine in the 2007 NHIS, indicating rising prevalence rates in the United States (Barnes et al. 2008).

User Characteristics

Research indicates that CAM users have been consistently female, young adult to middle ages, reporting higher education and income, chronic medical conditions, and living in states located in the western part of the country (Barnes et al. 2008). There is a high prevalence of CAM use among American-born groups such as non-white Hispanics and Native American/ Alaskans (Barnes et al. 2008). Interestingly, CAM use is *not* associated with foreign birth (Misra et al. 2010). A possible explanation for this may be under-reporting of CAM use by foreign-born participants.

Gender

Qualitative and quantitative studies across North America have replicated the NHIS finding that women are more likely than men to practice CAM therapies (Choudry 1998, Hilton et al. 2001, Misra et al. 2010, Rao 2006). This greater occurrence in women can be explained by women's greater tendency towards self-care rituals and practices (Fouladbakhsh and Stommel 2010). Another explanation may be that women are more likely to admit to using alternative methods to achieve health and healing compared to men. The one exception to this is that in the Asian Indian community there is an insignificant difference between men and women using Ayurveda, reflecting its widespread influence (Satow et al. 2008).

Ethnic Disparities

Data on the use of Ayurveda in the general population of the United States is almost non-existent and estimates of use may be made from research and reviews of CAM use. Similarly, information about use of Ayurvedic practices among ethnic subgroups is also non-existent (Misra et al. 2010). In an analysis of the 2002 NHIS data (Mehta et al. 2007), researchers found that the likelihood of CAM use among Asian adults was similar to levels of CAM use among Non-Hispanic white Americans. This study also indicated that CAM is used among Asian Americans for health maintenance rather than treatment of a specific ailment. Subsequent studies have not only confirmed the high prevalence of Ayurveda and other CAM usage among Asian Americans, but also indicate that user characteristics within the Asian American community are similar to user characteristics reported in the general population (Mehta et al. 2007, Misra et al. 2010, Satow et al. 2008).

Estimates based on the 2007 NHIS data indicate that CAM use varies among ethnic groups. Notably, it was reported that American Indian or Alaska Native adults (50.3 percent) and non-Hispanic white adults (43.1 percent) were more likely to use CAM compared to Asian adults (39.9 percent) or black adults (25.5 percent) (Barnes et al., 2008). In addition, Asian Indians were more likely to report use of mind-body therapies (31 percent) over the use of herbal remedies (19 percent); Asian Indians were also more likely to report using mind-body therapies compared to Chinese (32 percent) and Filipinos (26 percent) (Barnes et al., 2008). Another study contradicts this finding, however, with Chinese Americans reporting higher CAM use (86 percent) compared to South Asians (67 percent) (Hsiao et al. 2006).

An important point about the data related to Asian Indians is that first generation Asian Indians may be using Ayurvedic principles and practices that they have grown up with but not label them as such. For example, turmeric is used in Indian cooking and is frequently used in herbal and home remedies to treat colds and upper respiratory infections and for wound healing. However, Asian Indians when asked about Ayurvedic medicine may not specifically associate it with the use of home remedies or spices in daily cooking.

Spirituality

Spirituality is intrinsically entwined in CAM treatments, which are a combination of treatments for the mind, body, and soul or spirit exemplified by practices such as Yoga or Native American medicine. However, research in CAM rarely addresses spirituality (Mackenzie et al. 2003). In one study where spirituality was assessed (Misra et al. 2010), respondents who reported themselves as being spiritual were 1.5–2.0 times more likely to use CAM and specific Ayurvedic treatments. One possible reason for increased CAM use among individuals who valued spirituality could be that spirituality is deeply embedded in not just treatment modalities but also in the philosophy of Ayurvedic medicine. Illness, in the Ayurvedic framework, represents an imbalance between the mind, body, and spirit and also implies a loss of faith in the Divine (Misra et al. 2010).

Health and Access to Care

The link between access to health care and use of traditional medical treatment or Ayurveda is complex, especially within the Asian Indian community. Individuals with limited English proficiency or individuals who face significant barriers in accessing health care are more likely to use Ayurveda (Hsiao et al. 2006), Among Indians who are able to easily access conventional health care, treatment choices are based on availability of resources and cost (Rao 2006). In other words, Asian Indians will rely on conventional medicine that is covered by insurance providers when insurance is available rather than seek Ayurvedic treatment. Data from this study also indicated that homeopathic treatments were sought when participants visited India; participants also reported bringing back medicines for minor ailments (Rao 2006).

Additionally, Asian Americans and Asian Indians in particular are less likely than non-Hispanic whites to disclose CAM use to their primary health care practitioners compared to other ethnic groups (Mehta et al. 2007, Satow et al. 2008). Low disclosure rates are often attributed to concerns about perceived stigma and acceptance from practitioners. South Asians lacking in English proficiency are also less likely to use CAM in general, a finding that is inconsistent in other Asian American communities.

Acculturation

Data on CAM/Ayurveda use and acculturation comes from the Asian Indian community in the United States Acculturation appears to play a role in the types of conditions that Asian Indians treat with Ayurveda. An exploratory study involving qualitative community-based interviews revealed a "hierarchy of resort" approach to choice of medicine and treatment (Rao 2006). Informants followed a pattern of choosing homeopathic and Ayurvedic treatments for minor concerns and allopathic medicine for more serious and chronic conditions. As previously mentioned, people with chronic medical conditions tend to supplement medical treatment with CAM practices (Barnes et al. 2008). On the other end of the "hierarchy of resort," people will rely on CAM where allopathic medicine proves unsatisfactory and ineffective (Rao 2006).

Training

Traditionally, knowledge of Ayurveda incorporated hymns and text in order to educate the new generation of practitioners, and only within the last 50 years has Ayurveda and its effects been recorded (Mukherjee et al.

2012). Although the United States has no national standard for training or certifying Ayurvedic practitioners (NCCAM 2009), there are a number of schools that offer education and training programs in Ayurveda in the United States (National Ayurvedic Medical Association, [NAMA] 2013). The National Ayurvedic Medical Association (NAMA), founded in 1998, represents the Ayurvedic profession in the United States, and its purpose is to provide leadership within the Ayurvedic community and to promote a positive vision for Ayurveda and its holistic approach to health and wellness (NAMA 2013). The NAMA's vision statement is that this institution is the voice of the Ayurvedic community that empowers individuals, communities and humanity to achieve health and well-being through Ayurveda (NAMA 2013), and in line with this vision statement, a list is provided by NAMA of the institutions that have training programs for professional practitioners and laypersons.

In a survey of 85 Ayurvedic practitioners in the United States (Mean Age=49 years, 72 percent Female; 58 percent white and 31 percent Asian), 94 percent had a bachelor's degree and 43 percent had a masters or doctoral degree. Only 20 percent had a bachelor of Ayurvedic medicine and surgery degree (5 ½ year degree from India). One-third received their education in India and the rest in the United States. Average length of training in Ayurveda in India was 66 months, and in the United States it ranged from one-day seminars to 30 months of training (Brar, Norman and Dasanayake 2012). Most Ayurvedic practitioners practiced part-time (2/3), had been practicing for 7 years, and had treated about 35 patients per month.

Comparison of Ayurveda and "Mainstream Practice"

Differences between Ayurveda and Western medicine are illustrated in contrasting the treatment of presenting illnesses. The focus of modern medicine is on vigorous and immediate treatment of acute symptomatology. Precision in targeting and treating presenting conditions with a narrow scope of intervention are emphasized in allopathic medicine. The impact of this philosophy and its derivative method produces a Western system of medicine that focuses on treating manifest symptomology rather than the underlying disease/cause (Gupta and Katiyar 2012). A related impact is that Western medicine has been viewed as becoming reductionistic (Patwardhan 2010).

As an *alternative* to Western medicine's emphasis on diagnostic and treatment precision, Ayurveda's philosophy and treatment modalities are integrative and holistic (Mukherjee et al. 2012). The Ayurveda therapeutic orientation is to treat the ill person as a whole, going beyond only addressing the presenting disease, similar to Traditional Chinese Medicine (see chapter 9, this volume). One of Ayurveda's most notable strengths is its capacity to systematically engage multiple aspects of the individual in treatment simultaneously, through herbal medicine, diet, and lifestyle (Ramchandani et al. 2012). Ideal health, according to Ayurveda, is achieved through balancing different dimensions of human functioning. Hence the holistic perspective is critical to treatment and diagnosis in Ayurveda. Ayurvedic practitioners address multiple facets of health, which include prevention and treatment, lifestyle-related factors such as diet and behavior, and sometimes even spiritual discourse for individual health and social functioning (Gupta and Katiyar 2012). Treatment, in the Ayurvedic tradition, is tailored to the illness presented and the individual being treated. This dual focus on both the nature of the disease and the person being treated leads to highly individualized treatment (Gupta and Katiyar 2012, Mamtani and Mamtani 2005).

A related key difference between Ayurveda and western medicine is that Ayurveda emphasizes illness prevention, health promotion, and integrating wellness techniques into daily life (Mukherjee et al. 2012, Ramchandani et al. 2012). This contrasts with modern medicine's technology and sophistication in diagnosis and treatment approach. Ayurveda promotes integrating one's mind, body, consciousness, behavior, and reality as a means of fostering optimum health and wellbeing (Mamtani and Mamtani, 2005; Sharma et al. 2007, Sharma et al. 1991). In its integrative, holistic approach to individual health, Ayurveda looks at the body, mind, and spirit as indivisible (Patwardhan 2010). Within this framework, health is not simply a state of *not* being ill or a *lack* of symptomology; instead, *health* represents the balanced states of equilibrium that exist within an individual (Sharma et al. 2007).

Illness in the Ayurvedic perspective results from an imbalance in diverse aspects of human functioning—physiological, mental, social, spiritual—and treatment should focus on restoring an individual's idiosyncratic balance (Ramchandani et al. 2012). However, prevention is considered a primary goal and homeostatic balance between mind, body, and spirit is considered as an ideal way to achieve optimal functioning and health (Sharma et al. 2007).

Specific Treatments, Evidence-Base, and Disparity

It is difficult to describe specific treatments associated with Ayurveda since it is a complex system of medicine. Treatment strategies in Ayurveda derive from its philosophical underpinning, which focuses on the whole person rather than treating a particular disease. The whole person based on Ayurvedic conceptualization includes mind, body, past and present experiences, external influences ranging from the environment and climate to interpersonal and social factors, and includes systems and interaction between systems. Based on this conceptualization, Ayurvedic intervention and prevention are highly individualized. Specific Ayurvedic practices include herbs, massage, and specialized diets (Roehm, Tessema, and Brown 2012); treatment in Ayurveda emphasizes creating and restoring balance and cleansing the body (NCCAM 2009). All aspects of treatment in Ayurveda emphasize synergizing the body's ability to heal itself and restore homeostasis (Schneider et al. 2006).

Historically, Ayurveda was passed down to future practitioners using a method known as *Parampara,* in which the student would follow a guru—master of the art—and would often integrate into the guru's family in order to acquire knowledge and experience (Mukherjee et al. 2012). These practices, though traditional, did not meet today's standard of empirically validated medicine. Recent attempts to standardize and empirically validate Ayurveda as an established practice include research involving identifying particular components of plants that create therapeutic effects on a series of medical ailments (Mukherjee et al. 2012). Similar to the United States, India has established more rigorous testing and institutions, often including policy changes, towards research with Ayurveda. Clinical trials, modern research methods such as marker analysis and chromatographic techniques, and longitudinal effects of medication have been implemented in order to promote and establish Ayurveda as a modern medical practice (Mukherjee et al. 2012). Outcomes typically observed in the scientific study of Ayurveda include the reduction of symptoms, lower medication use among patients, and reducing the iatrogenic effects of treatment including inflammation (Donepudi et al. 2012, Nader et al. 2000).

Herbal preparations in some sections of Ayurvedic medicine include the use of heavy metals, which are considered to have therapeutic properties. Recent evidence indicates that some of these heavy metals such as lead are associated with serious side effects including neurologic effects. A Boston survey indicated that one of five herbal medicinal products available in local ethnic grocery stores contained potentially harmful amounts of lead, mercury, and arsenic (Saper et al. 2004). In 2004, nine cases of lead poisoning were documented resulting from the use of Ayurvedic medicine (Centers for Disease Control and Prevention [CDC] 2004). More recent data from the CDC (2012) comes from 10 pregnant women with lead poisoning. In all 10 cases, consumption of Ayurvedic preparations was implicated. The CDC, based on these data, has recommended increased education about the components of herbal preparations and their effects on health and function.

Evidence-Base

The evidence base in Ayurveda in the United States is sparse. Part of this derives from the difficulty of translating the scientific method with its reductionistic approach and randomized clinical trials perspective to study complex holistic systems with dynamic and synergistic interactions between its components (Bell, Koithan, and Pincus 2009). Nonlinear dynamical systems models have been proposed as a viable system of analysis to accumulate an evidence-base for holistic systems of health such as Ayurveda. The fundamental principle of treatment in Ayurveda and other CAM modalities that differs from biomedical theories is that illness and disease and treatment are not a function of a cause-effect relationship. Rather, illness results from an imbalance in individuals' functioning and a re-balancing or adjustment of functioning can create an optimal environment for health and wellbeing (Bell et al. 2009). This rebalancing is done taking into account individuals' innate tendencies, upbringing, and environment. In other words, dietary adjustments would be made taking into account a person's innate constitution, upbringing (e.g., grew up vegetarian), and environment (e.g., certain foods are better eaten when the weather is hot versus when cold). The implication of taking these factors into account is that when changes in diet are consistent with other factors such as innate constitution and environment, the efficacy of the treatment is greater because of synergistic interaction among factors. Despite these difficulties, randomized control trials and double blind studies have been conducted comparing conventional treatment with Ayurvedic treatments and found Ayurvedic treatments to be equally effective as conventional treatment in treating chronic disease (Furst et al. 2011).

A related difficulty associated with assessing the use of Ayurveda and other CAM therapies stems from unwillingness on the part of practitioners to admit to using CAM therapies to their physicians. For example, half of the 40 percent of the U.S. population that uses CAM does not admit that they have used alternative remedies to their physicians (Roehm et al. 2012) making it difficult to assess use or efficacy of CAM treatments.

A recent survey of Ayurvedic practitioners in the United States indicated the variety of ailments and diseases that are treated by Ayurvedic practitioners including loss of energy (76 percent), obesity (64 percent), osteoarthritis (53 percent), peptic disorders (51 percent), diabetes (42 percent), rheumatoid arthritis (42 percent), asthma (41 percent), and other conditions (65 percent); Other maladies include diverse conditions such as migraine, insomnia, infertility, menopause-related issues, skin conditions, fibromyalgia, chronic pain, high blood pressure, elevated cholesterol, constipation and mental health issues including anxiety, depression, and stress and distress (Brar et al. 2012). Treatment modalities utilized by Ayurvedic practitioners included instructions and information for leading a healthy lifestyle (89 percent), dietary education (81 percent), herbal medication (74 percent), yoga (76 percent), and massage (57 percent) Adverse events were reported by 58 of 85 respondents; forty-eight percent indicated serious adverse effects of Ayurvedic treatment.

Chronic Ailments

Although there are specific Ayurvedic remedies that are considered appropriate for particular disease conditions, research on a key spice/herb, turmeric, used in Ayurvedic medicine, food, and cosmetics is thought to have significant healing effects on a wide variety of conditions that range from various types of cancer, metabolic conditions, Parkinson's disease, respiratory conditions, liver disorders, wound healing, etc. (Goel, Kunnumakkara, and Aggarwal 2008, Irving et al. 2011, Johnson and Mukhtar, 2007; Shishodia, Chaturvedi, and Aggarwal 2007). These diverse effects stem from multi system effects of turmeric consumption (Goel et al. 2008).

One hypothesized pathway through which turmeric and other herbal agents influence diverse chronic conditions such as cancer, cardiovascular diseases, diabetes, pulmonary diseases, neurological diseases and related chronic diseases is through their anti-inflammatory properties. Inflammation is thought to play a significant role in the etiology and morbidity of these and other chronic disease (Aggarwal et al. 2011). This hypothesis has generated research on the anti-inflammatory properties of herbs such as turmeric and a combination of herbs (e.g., turmeric and black pepper) conventionally used in food preparation. In other words, informal observations have touted the benefits of turmeric and various other spices and have even alluded to their anti-inflammatory effects. Research is now "catching up" with Grandma's conventional wisdom.

A review of the Ayurvedic medicine literature investigating Triphala, an herbal concoction of three fruits—*Terminalia chebula, Terminalia bellirica, and Phyllanthus emblica*—found it had multiple effects on a variety of conditions (Baliga et al. 2012). These authors found empirical validation for its use to protect against certain kinds of cancers in rats; Triphala was found to protect against radioactive damage to cells in chemotherapy patients, was found useful in alleviating inflammation, helps reduce cataractogenesis (cataracts in the eye), and even had therapeutic effects as a skin care agent (Baliga et al. 2012). Triphala is a mixture of three medicinal myrobalans and it is difficult to assess which component has the beneficial effect. Most studies with Triphala have used an equal ratio of its three ingredients and therefore more research should take this under consideration (Baliga et al. 2012).

Metabolic Syndrome Disorders

Cardiovascular Disorders, Diabetes, and Obesity: Ayurvedic treatments, including salacia roots, target multiple systems in the body and may be particularly effective for treating complex conditions which implicate multiple biosystems in the body such as Cardiovascular Disease, Diabetes, and Obesity. In more recent times, research has investigated causal relationships of plant based treatments and recent findings have discovered the use of Ayurvedic medicine in controlling blood pressure with Reserpine (Mukherjee et al., 2012). Data indicates that salacia roots may lead to improvement of cardiovascular health, Type II diabetes, and obesity-associated dyslipidemia and hyperglycemia among humans and in animal studies (Li, Huang, and Yamahara 2008).

In addition to Salacia root, there is a significant and growing evidence-base for the use of various aspects of Ayurvedic medicine such as exercise, cleansing of toxins from the body, meditation, yoga, and various herbal remedies in the treatment of cardiovascular disease and risk factors associated cardiovascular disease (Schneider et al. 2006). Additional benefits of Ayurvedic treatment include the reduction of psychosocial risk factors including stress, depression, anxiety, and fatigue and enhanced well-being.

Ayurveda has been successfully used for the treatment of diabetes for a long time and an early review summarizing the use of Ayurvedic treatments concluded that herbal remedies, rather than other aspects of Ayurveda, were most frequently used (Hardy et al. 2001). The methodological variability of the studies reviewed and the diverse combination of herbs used in various studies limit any scientific conclusions about the evidence base for treating diabetes with Ayurveda. Ayurvedic treatment for diabetes typically results in reductions in symptoms and medication use (Nader et al. 2000).

A review investigating research included in the Cochrane database in the treatment of type II diabetes mellitus with Ayurvedic medication found that herbal mixtures had a significant impact in lowering glucose levels (Shridharan et al. 2011). However promising these results, many studies in this review experienced limitations, including insufficient sample size and methodology, which provide an obstacle towards inferring conclusions and prevent its application in a world market (Shridharan et al. 2011).

Cancer

Ayurvedic treatment of cancer includes various conventional practices such as surgery, herbs, and dietary changes and treatments that are more specific to holistic Ayurvedic formulations such as spiritual practices, prayer, gem therapy, aroma therapy, and detoxification and rejuvenation (Aggarwal et al. 2006).

In cancer research, Ayurvedic medications have been put to the test only within approximately the last decade; only a handful has been heavily researched (Sun et al. 2013). These authors isolated a water extract fraction from a Clerodendrum viscosum (CV) root and have found that when administered on cervical cancer cells, apoptotic effects result, indicating that a readily available Ayurvedic weed may be pivotal in the fight against cervical cancer (Sun et al. 2013). In another study, researchers found that *Eugenia jambolana* extract was shown to exhibit pro-apoptotic effects on breast cancer cells, but not on normal breast cells (Li et al. 2009).

Rheumatoid Arthritis

Patients suffering from arthritis and related conditions which are chronic and can be debilitating are often dissatisfied and frustrated with conventional treatment and seek alternative therapies including Ayurvedic remedies as adjuvant treatment (Chen and Schumacher 2005). In a double blind randomized control trial comparing Ayurvedic herbal remedies with conventional allopathic treatment, Ayurvedic and conventional treatment were equally efficacious in treating the condition. Although not statistically significant, fewer adverse events were reported in the Ayurvedic treatment condition (Furst et al. 2011).

In recent research initiatives, research has empirically supported successful outcomes in treatment with the use of Ayurveda. For instance, one study using more modern methods of clinical research, compared the effects of RA-11, a plant based Ayurvedic drug commonly used in the treatment of arthritis, in individuals suffering from symptomatic osteoarthritis of the knees to a placebo over a 32-week period (Chopra et al. 2004). In terms of therapeutic effect, RA-11 was significantly greater than the placebo and although there were sizeable limitations, this pilot study posited clinically significant results beneficial to research in treatment of OA with Ayurvedic medicine (Chopra et al. 2004). A similar and more recent study, six-month controlled, of the knee in OA patients found that an Ayurvedic formulation using a variety of Ayurvedic herbs significantly impacted pain and function, increasing mobility and lowering pain levels, equating its effects to common drugs on the market for the treatment of OA (Chopra et al. 2013).

Liver Diseases

Ayurvedic herbs are effective in treatment of liver disorders (Goel et al. 2008) and in reducing the iatrogenic effects of treatment for liver disorders including inflammation and fibrosis (Donepudi et al. 2012). In particular, *Eugenia jambolana*, which has also been shown to inhibit cancer growth

(Li et al. 2009), shows potential as an antioxidant/anti-inflammatory therapy for cholestasis (Donepudi et al. 2012).

Rhinology

Almost 17 percent of the total CAM use in the United States is for the treatment of ear, nose, and throat ailments. Ayurvedic herbal remedies have also been used for rhinologic ailments as there is some evidence of its efficacy in reducing inflammation (Roehm et al. 2012).

Oral Disease

Dentistry is not a specialized branch of Ayurveda, but practitioners acknowledge the importance of oral health care in maintaining overall health (Brar et al. 2012). Common Ayurvedic treatments for oral health care, such as neem chewing sticks, mango leaves and sesame oil mouth rinses have significant preventative and curative effects (Purohit and Singh 2011). Turmeric, which has known to have multi-systemic benefits, also can be used in relieving dental pain (Chaturvedi 2009).

In Conclusion

Given the increasing prevalence of chronic diseases and difficulty in accessing modern allopathic treatment, populations in the United States are increasingly turning to complementary and alternative medicines, including the ancient holistic system of Ayurvedic medicine. Currently, Ayurveda is predominantly used in the South Asian American community as a first resort treatment for minor ailments and for reducing chronic symptoms. The holistic, balanced perspective of Ayurveda has made it difficult to develop an evidence base for treatment; nevertheless, the existing body of research has shown that many Ayurvedic treatments have multi-systemic medicinal effects. As the research base grows, Ayurvedic treatments should be promoted not just in specific ethnic communities, but also in populations facing specific ailments or limited access to care.

References

Aggarwal, B. B., H. Ichikawa, P. Garodia, P. Weerasinghe, G. Sethi, I. D. Bhatt, M. G. Nair. 2006. "From Traditional Ayurvedic Medicine to Modern Medicine: Identification of Therapeutic Targets for Suppression of Inflammation and Cancer." *Expert Opinion on Therapeutic Targets* 10(1): 87–118.

Aggarwal, B. B., S. Prasad, S. Reuter, R. Kannappan, V. R. Yadev, B. Park, and B. Sung. 2011. "Identification of Novel Anti-Inflammatory Agents from Ayurvedic

Medicine for Prevention of Chronic Diseases: 'Reverse Pharmacology' and 'Bedside to Bench' Approach." *Current Drug Targets* 12(11): 1595–1653.

Baliga, M. S., S. Meera, B. Mathai, M. P. Rai, V. Pawar, and P. L. Palatty. 2012. "Scientific Validation of the Ethnomedical Properties of the Ayurvedic Drug Triphala: A Review." *Clinical Journal of Integrative Medicine* 18(12): 946–954. doi: 10.1007/s11655-012-1299-x.

Barnes, P. M., B. Bloom, and R. Nahin. 2008. "Complementary and Alternative Medicine Use among Adults and Children: United States, 2007." *CDC National Health Statistics Report #12*. Hyattsville, MD: National Center for Health Statistics.

Bell, I. R., M. Koithan, and D. Pincus. 2009. "Methodological Implications of Nonlinear Dynamical Systems Models for Whole Systems of Complementary and Alternative Medicine." *Forsch Komplementmed* 19: 15–21. doi: 10.1159/000335183.

Brar, B. S., R. G. Norman, and A. P. Dasanayake. 2012. "Involvement of Ayurvedic Pactitioners in Oral Health Care in the United States." *Journal of the American Dental Association* 143(10): 1120–1126.

Centers for Disease Control and Prevention (CDC). 2004. "Lead Poisoning Associated with Ayurvedic Medications—Five States, 2000–2003." *Morbidity and Mortality Weekly Report* 53(26): 582–584.

Centers for Disease Control and Prevention (CDC). 2012. "Lead Poisoning in Pregnant Women Who Used Ayurvedic Medications from India—New York City." *Morbidity and Mortality Weekly Report* 61(33): 641–646.

Chaturvedi, T. P. 2009. "Uses of Turmeric in Dentistry: An Update." *Indian Journal of Dental Research* 20(1): 107–109.

Chen, L. X. and H. R. Schumacher. 2005. "West Meets East in Rheumatology." *Current Rheumatology Reports* 7(4): 251–253.

Chopra, A., P. Lavin, B. Patwardhan, and D. Chitre. 2004. "A 32-Week Randomized, Placebo-Controlled Clinical Evaluation of RA-11, an Ayurvedic Drug, on Osteoarthritis of the Knees." *Journal of Clinical Rheumatology* 10(5): 236–245.

Chopra, A., M. Saluja, G. Tillu, S. Sarmukkaddam, A. Venugopalan, G. Narsimulu, and B. Patwardhan. 2013." Ayurvedic Medicine Offers a Good Alternative to Glucosamine and Celecoxib in the Treatment of Symptomatic Knee Osteoarthrititis: A Randomized, Double-Blind, Controlled Equivalence Drug Trial." *Rheumatology.* doi: 10.1093/rheumatology/kes414.

Choudry, U. K. 1998. "Health Promotion among Immigrant Women from India Living in Canada." *Image: The Journal of Nursing Scholarship* 279: 1548–1553.

Donepudi, A. C., L. M. Aleksunes, M. V. Driscoll, N. P. Seeram, and A. L. Slitt. 2012. "The Traditional Ayurvedic Medicine, Eugenia Jambolana (Jamun Fruit), Decreases Liver Inflammation, Injury and Fibrosis During Cholestasis." *Liver International* 32(4): 560–73. doi: 10.1111/j.1478-3231.2011.02724.x.

Eisenberg, D. M., R. C. Kessler, C. Foster, F. E. Norlock, D. R. Calkins, and T. L. Delbanco. 1993. "Unconventional Medicine in the United States. Prevalence, Costs, and Patterns of Use." *The New England Journal of Medicine* 328: 246–252.

Fouladbakhsh and M. Stommel. 2010. "Gender, Symptom Experience, and Use of Complementary and Alternative Medicine Practices among Cancer Survivors in the U.S. Cancer Population." *Oncology Nurse Forum* 37(1): E7–15.

Furst, D. E., M. M. Venkatraman, M. McGann, P. R. Manohar, C. Booth-LaForce. R. Sarin, and P. R. Kumar. 2011. "Double-Blind, Randomized, Controlled, Pilot Study Comparing Classic Ayurvedic Medicine, Methotrexate, and Their Combination in Rheumatoid Arthritis." *Journal of Clinical Rheumatology* 17(4): 185–192. doi: 10.1097/RHU.0b013e31821c0310. Erratum in: *Journal of Clinical Rheumatology* 27(7): 407.

Goel, A., A. B. Kunnumakkara, and B. B. Aggarwal. 2008. "Curcumin as 'Curecumin': From Kitchen to Clinic." *Biochemical Pharmacology* 75(4): 787–809.

Gupta, A. and C. K. Katiyar. 2012. "Evaluation of Efficacy and Safety of Herbal/ Ayurvedic Medicines." In *The Modern Ayurveda: Milestones Beyond the Classical Age,* edited by C. P. Khare and C. K. Katiyar, 317–336. CRC Press: Florida. doi:10.1201/b11722-12

Hankey, A. 2001. "Ayurvedic Physiology and Etiology: Ayurvedo Amritanaam: The Doshas and Their Functioning in Terms of Contemporary Biology and Physical Chemistry." *Journal of Alternative and Contemporary Medicine* 7(5): 567–574.

Hardy, M. L., I. Coulter, S. Venuturupalli, E. A. Roth, J. Favreau, S. C. Morton, and P. Shekelle. 2001. "Ayurvedic Interventions for Diabetes Mellitus: A Systematic Review." *Evidence Report/Technology Assessment* 41.

Hilton, A. B., S. G. Grewal, N. Popatia, J. L. Bottorff, J. L. Johnson, H. Clarke, et al. 2001. "The Desi Ways: Traditional Health Practices of South Asian Women in Canada." *Health Care for Women International* 22: 553–567.

Hsiao, A., M. D. Wong, M. S. Goldstein, L. S. Becerra, E. C. Cheng, et al. 2006. "Complementary and Alternative Medicine Use among Asian-American Subgroups: Prevalence, Predictors, and Lack of Relationship to Acculturation and Access to Conventional Health Care." *Journal of Alternative and Contemporary Medicine* 12(10): 1003–1010.

Irving, G. R. B., A. Karmokar, D. P. Berry, K. Brown, and W. P. Steward. 2011. "Curcumin: The Potential for Efficacy in Gastrointestinal Diseases." *Best Practices and Research in Clinical Gastroenterology* 25(4): 519–534.

Islam, N. 2010. "Indigenous Medicine as Commodity: Local Reach of Ayurveda in Modern India." *Current Sociology* 58(5): 777–798. doi:10.1177/0011392110372739

Islam, N. 2012. "New Age Orientalism: Ayurvedic 'Wellness and Spa Culture.'" *Health Sociology Review* 21 (2): 220–231. doi:10.5172/hesr.2012.21.2.220

Johnson, J. J. and H. Mukhtar. 2007. "Curcumin for Chemoprevention of Colon Cancer." *Cancer Letters* 255(2): 170–181.

Li, L., L. S. Adams, S. Chen, C. Killian, A. Ahmed, and N. P. Seeram. 2009. "*Eugenia Jambolana Lam.* Berry Extract Inhibits Growth and Induces Apoptosis of Human Breast Cancer but Not Non-Tumorigenic Breast Cells." *Journal of Agricultural and Food Chemistry* 57: 826–831.

Li, Y., T. H. Huang, and J. Yamahara. 2008. "Salacia Root, a Unique Ayurvedic Medicine, Meets Multiple Targets in Diabetes and Obesity." *Life Sciences* 82(21–22): 1045–1049. doi: 10.1016/j.lfs.2008.03.005

Mackenzie, E.R., L.Taylor, B. S. Bloom, D. J. Hufford, and J. C. Johnson. 2003. "Ethnic Minority Use of Complementary and Alternative Medicine (CAM): A

National Probability Survey of CAM Utilizers." *Alternative Therapies in Health and Medicine* 9: 50–56.

Mamtani, R. and R. Mamtani. 2005. "Ayurveda and Yoga in Cardiovascular Diseases." *Cardiology in Review* 12(5): 155–162. doi:10.1097/01.crd.0000128730.31658.36

Manohar, P. R. 2012. "Clinical Evidence in the Tradition of Ayurveda." In *Evidence-Based Practice in Complementary and Alternative Medicine,* edited by S. Rastogi, 67–78. Berlin, Heidelberg: Springer. doi:10.1007/978-3-642-24565-7

Mehta, D. H., R. S. Phillips, R. B. Davis, and E. P. McCarthy. 2007. "Use of Complementary and Alternative Therapies by Asian Americans. Results from the National Health Interview Survey." *Journal of General Internal Medicine* 22(6): 762–767.

Misra, R., P. Balagopal, M. Klatt, and M. Geraghty. 2010. "Complementary and Alternative Medicine Use among Asian Indians in the United States: A National Study." *Journal of Alternative and Complementary Medicine* 16(8): 843–852.

Mukherjee, P. K., N. K. Nema, P. Venkatesh, and P. K. Debnath. 2012. "Changing Scenario for Promotion and Development of Ayurveda-Way Forward." *Journal of Ethnopharmacology* 143(2): 424–434. doi:10.1016/j.jep.2012.07.036

Nader, T., S. Rothenberg, R. Averbach, B. Charles, J. Z. Fields, and R. H. Schneider. 2000. "Improvements in Chronic Diseases with a Comprehensive Natural Medicine Approach: A Review and Case Series." *Behavioral Medicine* 26 (1): 34–46.

National Ayurvedic Medical Association. 2013. Schools and Programs Listing. http://ayurvedanama.org/schools-programs/

National Center for Complementary and Alternative Medicine. 2009. "Ayurvedic Medicine: An Introduction." http://nccam.nih.gov/health/ayurveda/introduction.htm

Nemer, D. 2010. "Complementary and Alternative Medicine in the United States." ImproveHealthCare.org

Park, J. J., S. Beckman-Harned, G. Cho, D. Kim, and H. Kim. 2012. "The Current Acceptance, Accessibility and Recognition of Chinese and Ayurvedic Medicine in the United States in the Public, Governmental, and Industrial Sectors" *Chin J Integr Med* 18(6): 405–408.

Patwardhan, B. 2010. "Ayurveda and Integrative Medicine: Riding a Tiger." *Journal of Ayurveda and Integrative Medicine* 1(1): 13–5. doi:10.4103/0975-9476.59820

Purohit, B. A. and Singh. 2011. "Tooth Brushing, Oil Pulling and Tissue Regeneration: A Review of Holistic Approaches to Oral Health." *Journal of Ayurveda and Integrative Medicine* 2(2): 64.

Ramchandani, M. H., M. Dousti, A. Barkhordarian, and F. Chiappelli. 2012. "Translational Effectiveness in Ayurvedic Medicine: Implications for Oral Biology and Medicine." In *Evidence-Based Practice in Complementary and Alternative Medicine,* edited by S. Rastogi, 191–207. Berlin Heidelberg: Springer. doi:10.1007/978-3-642-24565-7

Rao, D. 2006. "Choice of Medicine and Hierarchy of Resort to Different Health Alternatives among Asian Indian Migrants in a Metropolitan City in the USA." *Ethnicity and Health* 11 (2): 153–167. doi:10.1080/13557850500460306

Roehm, C. E., B. Tessema, and S. M. Brown. 2012. "The Role of Alternative Medicine in Rhinology." *Facial Plastic Surgery Clinics of North America* 20(1): 73–81. doi: 10.1016/j.fsc.2011.10.008

Saper, R. B., S. N. Kales, J. Paquin, M. J. Burns, D. M. Eisenberg, R. B. Davis, and R. S. Phillips. 2004. "Heavy Metal Content of Ayurvedic Herbal Medicine Products." *Journal of the American Medical Association* 292(23): 2868–2873.

Satow, Y. E., P. D. Kumar, A. Burke, and J. F. Inciardi. 2008. "Exploring the Prevalence of Ayurveda Use among Asian Indians." *Journal of Alternative and Complementary Medicine* 14(10): 1249–1253. doi:10.1089/acm.2008.0106

Schneider, R. H., K. G. Walton, J. W. Salerno, and S. I. Nidich. 2006. "Cardiovascular Disease Prevention and Health Promotion with the Transcendental Meditation Program and Maharishi Consciousness-Based Health Care." *Ethnicity and Disease* 16(4):15–26.

Sharma, H., H. M. Chandola, G. Singh, and G. Basisht. 2007. "Utilization of Ayurveda in Health Care: An Approach for Prevention, Health Promotion, and Treatment of Disease. Part 1—Ayurveda, the Science of Life." *Journal of Alternative and Complementary Medicine* 13(9): 1011–1019. doi:10.1089/acm.2007.7017-A

Sharma, H., H. M. Chandola, G. Singh, and G. Basisht. 2007. "Utilization of Ayurveda in Health Care: An Approach for Prevention, Health Promotion, and Treatment of Disease. Part 2—Ayurveda in Primary Health Care." *Journal of Alternative and Complementary Medicine* 13(10): 1135–1150. doi:10.1089/acm2007.7017-B.

Sharma, H. M., B. D. Triguna, and D. Chopra. 1991. "Maharishi Ayur-Veda: Modern Insights into Ancient Medicine." *JAMA: The Journal of the American Medical Association* 265 (20): 2633–2637. doi:10.1001/jama.1991.03460200009001

Shishodia, S., M. M. Chaturvedi, and B. B. Aggarwal. 2007. "Role of Curcumin in Cancer Therapy." *Current Problems in Cancer* 31(4): 243–305.

Sridharan, K., R. Mohan, S. Ramaratnam, and D. Panneerselvam. 2011. "Ayurvedic Treatments for Diabetes Mellitus." *Cochrane Database of Systematic Reviews* 7 (12): CD008288. doi: 10.1002/14651858.CD008288.pub2.

Sun, C., S. Nirmalananda, C. E. Jenkins, S. Debnath, R. Balambika, J. E. Feta, and K. S. Raja. 2013. "First Ayurvedic Approach towards Green Drugs: Anti Cervical Cancer-Cell Properties of Clerodendrum Viscosum Root Extract." *Anticancer Agents in Medicinal Chemistry.* Epub ahead of print.

Varker, K. A., A. Ansel, G. Aukerman, W. E. Carson. 2012. "Review of Complementary and Alternative Medicine and Selected Nutraceuticals: Background for a Pilot Study on Nutrigenomic Intervention in Patients with Advanced Cancer." *Alternative Therapies in Health and Medicine* 18(2): 26–34.

CHAPTER EIGHT

Native American Medicine: The Implications of History and the Embodiment of Culture

Wendy M. K. Peters, Julii M. Green, and Pilar E. Gauthier

Prior to Columbus' arrival in North America, the continent had been populated by heterogeneous groups of indigenous peoples now collectively known as American Indians (AI). Subsequently, with geographical expansion into Alaska and Hawaii, the U.S. indigenous population has grown to include Alaska Natives and Native Hawaiians as well. Yet, for those in the United States who identify as American Indian, Alaska Native (AN), or Native Hawaiian (NH), the terms do not begin to convey the multitude of culturally diverse ethnicities and identities that exist among them. Currently, there are well over 500 federally recognized tribal entities in the United States, yet there are still other groups with roots indigenous to U.S. lands that remain unrecognized or disenfranchised (Barusch and TenBarge 2003).

This chapter focuses around the threads of common experience (history, acculturation, values) shared by Native peoples and explains how the unfolding of history and the development of culture over time have become embodied within the physical health and wellbeing of these peoples. Instead of reviewing the basic tenets of Native American medicine, which has been treated in detail before (e.g., Cohen 2003, Gurung 2014), we focus more on the societal complexities that exist for Native people and how those elements have impacted the health and health behaviors of Native people. Consequently, because culture is so significant to the well-being of Native peoples, we discuss considerations for treatment of Natives, including the significance of ceremony and rituals, and examples of traditional healing practices.

Cultural and Historical Perspectives Offer Context

According to ancient lore, every Hawaiian woman is considered a literal daughter of Haumea. The feminine Hawaiian deity of earth, nature, and sustenance, it is said that Haumea is reborn in each succeeding generation of her descendants. To the Hawaiian people, the parable of Haumea's promise is more than just a simple tale that accounts for natural phenomena, for them, it is both a truth and a fact. In this regard, the ancient stories of Native peoples and the supernatural personages of which they speak are not fictitious, but rather, they are the existents that originate from their collective memories, passed from generation to generation, and are indicative of the consciousness from which they have come forth (Allen 1992, Bopp 1989, Jensen 2005, Kameeleihiwa 1999, Kunnie and Goduka 2006, Mohawk 2006). In fact, all Native peoples have mythologies respective to their stories of origin that emanate from ancient cosmologies. Contained within those mythologies are the fundamental precepts that have informed Native peoples for countless generations (Allen 1992, Campbell 1978, De Landa 1997, Harden 1999, Kunnie and Goduka 2006, Liliuokalani 2001). At their very least, cosmologies were representative of the cycles, processes, and patterns present in nature and the environment. The integration of cosmological forms was the basis for their epistemology, and ultimately, comprised Native ways of knowing and cognition.

Similarly, perception and understanding also influenced Native conceptualizations of existence. For many, if not most Native peoples, the concept of monism, an ontological philosophy that all things emanate from a single source and are thereby connected, is central to their worldview. In Canada, First Nation Metis scholar Carl Urion stated that "native knowledge is an expression of life itself, of how to live, and of the connection between all living things" (Stewart-Harawira 2005, 35). Such connections, or relationships, are a primary driver for Native people's values, beliefs, behaviors, and actions. Valuing all life as sacred, Native people believe that all relationships should be approached in a good way, or honored, especially those relationships with family, ancestors, community, and the natural environment (Abrams and Primack 2001, Allen 1992, Hay 1998). This relational, collective view, unlike the individualism espoused by Western society, is something that becomes quite significant when looking at the health and well-being experienced by Native peoples. The point being made here is that the overall health and wellbeing experienced by Native peoples is predicated upon their belief systems, their cultural values, and their propensity toward communal forms of society. This assertion is substantiated in the literature related to the health and wellness of AIs/ANs/NHs and will be further explicated in the text that follows.

Subsequently, the health and wellbeing of Native peoples, both collectively and individually, has also been affected by the course of their respective histories. The process of colonization throughout the Western hemisphere impacted Native peoples by initiating a scenario of acculturation, that today has resulted in disastrous consequences clearly evident in the current biopsychosocial outcomes of Native descendants. A glimpse into most Native communities today reveals alarming rates in health disparities as compared to the dominant, mainstream populations and a dearth of prosperity that would rival most third-world countries (Cole 2006).

Alternately, much of the established scientific and scholarly research has attributed the disproportionate number and over representation of health disparities experienced by those of Native ancestry to individual dysfunction or deficiency. However, protracted understandings of Native culture and society, coupled with the data garnered in such research, arguably evidence a phenomenon with more collective attributes that, in turn, have varying manifestations at the individual level. Indeed such societal conditions were almost non-existent prior to Western integration (Brave Heart and DeBruyn 1998). Yet at present, such conditions are more the rule than the exception.

Current Conditions in Native Health and Disparities

According to the 2010 Census briefs, 308.7 million people reside in the United States. Yet, although growing at nearly twice the rate of the general U.S. population, AIs and ANs, including those who reported combination with another race, account for approximately 5.2 million, a mere 1.7 percent, of the total U.S. population (Humes, Jones, and Ramirez 2011). Native Hawaiians and other Pacific Islanders presented even smaller in numbers, being approximately 1.2 million, or .4 percent, of the total U.S. population. Due to being so few in number, there is a lack of accurate epidemiological data that undermines the general visibility and severity of Native public health issues. Furthermore, there is a severe paucity in statistically significant outcome studies for native populations (Gone and Trimble 2012, IHS 2013; Satcher 2001). Similarly, no large-scale outcome studies, and only a few evidence-based programs regarding mental health disorders among AI/ANs, have been documented or adapted for treating AI or AN populations (Satcher 2001, Suicide Prevention Resource Center 2005). What is known, and can be asserted about Native people's health, is that they are greatly over represented in issues related to: a) alcohol and substance abuse, b) mental health disorders, c) suicide, and d) violence (Campbell and Evans-Campbell 2011, Gone and Trimble 2012, IHS 2011, Kawamoto 2001).

Alcohol abuse has long plagued Native communities and AI/ANs are five times more likely to die due to alcohol-related incidents than Whites (IHS 2011). Another study demonstrated that the alcohol induced death rate for AI/ANs, aged 15–24, was 133 percent higher than their non-Native counterparts (Whitbeck et al. 2004b). Additionally, despite rates of alcohol use among AI/AN adults (43.9 percent) being lower than national averages (55.2 percent), AI/AN adults who reported drinking behaviors, reported that at least 11.2 percent of the time they binge drank or drank to excess as compared to 7.9 percent of non-Native adults who reported similar drinking behaviors. As a consequence, Natives also reported the need for alcohol-related treatment twice as often as non-Native adults (Office of the Surgeon General [U.S.], Center for Mental Health Services [U.S.], National Institute Mental Health [U.S.], 2001). Drug abuse rates, especially methamphetamine and prescription drugs, are comparable to alcohol rates with AI/ANs exhibiting the highest use percentages across all races. According to the Indian Health Service (IHS), AI/AN drug abuse issues threaten to surpass alcohol-related problems in the near future (2011).

David Satcher (2001) cited a 1988 community-based epidemiological report in which 70 percent of a sample of respondents (N=131) from a small Northwest Coast village reported experiencing a mental health disorder in their lifetime. A 20-year follow-up study of those respondents, found that 30 percent continued to experience a clinically diagnosable disorder highlighting the prolonged existence of mental health issues for Native individuals (Satcher 2001). Research has also indicated that 13 percent of AI/ANs experienced mental health issues as compared to 9 percent of the general population (Gone and Trimble 2012, IHS 2011, Kawamoto 2001, Radin et al. 2012, Satcher 2001). Unfortunately, AI/ANs also tend to have significantly higher dropout rates from therapy than all other ethnic groups and are far less likely to respond to therapeutic interventions (Sue, 1977). More recently, however, research has shown that AI/ANs would access mental health care if it were readily available and culturally appropriate (Gone and Trimble 2012, IHS 2011, Kawamoto 2001, Radin et al. 2012, Satcher 2001). Some of the barriers preventing AI/ANs from accessing mental health services include: a) limited funding, b) fewer mental health professionals in service areas, c) social stigma, d) poverty, and e) the lack of culturally sensitive programs or intervention delivery (IHS 2011, Manson 2000).

According to the Suicide Prevention Resource Center (2005), AI/ANs suffer from the highest number of suicide deaths across all demographic groups. Yet, risk factors such as mental health disorders, abuse of alcohol or other substances, previous attempts, and life stressors are similar to that of any other population (Alcántara and Gone 2007, Wexler, Silveira, and Bertone-Johnson 2012). Distressingly, in 2009, suicide was the leading cause of death among Alaska Natives, aged 15–24, and the eighth leading cause of death for the entire AI/AN population (Wexler, Silveira, and Bertone-Johnson 2012). Suicide rates for AI/AN males, aged 15–24, are two and a half times higher than males of similar age in the U.S. general population. Comparatively, suicide rates among AN males, aged 15–24, are eight times higher than that of similar aged White males in the United States. Interestingly, when AI/AN socio-cultural values are factored into the mix, the risks of suicide diverge. For example, AI/AN tribes with less traditional values (i.e., high emphasis on individual versus community) and more socio-economic advantage, experience higher suicide rates than other tribes (Alcántara and Gone 2007, Wexler, Silveira, and Bertone-Johnson 2012). Yet, there are also a number of Tribal nations that report no suicides on an annual basis. Nonetheless, suicide rates in Indian Country have been relatively consistent for the last 25 years, a fact that has since sparked serious action among the IHS, along with other Native health serving organizations, to publish on-going strategies to help address this distressing issue (Gone and Trimble 2012, IHS, n.d.).

Native women also find themselves as victims of violence and other abhorrent life conditions far too often. Research also supports the idea that violence against Native women is directly connected to historical victimization as the balance of power between genders had been relatively equal prior to Western assimilation and colonization (Allen 1992, Brave Heart and DeBruyn 1998, Burbar and Thurman 2004, LaRocque 1994, 75, Malcoe and Duran 2004, McEachern, Van Winkle, and Steiner 1998). Consequently, Native victims of domestic violence are more likely than victims of all other races to be injured and need hospital care. Medical costs related to treatment of Native women abuse victims was more than $21 million over a four-year period in North Dakota alone (U.S. Department of Justice as cited in North Dakota Council on Abused Women's Services 2007). Furthermore, the hegemony and oppression of Native peoples increased both economic dependency and deprivation through the devaluation of tribal rights and sovereignty. Native peoples today are, therefore, even more susceptible to internalized oppression and victimization (Burbar and Thurman 2004).

Subsequently, Native women have had to contend with pressure from Native men who dominate through sexism and other behaviors that stem from the U.S. majority culture. In a cross-sectional study that examined the impact of domestic violence on Northern Plains and Upper Midwest mother and daughter relationships, it was found that a majority of the participants had relatives involved with boarding school experiences and other historical losses (Green 2012). Additionally, the Native mother-daughter relationships appeared to be impacted by domestic violence, especially when the participants had used substances during domestic violence incidences (Green 2012). Yet, while the outcomes of that particular study should be regarded with caution due to a small sample size (N=60), it should also be noted that similar findings related to substance use and domestic violence have also been found in larger scaled studies focused on Native peoples (Duran et al. 2009, U.S. Department of Justice 2008).

Increased complexity in diagnosis and treatment also arises with co-morbidity of issues, often complicating treatment and interventions. Focused on the connection between mental health disorders, alcohol, and substance abuse, a study with members of a Southwestern tribe (N=582) found that binge drinking was associated with multiple psychiatric disorders in both males and females (Robin et al. 1998). Consistent with findings from other AI/AN population studies, 95 percent of the respondents who fell into the "binge-drinker" category (46 percent of the total sample) were also alcohol dependent (Robin et al. 1998). Furthermore, binge drinkers were found to have significant problems, physically and socially, as well as in relation to work, violence, and lawlessness. Alcohol use related to suicide was higher in AI/AN populations than all other racial and ethnic groups (Olson and Wahab 2006).

Historical and Intergenerational Trauma

Recently, a phenomenon called Historical Trauma or Intergenerational Trauma (HT/IT) has emerged to become one of the most dominant narratives throughout Indian Country (Walters et al. 2011). Asserted as the etiological agent underpinning the widespread distress and impoverished life conditions in which many Native communities and individuals subsist today, HT/IT is typically denoted by the multitude of disparities and the decline in issues of health and well-being among the populace, economic inequity in relation to most other ethnic groups, and marginalization in matters pertaining to civil, social, and political affairs. However, the aforementioned characteristics are but symptoms that evidence a far greater, interrelated condition long recognized by indigenous elders as a wounding of the soul, a phenomenon so pervasive that it has been passed down through multiple generations and it has been shown to impact entire societies (Brave Heart 2003, Brave Heart-Jordan 1995, Brave Heart and DeBruyn 1998, Duran and Duran 1995, Duran 2006, Duran, Firehammer, and Gonzalez 2008).

Further, while some consider HT/IT a major etiological agent in relation to the social determinants of health and well-being among Native populations, others view it as an outcome of societal oppression and marginalization. Regardless of etiology or outcome, the symptoms of HT/IT continue to be diagnosed as individual pathologies and, as such, render current interventions insufficient or inappropriate to address the scope of complexity it represents. This widespread misunderstanding of pathology, as it relates to Native peoples, engenders and perpetuates misperceptions about them as a whole. In contrast, it should be stated that HT/IT does not preclude all other pathological occurrences of various health or mental health issues among the Native populace but HT/IT does go a long way in accounting for the considerable over representation of health disparities that persists among them.

Additionally, healing and mental wellness in Indian Country is impeded by other barriers such as inconsistent cultural competence of mainstream mental health professionals and limited numbers of Native mental health professionals. (Brave Heart 2013, Manson 2000). As a result, the wellbeing of Native people continues to decline and indicators of social dysfunction such as pandemic chronic health conditions, alcohol abuse (including binge drinking), illicit substance use, school dropout rates, and death rates from suicide, persist and even increase (Barnes, Adams, and Powell-Griner 2010). Too often marginalized by mainstream society and relegated to some of the most remote and isolated geographical areas, the life conditions for Native peoples across the United States continue to deteriorate, while the handful of organizations oriented to render aid and services (e.g. IHS) struggle to do what is possible in the face of ever dwindling funds, resources, and manpower.

Embodiment of Societal Complexity

Having asserted that the symptoms manifested by HT/IT are not necessarily or typically individual pathologies, it bears some explanation as to how entire societies can be impacted by historical events. Consequently, because so many of the issues related to HT/IT have their origins at the time of initial contact with Western culture and integration, a retracing of historical events is also warranted. A synopsis of history postulating the chronology from societal breakdown through recent scientific breakthroughs makes a case that supports the phenomenon that is HT/IT and how it has impacted the Native populace. Moreover, use of the term *embodiment* as it relates to culture and society is also discussed.

The U.S. vision of *Manifest Destiny* (Gura 1999), a quest for imperialism originating in the 1800s, was the primary impetus underlying the annexation of many Western lands and territories now possessed by the United States, including Hawaii. Based on the notion that the United States was destined to expand its democratic institutions and, as such, had a superior moral right to govern despite others' interests to the contrary, the Americans followed the lead of their European predecessors and forged into the West, seizing occupied lands and assimilating its native peoples, even by force where necessary. The ideals ascribed to Manifest Destiny were perpetrated on North America's First Peoples in a plethora of hegemonic actions such as forced assimilation and the outlaw and abolition of traditional and cultural practices, all of which devastated their longstanding social structures. The homelands, languages, and sovereignty of Native peoples were intentional targets of eradication in an effort to nullify Native culture (Lyons and Mohawk 1998, Niezen 2000, Poupart 2002, Wells 1994).

Lamentably, well-established cultural structures and mores were disregarded when early settlers who made first contact with the Natives operated under the assumption that Native people shared the same values and social structure (Campbell and Evans-Campbell 2011, Wasson 1973). White males subsequently assumed dominance, while Native females forfeited all rights, heritability to leadership, and were forcibly moved into passive roles of servitude (Wasson 1973). Additionally, the near genocide of the traditional family systems espoused by Native peoples brought about a loss of purpose to members within those familial compositions (Alfred 2005, Baldridge 2001, Campbell and Evans-Campbell 2011, Ross 2006). The communal, family-centric systems that had permitted Native peoples to thrive and sustain themselves within their natural environments ceased to function and were supplanted with Western approaches to *proper* child-rearing, *civilized* culture, and Christian missionary teachings (Marshall III 2005, Ross 2006, Wasson 1973).

The usurpation of cultural practice, traditional values, and family structures soon gave way to the forced removal of children from their families throughout the early 1800s to mid-1900s (Baldridge 2001, Barusch and TenBarge 2003, Szasz 2003). Native children were literally roped and dragged, like cattle, to Christian boarding schools and missions (Unger 1977). Many Native children were subjugated to foreign methods of teaching, language, and concepts (Barusch and TenBarge 2003). Seldom permitted contact with their families, thousands of Native children died under horrifying conditions that spawned physical illness, brutality, and heartbreak (Baldridge 2001, Cross, Day, and Byers, 2010, Unger 1977).

With the loss of their children, the cycle of imperialism was ensconced. Weeping mothers and grandmothers were left without purpose. The fear, hopelessness, and helplessness among the men, once warriors and protectors, rendered them powerless against the sheer numbers and weaponry of the U.S. government (Alfred 2005, Ross 2006, White, Godfrey, and Iron Moccasin 2006). The intergenerational family system that had once fostered relationships and cultivated sustainability had suffered a trauma of such magnitude that it wounded Native peoples to the depth of their souls, broke their Spirits, and annihilated their respective Indigenous nations (Duran 2006).

Among the first to identify this widespread phenomenon among Native peoples were Eduardo and Bonnie Duran (1995, 2006), who called it a *soul wound,* maintaining the vernacular expressed by Native Elders. Considered by Native Elders as "spiritual injury, soul sickness, soul wounding, and ancestral hurt" (Duran 2006, 15), Eduardo Duran (1995) initially characterized the native soul wound as:

> A common thread. . . that weaves across much of the pain and suffering found in the Native American community across the United States and perhaps the entire Western Hemisphere. (24)

Maria Yellow Horse Brave Heart (1995, 2003) was another such pioneer in recognizing the collective pain that was prevalent among Native peoples. Her research on Intergenerational Trauma, a phenomenon first noted in studies among Jewish holocaust survivors and their descendants, postulated that the Lakota people also suffered from widespread impaired grief as a result of cumulative massive group trauma associated with cataclysmic events. Furthermore, while similarities have been asserted between the two population groups, a pertinent fact remains clear in that, unlike the Holocaust experience, an event of a single catastrophic period, the traumatic events experienced by Native North American peoples have endured for nearly 400 years in epidemic proportions (Duran and Duran 1995, Duran 2006, Whitbeck et al. 2004a).

Brave Heart's research was ground-breaking in that it dispelled what had previously been attributed to cultural deficit in the abilities, achievements, and attitudes of Native peoples. Evidencing something far more complex, Brave Heart's work transformed how the mental health of Native people could now be contextualized, thus, positioning this long-standing systemic issue at the forefront of discourse and policy in mental health.

Subsequently, Brave Heart (1995, 2003), in collaboration with Lemyra DeBruyn (1998), asserted that unresolved grief and its associated attendants are intergenerational in nature. Specifically, the symptoms and effects of trauma extended beyond direct, individual experience. Additionally, the symptoms and effects of these widespread traumatic experiences were not only pervasive, but also persistent and would continue to pass from one generation to the next. Studies have also shown that HT/IT is persistent until, and unless, it is acknowledged and resolved in an appropriate manner (Brave Heart, 2003), specifically, one conducive to Native culture, beliefs, and values.

Another aspect in the aftermath of colonization was its adverse implications regarding gender. Western emphasis on patriarchy and views of masculinity served to disrupt the traditional and cultural roles of Native men and women, which in turn resulted in very different experiences of acculturation for both genders (Brave Heart 1999, Brave Heart and DeBruyn 1998, Collins and Mcnair 2002, Dodgson and Struthers 2005, Dressler, Bindon, and Gilliland 1996, Monopoli, and Alworth 2000, Sullivan and Brems 1997, Widmer 2010). Because so much had been lost and devastated by colonization, many of the traditional Native societal structures were supplanted with those of Western society and culture. Patriarchal subservience of women and single family households (as opposed to multi-generational) are common examples of difference that were not common to most Native cultures (Allen 1992).

Scientific evidence also supports and affirms the phenomenon of HT/IT through the biological processes of epigenetics. Defined as heritable changes in gene expression caused by functionally relevant modifications to the genome that do not involve altering the underlying DNA sequence, epigenetics show that these mechanisms can enable the effects of parents' experiences to be passed down to subsequent generations and may also last for multiple generations (Brave Heart and DeBruyn 1998, Hunter 2008). Similarly, social scientists account for HT/IT through the transference of memes, or cultural items transmitted by repetition in a manner analogous to the biological transmission of genes (Dawkins 1976). Memetics, the study of memes, as well as epigenetics, offer strong support in explaining how cultural elements such as trauma, have been passed on from generation to generation (Peters 2011, Walters et al. 2011). Further, the theory of Spiral Dynamics Integral, asserts that a particular set of values or an entire belief system may also be passed on through memetic transmission (Beck 2006). Propagated and transmitted across the ecologies of the mind, the memes and epigenetic character of their ancestors are still present within Native peoples (Peters 2011). Despite the physiological changes that may have taken place with interracial mixing or cultural assimilation, the societal complexity experienced by Native peoples throughout their respective histories are literally embodied within their descendants (Peters 2011, Walters et al. 2011).

From Breakdown to Breakthrough

Despite everything that Native peoples have been subject to and endured since the time of first Western contact and integration, they are finally beginning to make inroads toward sustainable change and transformation in their communities. What began as a revival of culture, with the few Natives courageous enough to challenge the dominance of the status quo, became a cultural renaissance circa 1960s. Spurred by their struggle to survive and to preserve their distinct cultures and traditions amidst global change, the few soon became many, and the revival became a movement of socially interested activists rather than passive bystanders (Smith 1999). Over that time, a generation has matured and the resistance continues still.

Having again shifted in form, an ever growing number of Native voices are now making themselves heard. These are the children of the 1960s who have grown up learning to walk in both worlds. They have created and fortified the bridges of social change that will finally allow healing to occur. These Native voices have reached across the cultural divides to educate and inform their own and non-Native peoples through writing and speaking about indigenous ways of knowing, feminine knowing, healing traditions, and, of course, the many ramifications of HT/IT, the indigenous soul wound. The same Native voices, although not all scholars, are in turn conferring their experience upon Native youth. Unlike prior Western characterizations of Native peoples, these voices offer first person perspectives as perceived through an authentic Native worldview (Bastien 1999, 2003, Bin-Sallik 2000, Edwards 2002, Jacobs 2008, Kunnie and Goduka 2006, Smith 1999).

Western Academic Institutions have also become important tools for the revitalization of culturally relevant Native healing and treatment methods. Prior to Western contact, those who rendered care when needed were community Elders, or experts in the healing arts. However, the hegemony imposed in the course of colonization and assimilation completely overturned the ways in which knowledge was transmitted, resulting in the disruption of the traditional systems and methods that were far more congruent with Native worldviews and belief systems. Fortunately, Indigenous methods of scholarship have become key resources in the revitalization of some forms of knowledge. Moreover, Elders in many Native communities have also begun to tell their stories and share the teachings passed to them by their Elders. The Native lifecycles of yesteryear are being revitalized to usher in yet another generation.

Cultural Considerations for Healing and Wellness

Retraditionalization is about the return to traditional cultural forms (Arndt 2004, Edwards 2002, Hermes 2001, Menzies 2005). Unlike efforts of activism, used as a means of political protest, retraditionalization is about healing. It is a form of healing that endeavors to replace, reconstruct, and re-acculturate things long ago lost or harmed at the time of the original trauma. Consequently, to be most effective, the theoretical perspectives applicable to the assessment, diagnosis, and mental health treatment of Native people in the therapeutic setting should also incorporate notions of retraditionalization. To the dismay of many Native people, however, systems of care in most Native communities remain predominantly conventional.

In terms of mental health care as it relates to Native peoples, Western methods of counseling and therapy still hold sway over practice and theory. Behavioral health care delivery, as well as training programs, tends to be dissimilar from traditional Native methods of healing and potentially results in another form of colonization (McCabe 2007). Furthermore, history and hegemony have also propagated suspicion, mistrust, and even hostility in regard to Non-native health practitioners (Heinrich, Corbine, and Thomas [1990] 2011, King 1999). An individual's levels of acculturation, from traditional to fully assimilated, should also be considered in the assessment, diagnosis, and treatment of Native people (Trimble 2005).

Native culture and societies can often be distinguished by their value systems which, in many respects, have been found to be in direct contrast to those of Western society (Heinrich, Corbine, and Thomas, [1990] 2011). Examples of such juxtapositions in values are: subjugation of nature versus harmony with nature, focus on the future and progress versus focus on the present and traditions, competition versus conscious submission of self for the welfare of others, and verbal expression versus keeping to oneself. Additionally, Native value systems are deeply rooted in spirituality. Consequently, despite constant attempts by well-intentioned Christians or unconscionable politicians, Native people have been unwavering in their resistance to forsake their spiritual foundations, more so than any other minority group (Herring 1990, McCabe 2007). Likewise, situations where spiritual conversion appears to have taken hold may not be as straightforward as it would seem. Upon close examination, vestiges of Native values and spiritual foundations can still be found. Syncretism, or the blending of belief systems, is something so commonplace among Native peoples that it is rarely recognized as being anything out of the ordinary. From a Native person's perspective, or from the inside looking outward, syncretism was, arguably, a way to reconcile the incongruence and incompatibility of imposed values and foreign beliefs.

The Native person's view of health and healing is an extension of their influential value system and has been generalized across Native communities as embedded within oral histories (Garrett and Herring 2001). However, the concepts of balance and harmony, each stemming from monistic philosophy, are fairly widespread values among Native people. In general, believing that each individual is responsible for maintaining his/her own harmony with the universe, illness might often be regarded as a consequence of being out of balance (Garrett and Herring 2001, Heinrich, Corbine, and Thomas 1990). For example, diabetes, a Western derived disease, must be properly healed by using the total system of cause; that is, one must adhere to both western and traditional treatments, the first as the source of the problem and the latter as the power of the mind and body (Garrett and Herring 2001). In contrast, it could be interpreted that Native elders often minimize their need for Western health services due to secular barriers or access to care; however, their aversion to care may well be attributed to their value of harmony, self-help, and universal balance (Jervis, Jackson, and Manson 2002).

Miscommunication due to cultural difference is also a common problem experienced between Native people and Non-native practitioners. Behaviors and processes that are not necessarily traditional or cultural but, rather, are those that are intuitive, instinctive, enacted subconsciously and even unconsciously occur as often, if not more, than verbal exchanges. In fact, the use of silence produces optimal learning through observation and modeling methods among traditional teaching standards (Garrett and Herring 2001). Thus, actions and behaviors such as knowing when to speak or not, when to listen or follow, even when and how to make eye contact, are the types of inconspicuous, unspoken cues that permeate all communications. However, it is the fluency with which these cues are applied that typically highlights cultural difference. Further, these types of social protocols are seldom taught. Instead, they are the cues and subtleties that imbue culture and ethnicity with distinction and are acquired mainly through lived experience.

The lack of culturally competent communication styles are also a huge issue for Native people in mainstream healthcare settings. Many Natives, particularly Elders and their family members, perceive cultural incompetence as insensitivity and even disrespect (Jervis, Jackson, and Manson 2002). Although largely dependent on their degree of acculturation, many Native Elders often retain their native language and may speak little to no English and this is just one more salient barrier that impacts access and quality of care and services for Native people (John, Kerby, and Hennessy 2003).

While trends in Native communities have shifted toward more culturally informed alternatives, initiatives based on aspects of retraditionalization are those that have shown the greatest promise for healing, wellness, and transformative change for Native peoples (Bell and Lim 2005, Brave Heart Society 2006, Edwards 2002, Ole-Henrik 2005, Pihama, Cram, and Walker 2002, Ridenour-Wildman 2004, Short 1999, Smylie, Williams, and Cooper 2006). Likewise, cultural adaptation or enhancement of various instruments, diagnostic tools, and even therapeutic interventions are also especially important because they help to decolonize those practices based solely on Western methodologies (Lucero 2011) and encourage congruence with Native cultural experience and traditions (Morgan 2006).

Implementation of community-based, grassroots initiatives, founded upon traditional values, orientations, and principles have begun to yield some positive results. The Brave Heart Society, an initiatory youth program; White Bison and Journey to Forgiveness, both are community wellbriety programs; Dakota Fathering, an initiative offering a number of different life skills training programs; and Dakota 38, a video campaign to promote healing in Native individuals and communities, are all culture-based interventions that have made positive inroads through the implementation of culturally relevant models (Brave Heart Society 2006, Coyhis and Farley 2011, Dana 2000, White Bison, Inc. 2002). While not an exhaustive listing of culturally based programs, there are most assuredly more equally worthwhile programs, with more in development and yet to be implemented, but much more work remains to be done.

Cultural Practice: Healing Traditions, Ceremony, and Rituals

Healing traditions, along with cultural ceremonies and rituals are the domain of the sacred, and as such must be approached with great respect and caution as to what may be disclosed. Moreover, there are a few clarifications that should be made at the outset. Much about Native healing and traditions has been misconstrued since the time of first Western contact. One major reason for this is because much of what has been experienced by, or exposed to non-Natives or outsiders to a particular culture, was perceived through a different lens. Consequently, differing value and belief systems effectively develop different worldviews, and thus, cognitive perceptions and interpretations will vary. As such, much of what has been chronicled in Western literature to date has the potential for misinformation and inaccuracies because it lacks the credibility of interpretation from a bona fide Native worldview, despite the scientific rigor or objectivity it may carry. Therefore, what follows is a commentary regarding prevalent cultural forms that are fairly well known outside Native circles and that are still observed and practiced throughout Native communities today.

Medicine men are one of the prominent icons and a typical example of the patriarchal values and views introduced with Western integration. For thousands of years, medicine people, more popularly called shaman, have served as healers, counselors, advisors, and community leaders (Topper 1987). Both men and women may be gifted with the power to heal. Gender, however, is mostly determined by tribal protocols and traditions. What is common among those of the vocation is the spiritual predisposition from which their healing prowess is derived. Though usually not chieftain or matriarch, Medicine people are greatly revered by the tribe and its elders for their acquisition of ritual knowledge and skill and because it is considered a sacred responsibility (Topper 1987).

Usually well known to their communities, Medicine people may be called upon to treat anything from the common cold, to relationship issues, to exorcisms. They also do not simply opt to become medicine people or acquire their training through conventional means. The role of Medicine person is usually conferred and sanctioned by community elders or is a vocation transmitted through family heritage. Frequently, Medicine people will have an inherent propensity toward the spiritual and tend to hone and develop their abilities and wisdom throughout their lifetime (Topper 1987, Topper and Schoepfle 1990). Reiterating that Native people believe they are responsible for maintaining harmony with the universe through physical, mental, and spiritual balance, and because they regard illness as imbalance, the Medicine person's role is really to facilitate in the restoration of the patient's physical, mental, or spiritual balance (Garrett and Herring 2001, Heinrich, Corbine, and Thomas 1990, Topper 1987).

Healing, however, generally falls into two categories. The first would be things of a physiological nature such as injury or illness. The second type of healing would be for things of a more spiritual nature. Maladies in this category are what may be considered psychological or behavioral by contemporary standards. While the same Medicine person would be called upon to treat conditions of either category, the manner of treatment may vary widely. Suffice it to say, Medicine people may also specialize in particular styles or utilize specific methods of healing such as with herbs, tinctures, or poultices, while others may simply pray, recite incantations, converse with spirits, or possibly even travel to other realms of consciousness to obtain a healing remedy. The key for every healer is the capacity for spiritual guidance, a necessary component of the healing process and especially effective when the ill, injured, or troubled person is open to the remedy posed by the healer (Harris 1998, King 1999, McCabe 2007). Some Medicine people have even been known to treat cancer and other serious illnesses successfully (Topper 1987, Topper and Schoepfle 1990).

Ceremonies and rituals, some quite ancient, provide a means for physical and spiritual interconnectedness with community and environment. They also offer the opportunity for healing and reconciliation with Sprit, of self, and with others (McCabe 2007). Of course each ceremony or ritual has a specific purpose, and there are far too many to list. Fundamentally, however, ceremonies and rituals are all about spiritual communion in one way or another. There are ceremonies for the sick, for the newborn, for coming of age, or being a woman. There are naming ceremonies, and seasonal ceremonies, and rituals for fishing, hunting, planting, and harvesting. There are vision quests for those in search of their own messages from the Creator. All are considered momentous occasions and not undertaken lightly. Yet, there are as many ceremonies and rituals as there are tribes, cultures, and languages, and they all have one thing in common. Ceremony and ritual is the framework of Native culture and lends structure to everyday life.

Sweat lodges are a type of ceremony that have garnered much debate in recent years and been popularized with non-Natives through New Age practices. An ancient tradition, sweats are primarily used for physical detoxification (much like a European sauna) and spiritual purification. Sweat lodges are usually a low rounded framework constructed of branches and covered by burlap or blankets or canvas. There is a small fire pit in the center of the lodge for the placement of heated stones that generate steam when water is poured over them or smoke when different herbs are added. Most sweats are presided over by a Medicine person while those in attendance generally take part in songs, prayers, and sometimes discussions.

Smudging with herbs is also a ritual that has gained popularity beyond Native culture and communities. Smudging is accomplished by burning dried herbs down to smoldering embers, then fanning the smoke (usually with a feather or feather wand) toward the object of the ritual (usually a person or thing) or toward a certain space or area. Although the different herbs and plants used for smudging have different spiritual properties, smudging is primarily done to cleanse or bless the object being smudged.

Consequently, an entire book, if not several of them, could be written about the various rituals and ceremonies practiced and observed by native peoples (e.g, Cohen 2003). However, it should be again reiterated that ceremonies and rituals are the domain of the sacred, and as such must be approached with great respect and caution as to what may be disclosed. On this note it should also be said that even the traditional names of practices, ceremonies, and rituals have intentionally been omitted due to the sensitivity that many Native people may have in regard to the sharing of their sacred traditions.

As a final note relating to Native healing traditions, research has highlighted the need for traditional healing in conjunction with biomedical treatment (Shore, Shore, and Manson 2009). Furthermore, culturally adapted psychotherapy has also been reported as more effective in the treatment of ethnic and racial minorities (Griner and Smith 2006). As a consequence, although still few and far between, culturally-based healing modalities considered as complementary and alternative are now being utilized in conjunction with conventional treatment and it's making a difference (Park 2013). Primarily being implemented by Native serving health organizations, it is still too soon to say how much of a difference the culturally appropriate models for care and delivery of care will have on health outcomes for Native people.

Conclusion

Every culture holds a particular worldview that is comprised of the established patterns, protocols, and values that make them unique to a society. Considering the varying degrees of enculturation and acculturation that Native people have encountered, this chapter was about providing a cultural context for the complex myriad of biopsychosocial disparities that have become commonplace for most Native people and their communities. In summary, this chapter is about affirming the identity of Native peoples and the validity their values hold for them. It is also hoped that this explanation will inform Natives and non-natives alike of the history and rationale behind the suffering that so rampantly abounds in the children, homes, and communities of Natives. As new times have spawned new ways of thinking and scientific evidence is yielding fresh knowledge and theory, emancipatory initiatives are, at long last, advancing Native interests.

References

Abrams, N. E. and J. R. Primack. 2001. "Cosmology and 21st-Century Culture." *Science* 293(5536): 1769–1770. http://proquest.umi.com/?did=80827478 andsid=2andFmt=4andclientId=45836andRQT=309andVName=PQD

Alcántara, C. and J. P. Gone. 2007. "Reviewing Suicide in Native American Communities: Situating Risk and Protective Factors within a Transactional-Ecological Framework." *Death Studies* 31(5): 457–477. doi:10.1080/07481180701244587

Alfred, G. R. 2005. *Wasáse: Indigenous Pathways of Action and Freedom.* Peterborough, ON: Broadview Press.

Allen, P. 1992. *The Sacred Hoop: Recovering the Feminine in American Indian Traditions* (with a New Preface). Boston: Beacon Press.

Arndt, L. M. R. 2004. "Soul Wound, Warrior Spirit: Exploring the Vocational Choice of American Indian Law Enforcement Officers Working for Non-Tribal Agencies." Doctoral dissertation, University of Wisconsin, Madison, Wisconsin. ProQuest Dissertations and Theses, http://search.proquest.com/docview/305113196?accountid=25304

Bachman, R., H. Zaykowski, R. Kallmyer, M. Poteyeva, and C. Lanier. U.S. Department of Justice, Office of Justice Programs. 2008. *Violence against American Indian and Alaska Native women and the criminal justice response: What is known* (NCJ 223691). Retrieved from National Institute of Justice website: https://www.ncjrs.gov/pdffiles1/nij/grants/223691.pdf

Baldridge, D. 2001. "Indian Elders: Family Traditions in Crisis." *American Behavioral Scientist* 44(9):1515–1527. doi:10.1177/00027640121956953

Barnes, P. M., P. F. Adams, and E. Powell-Griner. National Center for Health Statistics, National Health Statistics Reports. 2010. *Health characteristics of the American Indian or Alaska native adult population: United states, 2004–2008* (no. 20). Retrieved from Centers for Disease Control and Prevention website: http://www.cdc.gov/nchs/data/nhsr/nhsr020.pdf

Barusch, A. and C, TenBarge. 2003. "Indigenous Elders in Rural America." *Journal of Gerontological Social Work* 41(1–2): 121–136. doi:10.1300/J083v41n01_07

Bastien, B. J. 1999. *Blackfoot ways of knowing: Indigenous science.* (Order No. 9955003, California Institute of Integral Studies). *ProQuest Dissertations and Theses*, 200-200. http://search.proquest.com/docview/304548503?accountid=40810. (304548503).

Beck, D. 2006. *Spiral Dynamics: Mastering Values, Leadership and Change : Exploring the New Science of Memetics.* Oxford: Blackwell.

Bell, J. and N. Lim. 2005. "Young Once, Indian Forever: Youth Gangs in Indian Country." *American Indian Quarterly* 29(3): 626–650, 744–745. Retrieved from http://proquest.umi.com/?did=986382131andsid=2andFmt=3andclientId=45836andRQT=309andVName=PQD

Bin-Sallik, M. 2000. *Aboriginal Women by Degrees : Their Stories of the Journey towards Academic Achievement.* St. Lucia Qld., Australia; Portland, OR.: University of Queensland Press; Distributed in the USA and Canada by International Specialized Book Services.

Bopp, J. 1989. *The Sacred Tree* (3rd ed.). Wilmot WI: Lotus Light.

Brave Heart, M. Y. H. 1999. "Gender Differences in the Historical Trauma Response among the Lakota." *Journal of Health and Social Policy* 10(4): 1–21. doi: 10.1300/J045v10n04_01

Brave Heart, M. Y. H. 2003. "The Historical Trauma Response among Natives and Its Relationship with Substance Abuse: A Lakota Illustration." *Journal of Psychoactive Drugs* 35(1): 7–13. http://proquest.umi.com/?did=338232111andFmt=3andclientId=45836andRQT=309andVName=PQD

Brave Heart, M. Y. H. 2013. "Incorporating Historical Trauma Informed Interventions with Evidence Based Practice." Unpublished manuscript.

Brave Heart, M. Y. H. and L. M. DeBruyn. 1998. "The American Indian Holocaust: Healing Historical Unresolved Grief." *American Indian and Alaska Native Mental Health Research* 8(2): 56–80. http://proquest.umi.com/?did=36164473andFmt =3andclientId=45836andRQT=309andVName=PQD

Brave Heart Society. 2006. *Cante Ohitika Okodakiciye* [Brave Heart Society Winter Count]. Lake Andes, SD: Author.

Brave Heart-Jordan, M. Y. H. 1995. "The Return to the Sacred Path: Healing from Historical Trauma and Historical Unresolved Grief among the Lakota." (Doctoral dissertation). http://proquest.umi.com/?did=741209551andFmt=2andclientId =45836andRQT=309andVName=PQD

Burbar, R. and P. J. Thurman. 2004. "Violence against Native Women." *Social Justice* 31(4): 70–86.

Campbell, C. D. and T. Evans-Campbell. 2011. "Historical Trauma and Native American Child Development and Mental Health: An overview." In *American Indian and Alaska Native Children and Mental Health: Development, Context, Prevention, and Treatment,* edited by M. C. Sarche, P. Spicer, P. Farrell, H. E. Fitzgerald, 1–26. Santa Barbara, CA: Praeger/ABC-CLIO.

Campbell, K., ed. 1978. *The Kumulipo: An Hawaiian Creation Myth.* Kentfield, CA: Pueo Press. (Original work published, 1897)

Center for Disease Control and Prevention. 2001. *Chronic Disease Overview.* http:// www.cdc.gov/nccdphp/aag/aag_reach.htm.

Cohen, K. 2003. *Honoring the Medicine: The Essential Guide to Native American Healing.* New York: Ballantine.

Cole, N. 2006. "Trauma and the American Indian." In *Mental Health Care for Urban Indians: Clinical Insights from Native Practitioners,* edited by T. M. Witko, 115–130. Washington, DC: American Psychological Association. doi:10.1037/11422-006

Collins, R. L. and L. D. Mcnair. 2002. "Minority Women and Alcohol Use." *Alcohol Research and Health* 26 (4): 251–256.

Coyhis, D. and M. Farley. 2011. "The Wellbriety Journey to Forgiveness." [Documentary]. United States: White Bison.

Cross, S. L., A. G. Day, and L. G. Byers. 2010. "American Indian Grand Families: A Qualitative Study Conducted with Grandmothers and Grandfathers who Provide Sole Care for Their Grandchildren." *Journal of Cross-Cultural Gerontology* 25(4): 371–383. doi:10.1007/s10823-010-9127-5

Dana, R. H. 2000. "The Cultural Self as Locus for Assessment and Intervention with American Indians/Alaska Natives." *Journal of Multicultural Counseling and Development* 28(2): 66. http://search.proquest.com.ezproxy.undmedlibrary .org/docview/235958081?accountid=40810

Dawkins, R. 1976. *The Selfish Gene.* New York: Oxford University Press.

De Landa, M. 1997. *A Thousand Years of Nonlinear History.* Brooklyn: Zone Books.

Dodgson, J. E. and R. Struthers. 2005. "Indigenous Women's Voices: Marginalization and Health." *Journal of Transcultural Nursing* 16(4): 339–346. doi: 10 .1177/1043659605278942

Dressler, W. W., J. R. Bindon, and M. J. Gilliland. 1996. "Sociocultural and Behavioral Influences on Health Status among the Mississippi Choctaw." *Medical Anthropology: Cross Cultural Studies in Health and Illness* 17(2): 165–180.

Duran, E., J. Firehammer, and J. Gonzalez. 2008. "Liberation Psychology as the Path Toward Healing Cultural Soul Wounds." *Journal of Counseling and Development* 86(3): 288–288.

Duran, B., J. Oetzel, T. Parker, L. H. Malcoe, J. Lucero, and Y. Jiang. 2009. "Intimate Partner Violence and Alcohol, Drug and Mental Disorders among American Indian Women from Southwest Tribes in Primary Care." *American Indian and Alaska Native Mental Health Research: The Journal of the National Center* 16(2): 11–26.

Duran, E. 2006. *Healing the Soul Wound: Counseling with American Indians and Other Native Peoples.* NY, NY: Teachers College Press.

Duran, E. and B. Duran. 1995. *Native American Postcolonial Psychology.* Albany: State University of New York Press.

Edwards, Y. 2002. "Healing the Soul Wound: The Retraditionalization of Native Americans in Substance Abuse Treatment" (Doctoral dissertation). http://proquest.umi.com/?did=726390871andsid=2andFmt=2andclientId=45836andRQT=309andVName=PQD

Garrett, M. T. and R. D. Herring. 2001. "Honoring the Power of Relation: Counseling Native Adults." *Journal of Humanistic Counseling, Education, and Development* 40: 139–160.

Gone, J. P. and J. E. Trimble. 2012. "American Indian and Alaska Native Mental Health: Diverse Perspectives on Enduring Disparities." *Annual Review of Clinical Psychology* 8: 131–160. doi:10.1146/annurev-clinpsy-032511-143127

Green, J. 2012. "Intimate Partner Violence: Implications for Northern Plains and Upper Midwestern American Indian Mother-Daughter Dyads' Attachment Relationships." (Unpublished dissertation, University of North Dakota, 2012).

Griner, D. and T. B. Smith. 2006. "Culturally Adapted Mental Health Intervention: A Meta-Analytic Review." Special Issue: Culture, Race, and Ethnicity in Psychotherapy. *Psychotherapy* 43(4): 531–548. doi:10.1037/0033-3204.43.4.531

Gura, P. F. 1999. "Making America's Destiny Manifest." *Reviews in American History* 27(4): 554–559.

Gurung, R. A. R. 2014. *Health Psychology: A Cultural Approach* (3rd ed.). San Francisco: Cengage.

Harden, M. J. 1999. "Introduction." *Voices of Wisdom: Hawaiian Elders Speak.* Kula, HI: Aka press.

Harris, H. L. 1998. "Ethnic Minority Elders: Issues and Interventions." *Educational Gerontology* 24(4): 309–323. doi:10.1080/0360127980240402

Hay, R. 1998, Fall. "A Rooted Sense of Place in Cross-Cultural Perspective." *Canadian Geographer* 42 (3): 245-266. Retrieved from http://proquest.umi.com/?did=38677956andsid=1andFmt=4andclientId=45836andRQT=309andVName=PQD

Heinrich, R. K., J. L. Corbine, and K. R.Thomas. 2011. "Counseling Native Americans." *Journal of Counseling and Development* 69(2): 128–133. (Originally published 1990)

Hermes, S. S. 2001. *A Cosmological and Psychological Portrayal: An Integration of Psyche, Culture, and Creativity*. (Order No. 3015810, Pacifica Graduate Institute). *ProQuest Dissertations and Theses*, 280-280. http://search.proquest.com/docvi ew/252112071?accountid=40810. (252112071).

Herring, R. D. 1990. "Understanding Native-American Values: Process and Content Concerns for Counselors." *Counseling and Values* 34(2): 134–137.

Humes, K. R., N. A. Jones, and R. R Ramirez. 2011. "Overview of Race and Hispanic Origin: 2010 Census Brief." www.census.gov/prod/cen2010/briefs/c2010br-02.pdf

Hunter, P. 2008. "What Genes Remember." *Prospect Magazine* 146.

Indian Health Service. 2011. *American Indian/Alaska Native Behavioral Health Briefing Book*. Rockville, MD: Indian Health Service. *www.ihs.gov/behavioral/documents/AIANBHBriefingBook.pdf*

Indian Health Service. 2013. *Indian Health Service: A Quick Look*. Rockville, MD: Indian Health Service. http://www.ihs.gov/factsheets/index.cfm?module=dsp_fact_quicklook

Jacobs, D. T. 2008. *The Authentic Dissertation: Alternative Ways of Knowing, Research, and Representation*. London: Routledge.

Jensen, L. 2005. *Daughters of Haumea = Nā kaikamahine 'o Haumea: Women of Ancient Hawai'i*. San Francisco CA.: Hawai'i: Pueo Press: Anima Gemella.

Jervis, L. L., M. Jackson, and S. M. Manson. 2002. "Need for, Availability of, and Barriers to the Provision of Long-Term Care Services for Older American Indians." *Journal of Cross-Cultural Gerontology* 17(4): 295–311. doi:10.1023/A:1023027102700

John, R., D. S. Kerby, and C. H. Hennessy. 2003. "Patterns and Impact of Comorbidity and Multimorbidity among Community-Resident American Indian Elders." *The Gerontologist* 43(5): 649–660.

Kameeleihiwa, L. 1999. *Nā wāhine kapu = Divine Hawaiian Women*. [Honolulu]: 'Ai Pōhaku Press.

Kawamoto, W. T. 2001. "Community Mental Health and Family Issues in Sociohistorical Context." *American Behavioral Scientist* 44(9): 1482–1491.

King, J. 1999. "Denver American Indian Mental Health Needs Survey." *American Indian and Alaska Native Mental Health Research* 8(3): 1–12.

Kunnie, J. E. and N. I. Goduka, eds. 2006. *Native Peoples' Wisdom and Power: Affirming Our Knowledge through Narratives*. Hampshire, England: Ashgate.

LaRocque, E. D. 1994. *Violence in Aboriginal Communities*. Ottawa, Canada: National Clearing house on Family Violence.

Liliuokalani. 2001. *Hawaii's Story by Hawaii's Queen*. Honolulu (T.H.): Mutual.

Lucero, E. 2011. "From Tradition to Evidence: Decolonization of the Evidence-Based Practice System." *Journal of Psychoactive Drugs* 43(4): 319–324. doi:10.1080/02791072.2011.628925

Lyons, O. and J. Mohawk, eds. 1998. *Exiled in the Land of the Free: Democracy, Indian Nations and the U.S. Constitution*. Santa Fe, NM: Clear Light Pub.

Malcoe, L. H. and B. Duran. 2004. "Intimate Partner Violence and Injury in the Lives of Low Income Native American Women." U.S. Department of Justice.

Violence Against American Indian and Alaska Native Women and the Criminal Justice Response: What is Known. 45.

Manson, S. M. 2000. "Mental Health Services for American Indians and Alaska Natives: Need, Use, and Barriers to Effective Care." *The Canadian Journal of Psychiatry / La Revue Canadienne de Psychiatrie 45*(7): 617–626.

Marshall III, J. M. 2005. *Walking with Grandfather: The Wisdom of Lakota Elders.* Boulder, CO: Sounds True Inc.

McCabe, G. H. 2007. "The Healing Path: A Culture and Community-Derived Indigenous Therapy Model." *Psychotherapy: Theory, Research, Practice, Training 44*(2): 148–160. doi:10.1037/0033-3204.44.2.148

McEachern, D., M. Van Winkle, and S. Steiner. 1998. "Domestic Violence among the Navajo: A Legacy of Colonization." *Journal of Poverty 2*: 31–46.

Menzies, P. M. 2005. "Orphans within our Family: Intergenerational Trauma and Homeless Aboriginal Men." (Doctoral dissertation, University of Toronto, Canada). Retrieved from ProQuest database.

Mohawk, J. 2006, Summer. "Surviving Hard Times: It's Not for Sissies." *Yes Magazine.* http://www.yesmagazine.org

Monopoli, J. and L. L. Alworth. 2000. "The Use of the Thematic Apperception Test in the Study of Native American Psychological Characteristics: A Review and Archival Study of Navaho Men." *Genetic, Social, and General Psychology Monographs 126*(1): 43–78.

Morgan, R. F. 2006. "Native American Postcolonial Psychology/in Redface/the Soul Wound: Counseling with American Indians and Other Native Peoples" [Review of the books *Native American Postcolonial Psychology/Buddha in Redface/ Healing the Soul Wound*]. *Journal of Transpersonal Psychology 38*(2): 242–245. Retrieved from ProQuest database. (Document ID: 1257711941

Niezen, R. 2000. *Spirit Wars: Native North American Religions in the Age of Nation Building.* Berkeley: University of California Press.

Office of the Surgeon General (U.S.), Center for Mental Health Services (U.S.), National Institute of Mental Health (U.S.). 2001. *Mental Health: Culture, Race, and Ethnicity: A Supplement to Mental Health: A Report of the Surgeon General.* Rockville, MD: Substance Abuse and Mental Health Services Administration (U.S.), 2001 Aug. http://www.ncbi.nlm.nih.gov/books/NBK44243/

Ole-Henrik, M. 2005. "Native Education." *Childhood Education 81*(6): 319–320. http://proquest.umi.com/?did=885976151andFmt=3andclientId=45836andR QT=309andVName=PQD

Olson, L. M. and S. Wahab. 2006. "American Indians and Suicide: A Neglected Area of Research." *Trauma, Violence, and Abuse 7*(1): 19–33. doi:10.1177/ 1524838005283005

Park, C. 2013. "Mind-Body CAM Interventions: Current Status and Considerations for Integration into Clinical Health Psychology." *Journal of Clinical Psychology 69*(1): 45–63. doi: 10.1002/jclp.21910

Peters, W. 2011. "The Indigenous Soul Wound: Exploring Culture, Memetics, Complexity and Emergence." Institute of Transpersonal Psychology. ProQuest

Dissertations and Theses, http://search.proquest.com/docview/898334092?acc ountid=25304

Pihama, L., F. Cram, and S. Walker. 2002. "Creating Methodological Space: A Literature Review of Kaupapa Maori Research." *Canadian Journal of Native Education* 26(1): 30.

Poupart, L. M. 2002. "Crime and Justice in American Indian Communities." *Social Justice* 29 (1/2): 144–159. http://proquest.umi.com/?did=208056261andsid=1 andFmt=3andclientId=45836andRQT=309andVName=PQD

Radin, S. M., C. J. Banta-Green, L. R. Thomas, S. H. Kutz, and D. M. Donovan. 2012. "Substance Use, Treatment Admissions, and Recovery Trends in Diverse Washington State tribal Communities." *The American Journal of Drug and Alcohol Abuse* 38(5): 511–517. doi:10.3109/00952990.2012.694533

Ridenour-Wildman, S. L. 2004. "A Comparative Study of Indigenous Content of Multicultural Teacher Education Textbooks in Canada and the United States." (Doctoral dissertation). http://proquest.umi.com/dweb?did=795938391and Fmt=6andclientId=45836andRQT=309andVName=PQD

Robin, R. W., J. C. Long, J. K. Rasmussen, B. Albaugh, and D. Goldman. 1998. "Relationship of Binge Drinking to Alcohol Dependence, Other Psychiatric Disorders, and Behavioral Problems in an American Indian Tribe." *Alcoholism: Clinical and Experimental Research* 22(2): 518–523. doi:10.1097/00000374 -199804000-00032

Ross, R. 2006. *Dancing with a Ghost: Exploring Aboriginal Reality.* Toronto, Canada: Penguin Group.

Satcher, David. 2001. *Mental Health: Culture, Race, and Ethnicity—A Supplement to Mental Health: A Report of the Surgeon General.* U.S. Department of Health and Human Services, Washington, D.C.

Shore, J. H., J. H. Shore, and S, M. Manson. 2009. "American Indian Healers and Psychiatrists." In *Psychiatrists and Traditional Healers: Unwitting Partners in Global Mental Health,* edited by M. Incayawar, R. Wintrob, L. Bouchard, G. Bartocci, 123–134. Wiley-Blackwell. doi:10.1002/9780470741054.ch10

Short, C. W. 1999. *The Cultural Metamorphosis of Cree Education.* (Order No. MQ38548, University of Calgary (Canada)). *ProQuest Dissertations and Theses,* 245–245. http://search.proquest.com/docview/304495454?accountid=40810 .(304495454).

Smith, L. T. 1999. *Decolonizing Methodologies: Research and Indigenous Peoples.* London, New York : Zed Books, Dunedin, N.Z, New York: University of Otago Press.

Smylie, J., L. Williams, and N. Cooper. 2006. "Culture-Based Literacy and Aboriginal Health." *Canadian Journal of Public Health* 97: S21-S25. Retrieved from http://proquest.umi.com/?did=1074629311andFmt=4andclientId=45836and RQT=309andVName=PQD

Stewart-Harawira, M. 2005. *The New Imperial Order: Native Responses to Globalization.* London, New York: Zed Books; Distributed in the USA exclusively by Palgrave Macmillan.

Sue, S. 1977. "Community Mental Health Services to Minority Groups: Some Optimism, Some Pessimism." *American Psychologist* 32 (8): 616–624. doi:10. 1037/0003-066X.32.8.616

Suicide Prevention Resource Center. 2005. *Registry of Evidence-Based Practices.* http://sprc.org/featured_resources/ebpp_factsheets.asp

Sullivan, A., and C. Brems. 1997. "The Psychological Repercussions of the Socio-cultural Oppression of Alaska Native Peoples." *Genetic Social, and General Psychology Monographs* 123(4): 411–440.

Szasz, M. C. 2003. *Education and the American Indian: The Road to Self-Determination since 1928.* Albuquerque, NM: University of New Mexico Press.

Topper, M. D. 1987. "The Traditional Navajo Medicine Man: Therapist, Counselor, and Community Leader." *Journal of Psychoanalytic Anthropology* 10(3): 217–249.

Topper, M. D. and G. Schoepfle. 1990. "Becoming a Medicine Man: A Means to Successful Midlife Transition among Traditional Navajo Men." In *New Dimensions in Adult Development,* edited by R. A. Nemiroff and C. A. Colarusso, 443–466. New York, NY: Basic Books.

Trimble, J. E. 2005. "An Inquiry into the Measurement of Ethnic and Racial Identity." In *Handbook of Racial-Cultural Psychology and Counseling, Vol 1: Theory and Research,* 320–359. doi:10.1177/0013164492052004028

Unger, S., ed. 1977. *The Destruction of American Indian Families.* New York, NY: Association on American Indian Affairs, Inc.

U.S. Department of Justice, Bureau of Justice Statistics. 2007. "American Indians and Crime Report." *North Dakota Council on Abused Women's Services* www .ndcaws.org/SharedFiles/NativeAmerican.asp

Walters, K. L., S. A. Mohammed, T. Evans-Campbell, R. E. Beltrán, D. H. Chae, and B. Duran. 2011. "Bodies Don't Just Tell Stories, They Tell Histories." *Du Bois Review: Social Science Research on Race* 8(01): 179. doi: 10.1017/S1742058X1100018X

Wasson, W. C. 1973. "Philosophical Differences between Europeans and Native Americans as an Explanation of the Alienation of Native American Students from the Educational System." (Doctoral dissertation). Oregon: Department of Curriculum and Instruction.

Wells, R. N., Jr. 1994. *Native American Resurgence and Renewal: A Reader and Bibliography.* Metuchen, NJ: The Scarecrow Press.

Wexler, L., M. L. Silveira, and E. Bertone-Johnson. 2012. "Factors Associated with Alaska Native Fatal and Nonfatal Suicidal Behaviors 2001–2009: Trends and Implications for Prevention." *Archives of Suicide Research* 16(4): 273–286. doi: 10.1080/13811118.2013.722051

Whitbeck, L. B., G. W. Adams, D. R. Hoyt, and X. Chen. 2004a. "Conceptualizing and Measuring Historical Trauma among American Indian People." *American Journal of Community Psychology* 33(3/4): 119–130. doi:10.1023/B:AJCP .0000027000.77357.31

Whitbeck, L. B., X. Chen, D. R. Hoyt, and G. W. Adams. 2004b. "Discrimination, Historical Loss and Enculturation: Culturally Specific Risk and Resiliency

Factors for Alcohol Abuse among American Indians." *Journal of Studies on Alcohol* 65(4): 409–418.

White, J. M., J. Godfrey, and B. Iron Moccasin. 2006. "American Indian Fathering in the Dakota Nation: Use of Akicita as a Fatherhood Standard." *Fathering* 4(1): 49–69. doi:10.3149/fth.0401.49

White Bison, Inc. 2002. *The Red Road to Wellbriety.* Colorado Springs, CO: White Bison, Inc.

Widmer, R. J. 2010. "The Rise, Fall, and Transformation of Native American Cultures in the Southeastern United States." *Reviews in Anthropology* 39(2): 108–126. doi: 10.1080/00938151003772850

CHAPTER NINE

Traditional Chinese Medicine: A Healing Approach from the Past to the Future

Chun Nok Lam and Soh-Leong Lim

The North American public's perception of complementary and alternative medicine (CAM) has evolved from skepticism to one of openness and increasing preference over the past decades. The demand for nonconventional therapies has extended beyond ethnic minority communities to the general American populace. Traditional Chinese Medicine (TCM), a cultural healing system originating from China, is one of the growing CAM fields in U.S. healthcare practices. This growth is largely aided by patients' testimonial of clinical effectiveness. However, TCM encounters criticism for its lack of scientific evidence in treatment efficacy. Further, standardization of herb production remains a challenging issue. The broad utilization of TCM among Chinese Americans, and increasingly among the American public, provides the impetus for medical professionals to carefully consider the benefits and potential dangers of this therapeutic approach. With an expanding consumer market for TCM treatments and products, including acupuncture, herbal medicine, and massage, researchers from both academia and the healthcare industry are showing greater interest in its efficacy. In this chapter we will provide an overview of the history, culture, theory, treatment, usage, research, efficacy, challenge, and prospect of TCM in the United States.

History, Theory, and Philosophy of TCM

Traditional Chinese Medicine (TCM) is an ancient medical system that originated in China. Signified as a cultural and historical heritage, its use dated back to the Shang Dynasty (17th to 11th century BC) (Burke et al. 2008). TCM was first developed as a search for edible foods. At the risk of ingesting toxic substances, early Chinese explorers were rewarded with the knowledge of foods and their curative effects against diseases (Kung and Tsim 2006). Their collective experiences on herbs became the foundation of herbal medicine. The knowledge of disease and illness was also developed early in ancient Chinese history. Archeologists have discovered partial records of epidemics from inscriptions on tortoise shells (i.e. oracle bones). In the Han Dynasty (4th century AD), the *Divine Farmer's Classic of the Materia Medica* (神農本草經) became the first publication compiling the medical applications of 365 plants and minerals (Kung and Tsim 2006).

The foundation of TCM was established on the principles of Chinese philosophy: Yin- Yang (陰陽), Five Elements (五行), Essence (精), Qi (氣) and Spirit (神). Yin-Yang (Figure 9.1) refers to the opposing, interchanging and interdependent nature of all existence in the universe. The Yin-Yang theory was introduced by Lao Zi in the *Book of Changes* and had a critical influence on how Chinese perceived the functioning of the human body. When Yin and Yang are in balance, the body is in a harmonious and healthy state. Yin refers to the dense, damp, and turbid

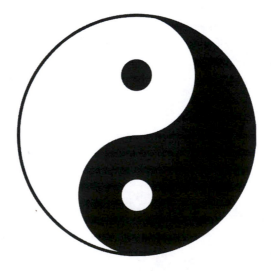

Figure 9.1   Yin-Yang

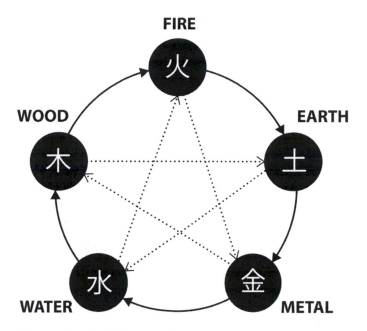

Figure 9.2 Five Elements Theory
Note: Solid line, create. Dotted line, control.

matter, which nourish the body (e.g. blood and body fluid); while Yang refers to the light, active, and clear matter, which keep the body in motion. TCM calls this matter Qi, widely known as the energy that flows within the body. The disruption of this harmony will result in an imbalanced state between the two forces, which makes a person susceptible to sickness.

The ancient Chinese first understood human anatomy and human functioning primarily through dissecting cadavers and later to develop a system to observe internal organs from the exterior of live persons. From these, the theory of visceral manifestation was formulated. In TCM, the human body is governed by five Zang (臟) visceral systems consisting of the Heart, Lungs, Spleen, Liver, and Kidney systems. These power centers, supported by six Fu (腑) viscera – the Bladder, Colon, Gall Bladder, Small Intestine, Stomach, and Triple Heater – are each responsible for specific functions to maintain bodily activities. The Zang viscera are guided by the Five Elements theory (Figure 9.2) formed around the Qin dynasty (2nd century BC). Each Zang is illustrated by a natural element, i.e. wood (木)-Liver, fire (火)-Heart, earth (土)-Spleen, metal (金)-Lungs, and water (水)-Kidneys. These elements are interrelated. They create and control (as symbolized by the interactive arrows in Figure 9.2) one another to maintain a proper balance for sustaining health. In TCM, the human body is viewed in broad functional units for diagnosis and treatment.

TCM views Essence, Qi, and Spirit as the basis of life. Essence is the crucial substances and nutrients that construct and supply the human body to sustain physiological activities and life. Essence is received in two forms: parental inheritance that is given to a newborn at birth; and replenishment in physical form from food, water and air in daily life. Essence and Qi, formerly introduced by philosophers in the Qin dynasty and further elaborated in Taoism, represent the origin and change of life. Essence and Qi are the same matter but appear in different forms. Qi's metamorphic activities serve to mobilize and maintain proper functioning of the body and the viscera. Spirit, from ancient Chinese's viewpoint, is the volatile, ever-changing power of nature and its creation. In the human body, Spirit refers to the manifestation of life that exerts upon the flesh. To further illustrate, life consists of two core materials: Essence that stores and Qi that flows. Spirit exists because of Essence and Qi; on the other hand, it manipulates the work of Essence and Qi. The theory of Essence, Qi, and Spirit guides the applications of TCM.

A healthy body is one where the Zang-Fu viscera functions properly. The Heart is in charge of the pathways of blood circulation and controls the Spirit, which masters consciousness and thinking. The Lungs control respiration by dominating the dispersion and descent of Qi, while regulating water passage in the body. The Spleen regulates digestion and absorption of food nutrients and governs the transportation and transformation of food Essence into Qi and blood. The Liver stores blood and arranges for the proper amount of blood to be circulated. Lastly, the Kidneys control water metabolism, storing Essence and controlling human reproduction, growth, and development. Each organ in the Zang viscera is supported by a Fu organ. Zang and Fu viscera are interrelated; Zang represents Yin, and Fu represents Yang. Fu processes the consumed raw materials (e.g., food, air, water), while Zang extracts and transforms the metabolites into useful nutrients that become Essence to power the body. The Zang-Fu system represents a complex relational net that imperatively maintains the activities of the human body.

Historical breakthroughs in TCM were underscored by four TCM classical literatures. The *Yellow Emperors' Classic of Internal Medicine* (Nei Jing – 內經) contains the fundamental principles of TCM. It represents the core of all medicinal achievements since the Zhou dynasty (11th century BC). Up until the Han dynasty (1st century BC), TCM's clinical theories and practices were consolidated and edited into this published work. This volume further established the application of Yin-Yang and Five Elements theories in medicine; in addition, it focuses on regimens, which suggest that humans can follow the structure of nature to achieve optimal health. The three other books that aided in the breakthrough of TCM are the *Treatise on Cold Damage Febrile Disorders* (傷寒論), the *Survey of Important Elements from the Golden Cabinet* (金匱要略), and the *Study of Warm Disease Theory* (溫病學). Another classical work, Li Shi Zhen's *Grand Compendium of Meteria Medica* (本草綱目, 14th to 17th AD), was a collection of medicinal substances and their applications and it also was a major contribution to TCM. This book, mainly focusing on herbology, also contains invaluable knowledge in biology, chemistry, astronomy, geography and geology. It is a collection of over 1,800 medicines and over 10,000 TCM decoction formulas. It remains one of the recognized works underpinning TCM education today.

TCM Diagnosis and Treatment Modalities

Why People Become Sick: Loss of Harmony

TCM views health as the manifestation of harmony between Yin and Yang. When the balance is disrupted, the body's defenses can be compromised; hence, people become sick. TCM has identified four sources of illnesses that potentially trigger this imbalance. These are: external, internal, miscellaneous, and lifestyle causes. Each source is sufficient to induce poor harmony in the body and lead to weakening of the body immune system.

External causes (外因) can be weather, environment or geographic location related. The causes are known as the "six excesses" (六淫), or "six devils" (六邪) and consist of: wind (風), cold (寒), heat (暑), moisture (濕), dryness (燥), and fire (火). From the perspective of modern medicine, there is no clear definition for these causes; they could be disease-inducing factors such as sudden temperature change, extreme weather condition, or pathogens that weaken the immune system. Second, internal causes (內因) are known as the "seven emotions" (七情). The seven emotions arise from unstable psychological states, such as excessive pleasure (喜), anger (怒), worry (怒), depression (憂), sorrow (悲), fear (恐), and shock (驚). Uncontrolled emotions disrupt the flow and quality of Qi, which in turn results in the imbalance between Yin and Yang. This imbalance puts an individual at risk of becoming sick. Third, miscellaneous causes refer to direct impacts, including injuries and accidents. Finally, lifestyle causes refer to poor diet or social habits and lack of exercise.

The Four Examinations

Diagnosis in TCM involves a comprehensive examination from a holistic point of view. TCM practitioners examine their patients with four diagnostic methods: observing (望), listening/ smelling (聞), questioning (問), and palpation (切). These same techniques have been practiced since ancient times when technological devices were still unavailable in medicine. Skills and expertise in TCM were honed over time and the standard of care in TCM was established through proof of success from years or generations of clinical experience.

A TCM practitioner first observes the appearance of the patient to find out the type and origin of the problem. This process includes: looking into the eyes and examining the complexion, skin color, nails, lips, and the appearance and coating of the tongue. The practitioner also observes the posture of the patient. Since many combinations of symptoms are possible, the practitioner then carefully listens to the patient's breathing and quality of his or her voice. The practitioner also notes any odors of the mouth and body. To further obtain the patient's subjective complaints, the practitioner inquires about the patient's presence of pain, sweat, appetite and thirst, frequency and condition of urine and stool, quality of sleep at night, discomforts, and for females, information related to their menstrual cycle. Finally, the practitioner performs the traditional pulse diagnosis, known as palpation. In the pulse diagnosis, which is usually performed on the wrist, the practitioner observes if the pulse is fast or slow, floating or sinking, long or short, empty or full, slippery or choppy, and soft or tense. With a complete consultation, the practitioner gains insight into the nature of the disease symptoms and can prescribe the right treatment to the patient.

TCM Treatment Modalities

TCM covers a variety of treatment methods that results in comprehensive care and healing. These therapeutic modalities include: acupuncture (針灸), moxibustion (艾灸), Chinese herbal medicine (中草藥), Chinese massage (Tui Na 推拿), Qi Gong (氣功), cupping (拔罐), bone setting (正骨), and food therapy (食療). Each modality can be its own distinct profession because mastering the sophisticated techniques associated with each modality require years of serious training and practice. Chinese practitioners often combine various traditional methods when treating patients to achieve optimal therapeutic results. The following outlines some of these common TCM treatments in the United States.

Acupuncture/Moxibustion

Acupuncture (針灸) is a popular healing modality among the many alternative therapies in the United States. The technique was first developed when the ancient Chinese discovered the use of sharp tools to cut open pustules for the relief of pain, which accelerated recovery. These sharp devices later evolved into steel needles through centuries of meticulous study and clinical practices.

In acupuncture treatment, practitioners systematically insert 12–15 needles into specific points on the body's surface, with the aim of manipulating and moving the flow of Qi. These points are openings of the meridians, an intricate system of channels for Qi movement throughout the body. There are approximately 365 points over the 14 major channels interconnecting various positions external and internal to the flesh. These acupuncture points are also used in moxibustion, a technique that applies burned, dried mugwort directly on the skin along these major channels. The penetrating heat moves and circulates stagnant masses of blood and Qi and works to clear out blockages. The average time for an acupuncture or moxibustion treatment is between 20–40 minutes and results vary according to health conditions. A common benefit is the management of pain arising from conditions as varied as arthritis to lower back pain.

Chinese Herbal Medicine

Chinese herbal medicine (中草藥) has been the primary TCM treatment in China. Today, approximately 12,000 types of mostly organic substances are classified as TCM herbs, including plants, minerals, and animal matter (Kung and Tsim 2006). The functions of these herbal materials were carefully studied and documented by Li Shi Zhen in his book, *The Grand Compendium of Meteria Medica* (本草綱目). Typical herbal ingredients in the U.S. market include plant roots, leaves, seeds, peels, barks, and twigs. The import of these is FDA regulated. Based on a patient's diagnosis, TCM practitioners prescribe from over 300 commonly used herbs that have significant clinical therapeutic effects in TCM treatments.

Most herbal formulas prescribed to patients combine multiple herbs with different treatment properties; these herbs target various symptoms to achieve a synergic effect. The therapeutic goal is to provide a comprehensive, curative result beyond the patient's primary complaint, and more importantly, take into account the root causes of the illness. This sophisticated combination of herbs is formulated according to the herbs' interrelated effects to optimize health outcome and minimize side-effects. Thus herbal medicine has great advantages of being a powerful personalized treatment because it customizes the patients' specific health needs. Herbal formulas are commonly prescribed in raw herbal form; the herbs are boiled with water and drunk in the form of a decoction. Since our body is a dynamic entity, there is a need to adjust the herbal formula over the course of sickness. While the medicine activates and unblocks Qi, it provides nourishment to strengthen the balance of the body at the same time.

Over-the-Counter Chinese Herbal Pills

Over-the-counter (OTC) Chinese herbal pills (中成藥) are herbal formulas in the form of compressed herbal tablets or herbal powder in capsules manufactured by pharmaceutical companies, both locally and overseas. They are made of granulated raw herbs selected from generic and commonly used TCM formulas. Many of these pills are patented in China and exported worldwide. Although the concentration per dosage of herbal pills is smaller than the decoction, pills come in handy when formula preparation is not convenient or the decoction is difficult to stomach. Note that even though herbal pills can be purchased without a prescription, in TCM they are drugs meant for specific treatment purposes and ingestion of wrong herbs can lead to adverse effects. Therefore, it is best to consult a TCM practitioner for guidance. Currently, OTC herbal pills are not FDA-approved for disease treatment or prevention in the United States, and they are sold mainly as dietary supplements.

Chinese Americans: History, Health Characteristics, and Healthcare Utilization

History of Chinese Americans in the United States

Chinese Americans refer to individuals of Chinese descent in the United States. The population is comprised of immigrants from mainland China, Hong Kong, Taiwan, and other countries where there are overseas Chinese such as Singapore, Malaysia, and Indonesia (Caring Connection 2009, Jang, Lee, and Woo 1998). Chinese Americans also include the American-born members of these immigrant families. In 2010, over 3.8 million Chinese Americans resided in the United States, representing about 1.2 percent of the U.S. population (U.S. Census Bureau 2012). Chinese Americans are mainly concentrated in the East and West Coast in metropolitan areas such as New York, Boston, San Francisco and Los Angeles. The Chinese American community comprises 26.5 percent of the entire Asian American population; it is the largest ethnic group of Asian-Americans in the United States.

Since the first entrance of the Chinese into the United States in 1840 as railroad workers until the 1900s, their population maintained at 0.2 percent of the total U.S. population (Hsu 2006). The Chinese population declined to 0.1 percent for the first half of the 20th century, and in 50 years it climbed to 1.1 percent of the U.S. population (U.S. Census Bureau 2012). The New York City Metropolitan Area has the largest Chinese American population in the United States, with over 0.6 million individuals. Chinese communities predominantly concentrate in Chinatowns or nearby neighborhoods; these communities are prominent in Los Angeles, San Francisco, Boston, Chicago, Washington D.C., Houston, and Seattle. In addition, Chinese Americans are also dispersed in rural towns and university-college towns across the United States.

In California, one out of five Chinese Americans lives in poverty (California Health Interview Survey 2007, Caring Connection 2009, University of Maryland 2001). Lack of health insurance is a major barrier for many to access healthcare and preventive health services (NICOS 2004, Dong et al. 2011). In the process of acculturation, Chinese Americans have, in many cases, been adapting to health behaviors practiced by the local Americans, which affect their disease patterns (Tom, n.d.). Cardiovascular diseases, diabetes mellitus, breast cancer, and prostate cancer are among the rising disease categories Chinese Americans experience more often than Chinese living in Asia (Lum n.d., Sadler et al. 2000, Tom, n.d., Yee and Weaver 1994). Other health-related problems including Hepatitis B, tuberculosis, osteoporosis, smoking, alcoholism, and mental conditions such as depression, suicidal intent, and dementia are also prevalent among the Chinese residing in the United States. (Chen 1995, Huff and Kline 1998, Institute of Community Health and Research 2007, Lassiter 1995, Lum n.d., National Alliance on Mental Illness 2011).

Chinese immigrant populations in the United States are known to underutilize healthcare (Jang et al. 1998, Ma 1999, Miltiades and Wu 2008, Pang, Jordan-Marsh, Silverstein, and Cody 2003). One major factor is being uninsured. In Jang et al.'s (1998) study, of 1,808 Chinese American residents in San Francisco, 22 percent reported having no insurance at the time of the survey. Factors associated with their uninsured status included low income (<$45,000), not being a U.S. citizen, lack of acculturation, and being only Chinese-speaking. Among these uninsured respondents, 56 percent reported not having a regular place of care compared to 11 percent among the insured. Twenty-five percent of the uninsured participants reported visiting a Chinese medicine doctor or herbalist when sick, compared to 7.7 percent among those insured. Other socio-economic factors such as inadequate formal education, limited English language fluency, restricted social network, financial, cultural and transportation barriers, shift in family relationship and support, and skepticism of Western medical treatments also negatively affected Western Medicine physician visits (Institute of Community Health and Research 2007, Ma 1999, Miltiades and Wu 2008, Mayeno and Hirota 1994, Pang et al. 2003). Interestingly, Chinese immigrants in these studies frequently reported using an integration of Western Medicine and TCM for their health needs. The reasons for their pluralistic healthcare approach included consistency with personal and cultural beliefs, patient dissatisfaction with Western Medicine, increasing medical cost associated with Western Medicine, and social and family influences (Wade, Chao, and Kronenberg 2007).

TCM Development

Historically, the general population in the United States has been skeptical of alternative medicine because of its limited scientific validation. However, in the last two decades, the number of American adults who are seeking out these therapeutic methods has rapidly increased. This growing demand makes CAM a viable treatment option among U.S. healthcare consumers. The Chinese immigrants, who retained their cultural health practices, introduced TCM to the American public. TCM's clinical effectiveness, specifically acupuncture, became noteworthy when a U.S. reporter, James B. Reston, was treated with acupuncture for his post-surgical pain during his visit to China during the Nixon era in 1970s (Hui, Yu, and Zylowska 2002, Prensky 1995).

TCM has further increased in popularity over the past two decades when scientific evidence began to become available to the American public. Acupuncture has the largest body of literature, followed by Chinese herbal medicine. Examples of research on these treatment modalities include those related to back pain, depression, osteoarthritis, cancer, heart disease, diabetes and HIV/AIDS (NCCAM 2011). According to the National Center for Complementary and Alternative Medicine (NCCAM), TCM is defined as a "whole medical system," which refers to a "complete system of theory and practice that has evolved independently from or parallel to allopathic (conventional) medicine" (Food and Drug Administration 2006). TCM consists of a variety of treatment modalities, and some are subjected to the Food and Drug Administration (FDA) regulations. FDA defines raw herbal materials and manufactured herbal products as dietary supplements. Acupuncture needles are regulated as CAM "devices" under Class II classification due to its minimally invasive nature and its intention to treat or prevent diseases (FDA 2006, FDA 2012). Even though acupuncture and TCM herbal medicine are considered safe according to FDA, their uses are advised with caution due to potentially undetermined side-effects (NCCAM 2010).

Acupuncture practice in the United States is regulated by state licensure. In 43 states and the District of Columbia, it requires the practitioner to pass the National Certification Commission for Acupuncture and Oriental Medicine (NCCAOM) examination. In California, one may qualify to take the exam when one fulfills any of the following two requirements: (a) graduating from a four academic-year program in acupuncture and oriental medicine offered by an Acupuncture Board-approved school, or 2) completing an equivalent foreign education (Dower 2003). There are 35 approved schools and training programs in the United States; nineteen of these are in California. Licensed acupuncturists (LAc's) are required to renew their license every two years with 30 continuing education unit hours. As of 2004, California had licensed more than 6,000 acupuncturists, accounting for at least one-third of the total U.S. acupuncture workforce (Dower 2003, Eisenberg et al. 2002). Most LAc professionals work in private practice due to limited institutional opportunities in the healthcare system. Nevertheless, the profession continues to grow and acupuncturists are now considered primary care physicians in many states.

Prevalence of TCM Utilization

Eisenberg et al. (1998) conducted two nationally representative telephone surveys to document trends in alternative medicine use in the United States during the 1990s. Their findings showed that the use of acupuncture was 0.4 percent in 1990 and increased to 1.0 percent in 1997 in a representative sample of American adults. The use of herbal medicine was 2.5 percent in 1990 and increased to 12 percent in 1997. In 2002, the National Health Interview Survey (NHIS) estimated the prevalence of acupuncture use to be 1.1 percent; this further increased to 1.4 percent in 2007 (Burke et al. 2006, Su and Li 2011). Furthermore, lifetime acupuncture users increased from 4.2 percent in 2002 to 6.3 percent in 2007, representing over 10 million users in the United States (Zhang et al. 2012). The increase in acupuncture use among American adults has been prominent and significant over the past two decades.

Among Asian Americans, the use of acupuncture was expectedly higher than the overall American public. Su and Li (2011) reported that Asian acupuncture users increased from 2.4 percent in 2002 to 3.7 percent in 2007, twice the rate of use compared to the Caucasian populations. However, studies providing national estimates of prevalence of TCM use among Chinese Americans are limited. Wade et al. (2007) studied the use of CAM, primarily TCM modalities, among a subsample of Chinese American women (n=804) from a nationally represented survey of American adult females in 2001. They found that 41 percent of subjects reported using CAM therapies; among these, 62 percent employed predominately TCM and 29 percent used only herbal treatments and acupuncture (Wade et al. 2007). Ahn et al. (2006) studied Chinese American patient cohorts on a national scale and collected convenience sampling from 11 health centers serving primarily Chinese and Vietnamese Americans across eight major cities in the United States. Two-thirds (68 percent) of the Cantonese- and over half (55 percent) of the Mandarin-speaking Chinese participants reported lifetime use of therapies including herbs, acupuncture, cupping, and massage. Ten to 17 percent of the respondents reported using these treatments during the week before visiting a health center.

Community-based studies focusing on TCM use were also conducted in major U.S. cities. A study in San Francisco reported that 80 percent of Chinese Americans used at least one type of TCM treatment in the two years prior to the survey (Lam 2010). Among the TCM users, 90 percent also reported seeking conventional treatments in the same time period. Wu, Burke, and LeBaron (2007) focused on two San Francisco federally funded health centers and their results suggested that the usage rate of TCM among Chinese American patient samples was up to 98 percent. A similar high prevalence rate of TCM use among Chinese Americans is also apparent in New York, Boston, Houston and Los Angeles (Chan and Chang 1976, Ma 1999, Pearl, Leo, and Tsang 1995, Young 1999). Furthermore, TCM use is prevalent among Chinese American cancer and mental health patients (Lee et al. 2000, Lin 2005).

Factors Associated with TCM Use

Few studies in the United States have examined factors associated with TCM use among American adults. Pagán and Pauly (2005) abstracted data from the National Health Interview Survey (NHIS) showing participants who reported any difficulty in getting needed medical care were 1.7 and 2.1 times more likely to have used herbal medicine and acupuncture, respectively. Among Chinese Americans, cultural and integration factors are thought to be closely related to their TCM utilization. Lam (2010) conducted a community survey in San Francisco and found that TCM use was associated with those who reported being from mainland China, recent immigration and noninsurance status. In Wade et al.'s paper (2007), the authors observed that Chinese American women often use Western Medicine and TCM simultaneously, adopting a pluralistic approach to medical care. They also found that acculturation and socioeconomic status did not predict the use of TCM in their sample; this result suggested that respondents practiced TCM across all socio-demographic levels. In addition, Ahn et al. (2006) found that being Cantonese, having family available in the United States, residing in the Western regions of the United States, and having poor self-perceived health status were significantly associated with TCM use. The same study also suggested that only 7.6 percent of CAM/TCM users had discussed their use of CAM/TCM therapies with their Western Medicine-trained clinicians.

Health Symptoms among TCM Users

A study in New York City's Chinatown reported that over 60 percent of respondents preferred using TCM for treating symptoms including stomachache, diarrhea, fracture, itching, anemia and rheumatism (Chan and Chang 1976). Preference for TCM also becomes apparent when patients found Western Medicine ineffective or experienced side-effects from pharmaceuticals in conditions, not limited to fatigue, digestive difficulties and long-term damage to internal organs (Lee et al. 2000, Ma 1999, Wong et al. 1998, Tabora and Flaskerud 1997). In addition, Chinese Americans relied on TCM for chronic conditions including asthma and arthritis, as well as musculoskeletal dysfunctions, mood care and wellness care (Cassidy 1998). Since TCM is an extensive treatment method for various health problems, specifically at a preventive level, Chinese Americans often use TCM to maintain their health-related quality of life (Cassidy 1998, Caring Connection 2009).

TCM Research Updates

In recent years, the National Institute of Health (NIH) has been increasing invested research funding in the field of Complementary and Alternative Medicine (CAM). Research areas cover basic and translational research, as well as observational studies and clinical investigations. The purpose is to develop a rigorous evidence base for CAM practices and to attend to areas of unmet healthcare needs. This global effort has significantly benefited the advancement and acceptance of TCM internationally, especially in Western nations. This section will provide an overview and updates on current TCM research in the United States and aboard.

Randomized Control Trials

The increasing demand of acupuncture in the United States has sparked tremendous interest in its efficacy. The National Center for Complementary and Alternative Medicine (NCCAM) has funded extensive research, which includes: 1) acupuncture's efficacy in treating specific health conditions, 2) the body's biological responses to acupuncture treatment, 3) neurological properties of meridians and acupuncture points, and 4) methods for improving research quality (NCCAM 2010, NCCAM 2011). Both NCCAM and independent research groups have summarized scientific evidence of acupuncture from rigorous review articles, which include systematic reviews and meta-analyses on randomized control trials that focus on pain conditions, such as carpal tunnel syndrome, headache, migraine, fibromyalgia, low-back pain, menstrual cramps, myofascial pain, neck pain, osteoarthritis, knee pain, postoperative dental pain, and tennis elbow (AHRQ 2003, Hui 1999, Manheimer et al. 2005, NIH 1998). Although study outcomes encompass mixed findings, which prompt further evaluations, a growing number of Western Medicine physicians have begun to recommend acupuncture as an adjunct treatment for some of these health conditions (Ernst and Fugh-Berman 2002).

Evaluations of Chinese herbal medicine remain controversial. Poor quality of trial designs, inconsistent outcomes and biased results are common criticisms of its scientific merit (Cheung et al. 2012, Ernst 2004, Liu and Douglas 1998, Pittler et al. 2000, Shang et al. 2007, Tang et al. 1998). In addition, research studies published in Chinese are inaccessible to most Western researchers, thus making literature searches difficult for a thorough appraisal. Nevertheless, these challenges have worked to enhance collaborations among TCM and Western Medicine scholars to develop new research ideas. In the United States, Shang et al. (2007) compared the quality of clinical trials between Chinese herbal medicine and Western Medicine. Cardiovascular, gynecological and obstetrical disorders were among the treatment focus in these studies, and the result suggested that the quality of the study of both medicines did not differ significantly from each other. Hanks (2000) summarized the effects of Chinese herbs in treating the side-effects of chemotherapy and radiation. The study focused on herb-induced immunologic parameters including T lymphocytes, monoclonal antibodies, natural killer cells, and leukocytes activities. The author concluded that Chinese herbal medicine improved the immune system when used in conjunction with conventional Western cancer interventions. *The Cochrane Reviews,* an international organization that conducts systemic reviews of primary research in healthcare, has also invested tremendous effort in building a robust evaluation on TCM-related research (The Cochrane Collaboration - Cochrane Reviews 2012). In addition, Chinese herbal medicine research is also tested with animal trials. Srivastava et al. (2009) treated an induced peanut allergic condition in rats using a customized Chinese herbal formula. Although the outcome of Chinese herbal medicine on human trials seems to remain inconclusive, there has been an increasing demand for its use and one cannot prejudge its potential impact on health and healthcare until it is properly evaluated.

The current clinical evaluation of TCM is framed primarily in the biomedical terms of conventional medicine. This has both advantages and limitations. An accurate measure of the patient-centered outcome in TCM has yet to be fully portrayed. Dedicated to the process of harmonizing traditional and modern medicine, Ka-Kit Hui, the director of UCLA Center of East-West Medicine suggested several assessment approaches that could benefit the understanding of TCM (Hui 1999). For example, clinical research should take the theoretical construct of TCM in designing trials with appropriate metrics. This includes assessing Chinese herbs efficacy through proper diagnosis and therapeutic strategies, guided by TCM principles, and testing acupuncture effects in conjunction with herbal medicine, massage and/or diet rather than solely the needling technique (Braverman, Baker, and Harris 2009). An assessment of the intrinsic value of TCM in society, not limited to political, economic and social factors, is also of great importance. Hui's recommendation offers a guideline for developing a model of integrative medicine for future healthcare in the United States.

Technology and Molecular Property

A new generation of TCM research has benefited tremendously from technological advancements in the past decades. Microscopic imaging uncovers Chinese herbal properties in a level unperceived by the ancient TCM founders. These innovative approaches enable a common ground between TCM and modern medicine. On the other hand, the technological-based research process might have overarched TCM principles that were originally established in a time without computing techniques. Nonetheless, all these efforts offer new insights to an ancient medicine of over 3000 years and herald a promising future of continued discovery and development.

Prescription of multi-herb recipes is routinely used in TCM. However, the scientific basis of TCM-defined herbal properties remains unclear. Research groups in Singapore and China have joined efforts to evaluate the distribution patterns of herbal properties using artificial intelligence (AI) methods (Chen et al. 2006, Ung et al. 2007). These AI systems were trained to distinguish TCM prescriptions from non-TCM recipes, and the systems correctly classified 80–90 percent of the formula from thousands of herbal ingredient combinations. These results are useful for formulating new TCM prescriptions for specific disorders; they also enhance the understanding of the physicochemical, pharmacological, and molecular mechanisms of the multi-herb, multiple-target intervention strategy of TCM therapies. The same research group has also established a comprehensive TCM online database to provide information about TCM prescriptions, herbs, herbal ingredients, molecular structure, therapeutic and side effects, and applications (Chen et al. 2006). In the United States, a research team led by Eisenberg and his colleagues has also developed a library of authenticated TCM plants for systematic biological evaluation (Eisenberg et al. 2011, Harris et al. 2011). The library collects the therapeutic contents of the most commonly prescribed TCM herbs and herbal prescriptions, including processed herb species, in addition to information on the locations where the herbs were grown, and any presence of heavy metal or pesticide contamination. These computer-based research techniques increase the accessibility of TCM information to researchers that foster TCM's development.

Advances in molecular biotechnology have set standards on utilizing genetic tools to authenticate the pharmacological components of herbs. Scientists use these tools to map out the blueprint of the herbal material at the DNA level. Hon, Chow, Zeng, and Leung (2003) proposed a large-scale TCM center to authenticate the botanical identities and origins of TCM herbs. The process uses microsatellite genotyping to differentiate the biological compounds and chemicals of Chinese herbs. It can help standardize and modernize Chinese herbal medicine and contribute towards quality control. Another study by Parekh, Liu, and Wei (2009) reported the application of TCM using the molecular basis approach in cancer treatments. They described the complex interplay of TCM on four cancer-targeted therapies: (a) inducing apoptosis, (b) inhibiting angiogenesis, (c) boosting the immune system, and (d) overcoming multi-drug resistance. The identification of potent bio-actives from TCM herbs may guide better personalized treatments for cancer patients. An article by Li (2007) reviewed the pharmacological mechanisms of TCM through proteomic technology. Proteomics provides the profiling of protein expression among patients following TCM treatments. It can measure the body's response to the treatment in quantifiable terms. Altogether, this generation of advanced technology will bring biomedical and clinical research in TCM to a new level.

Social Science and Healthcare

Traditional Chinese Medicine encompasses a complex health and healthcare system. Using a multi-level construct approach, social science researchers evaluate TCM beyond its clinical and medicinal values. A report by Braverman et al. (2009) examined the safety, cost-effectiveness, education requirements, and healthcare policy reform related to the development of TCM in the United States. The report presented evidence to support acupuncture in reference to its low adverse effects, improvement in quality of life and reduced use of prescriptions. Another report by Jabbour, Sapko, Miller, Weiss, and Gross (2009) pointed out that consumers' decision to pay for acupuncture treatment, regardless of reimbursement, further suggests the economic value and health benefits of the treatment. These evidences are in favor of appropriating the integration of TCM modality, specifically acupuncture, into the current healthcare system for treatments such as post-surgical healing, neurological rehabilitation, pain management, reproductive services, oncology, and anxiety (Braverman 2009). Dower (2003) summarized the acupuncture profession and its healthcare delivery in California. The data presents an on-going and increasing demand for this alternative therapy by the American public.

Another major component in TCM research is the focus on sub-health conditions. Sub-health is broadly described as the state between health and disease, where the individual experiences all kinds of discomfort but no abnormality is detected using medical equipment and indexes. Since many sub-health conditions have no clear laboratory markers for diagnosis, TCM offers a potentially effective intervention based on its syndrome differentiation diagnostic technique (Xue et al. 2009). Zou, Shi, and Cai (2008) applied an epidemiologic approach combined with TCM syndrome differentiation techniques to understand the TCM clinical manifestations of a sub-health population in China. This mixed-method offered a unique diagnostic and preventative strategy to health conditions that are yet to be fully detectable and understood by Western Medicine. Another major research topic in TCM is the evaluation of the health-related quality of life (HRQOL) of the study population. HRQOL refers to physical, mental, family and social health domains that constitute the well-being of an individual. A study in Hong Kong suggested that TCM offered the same level of improvement in HRQOL as Western Medicine and therefore supported the role of TCM as an alternative care to patients (Wong et al. 2011). In addition, researchers also studied TCM by using its principles in epidemiological studies to understand the relationship between dietary patterns and disease (Lee and Shen 2008).

The research foci being presented in this section are simply the tip of an iceberg; the idea is to provide readers an overview of some major research breakthroughs that are happening in the on-going field of TCM research.

Implications, Challenges, and Future Directions

Challenges of TCM Development in the United States

The development of TCM is an uphill battle in Western society. The mainstream medical system has set an inconceivable challenge for the growth of non-conventional medicine. In the United States, TCM encounters criticism of whether it can live up to scrutiny when justified by clinical research. Li (2009) summarized these concerns as: (a) the specificity of acupuncture point, (b) needling manipulation, (c) role of placebo in TCM, (d) advantage of TCM pattern differentiation, (e) quality control of Chinese herbs, (f) safety and toxicity of herbal medicine, (g) efficacy of herbal medicine, (h) drug-herb interaction, (i) application of Western diagnosis and techniques in TCM treatment, and (j) the best clinical model for modern TCM practice. These items provide a direction and guidance to help the understanding and development of TCM in Western nations. We will discuss some of the problems and progress of these critical challenges.

TCM has sparked debates on topics such as its status in the United States's pharmaceutical market, methods in determining its efficacy, and potential complications in cancer treatments. In the United States, TCM products are sold as dietary supplements according to their "structure and function" claim allowable under Dietary Supplement Health and Education Act (DSHEA) (Chang 1999). Scientific evaluation of how TCM products may affect the structure and functioning of the body is challenging due to TCM's multi-herb approach. The multi-herb approach produces synergic effects in herbal combinations that target multiple locations in the body. Current research methods that are capable of evaluating multi-level interventions similar to this remain limited. Whether TCM's putative health benefits may be of value for pharmaceutical development for disease treatment will depend on a research-based strategy suitable for the medicine's validation.

In Western society, clinical research is the gold standard in medical evaluation. Ernst (2004) suggested that randomized, placebo-controlled, and double-blind clinical trials should be the standard to evaluate the efficacy and effectiveness of alternative therapies. However, Paterson and Dieppe (2005) argued that these standards may not be appropriate for complex interventions with a basis in non-conventional medicine or in non-pharmaceutical trials. The authors questioned whether the underlying assumptions of placebo-controlled design hold true for treatments, such as acupuncture.

First, randomized controlled trials assume that the diagnostic process takes place before the trial intervention begins. In TCM, the diagnostic process is an integral part of the intervention, with repeated pulse taking and patient feedback about needle insertion. Second, in Western trials, incidental factors, such as talking and listening, are perceived to be independent of the treatment effect. Within acupuncture consultations, aspects of talking and being listened to can have subsequent effects on the interventions. Third, in drug trials the drug is a distinct, separate material entity from other aspect of the intervention. In acupuncture, however, the diagnostic process and the needling are interwoven into the whole intervention. The authors described the interactions between the characteristic effects of medications and incidental effects to be too complicated for the current model of randomized controlled trials. Therefore, TCM's therapeutic efficacy and effectiveness are yet to be ascertained until more accurate metrics and measurements become available (Paterson and Dieppe 2005).

The increasing use of TCM among cancer patients has perplexed oncologists. Evidence regarding the interaction of herbal products with conventional cancer treatments remains insufficient. A systemic review by Chiu, Yau and Epstein (2008) presented existing knowledge on this behalf to guide physicians and cancer caregivers. The article summarized categories of toxicity that could be directly or indirectly triggered by drug-TCM interaction. These observed toxic-induced syndromes included liver complications, bleeding tendency, kidney diseases, hypertension, or hearing impairment. Because few patients report their use of herbal products, these potentially TCM-induced complications are frequently under-detected by oncologists. Given that there are reasons favoring TCM usage or possible treatment effects, more studies are underway to determine its safety and efficacy in conventional anticancer treatments.

Potential Developments

While conventional medicine may have quicker responses in treating acute problems, TCM therapeutics is particularly advantageous in dealing with chronic conditions (Cassidy 1998, Hui, Hui, and Johnston 2006, Maciocia 2005, Wong et al. 2001, Wong, Sagar, and Sagar 2001). The integration of TCM into oncology practices has been a major research focus in China over the past decades. Hui et al. (2006) at UCLA extended this East-West integrative treatment to cancer patients in the United States. The authors utilized a patient-centered approach in cancer care to enhance efficacy of target therapies, prolong survival, decrease treatment side effects, and improve quality of life. TCM practitioners, in particular, recognize the role that psychosocial factors play in the etiology of diseases; therefore, they offer assistance to patients' emotions and stress management, in addition to biomedical regimens. TCM's global diagnosis and pathophysiological therapeutic approach to the entire patient thus have profound implications for cancer care practices (Hui et al. 2006). Wong et al. (2001) summarized the supportive role of TCM in cancer care by suggesting that TCM may supplement the deficiencies in the current biomedical model. By integrating TCM treatments into conventional cancer regimens, TCM is able to support patients in their biological response, psychoneuroimmunological function, symptom control, and psycho-spiritual well-being. Altogether, the synergic effect of TCM and Western Medicine can potentially increase patients' survival, while improving their quality of life.

Another major research effort worldwide is to foster common ground communication between TCM and Western Medicine. The goal is to develop an integrative approach linking the diagnostic theory and therapeutic method of traditional practice that is measurable by biomedicine. Pattern classification, which is also referred to as syndrome differentiation, is a key concept in TCM diagnosis. Hsiao, Tsou, Wu, Lin, and Chang (2008) proposed a statistical validation method to measure the performance of TCM in respect to the clinical endpoints for Western Medicine. This method uses numerical evaluation to determine the accuracy and precision of TCM assessment that is reported in qualitative terms. In another paper, Lu, Jiang, Zhang, and Chan (2012) demonstrated an evolving evaluation of integrative medicine in China. TCM information such as symptoms, signs, tongue appearance and pulse feeling are incorporated into biomedical disease diagnosis for a more comprehensive assessment. The TCM pattern classification method further categorizes patients into treatment sub-groups to determine treatment efficacy. Since TCM and Western Medicine are founded on different principles and fundamental theories, a combined diagnosis could lead to new findings in biomedicine.

The systemic structure of biomedicine has imposed substantial influence on standardizing TCM. Some areas of standardization focus on syndrome differentiation and herbal medicine. Wei, Ji and Zheng (2009) presented the concept of integrating the diagnoses of disease and relevant TCM syndromes. They proposed using clinical epidemiological methods, through study design, measurement and evaluation in population-based samples to standardize TCM research approach. In addition, the authors suggested using systemic biology as a guiding principle to strengthen an unequivocal diagnostic technique. Kung and Tsim (2006) discussed the modernization of TCM from the prospect of Western Medicine. Pharmaceutical drugs are subjected to international standards during production and processing. The authors agreed that the production and processing of herbal materials should also meet these standards, including Good Manufacture Practice (GMP), Good Clinical Practice (GCP), and Good Laboratory Practice (GLP). This is to ensure the reliability and safety of herbal treatments as well as more standardized results in clinical settings. The authors also advocated for Good Agricultural Practice of Medicinal Plants and Animals (GAP) for a robust management system for TCM development. Movements of these standardization approaches will lead TCM to a more recognizable and scientifically valid medical system in the near future.

Conclusion

Traditional Chinese Medicine, with a history of over 3,000 years and of having nurtured a nation that represents one-fifth of the world population, demonstrates a promising future in Western nations. Although TCM is rigorously scrutinized for its treatment efficacy based on the standard of biomedical science, the process toward developing TCM as an evidence-based medicine is legitimate for better healthcare development. Currently, TCM in the United States is heavily market-driven; it becomes a serious concern when consumer safety is directly involved. Even though numerous clinical studies examining its therapeutic effects are available, debates persist among field experts due to low quality of research design (Ernst 2012, White 2012, Ernst, Lee, and Choi 2011, Manheimer and Berman 2011, Henke 2011). In 2010, the European Union funded the first consortium dedicated to TCM research (Uzuner et al. 2012). This worldwide collaborative effort offers a systemic structure aiming to enhance good practice, set priorities, resolve challenges, and explore opportunities for TCM. The consortium represents a stepping stone for TCM to further promote health and healthcare to all.

The holistic approach of TCM has shed light on future healthcare. Its whole-person, person-centered therapeutic principles resemble the concept of individualized treatments in Western Medicine. Whether all health-related outcomes of this multi-foci strategy can be adequately assessed by current scientific methods remain questionable (Paterson et al. 2009). Nevertheless, the topic of integrative medicine has become a widely discussed subject in public, and in the field of medicine. In China, this bicultural medical system is already in practice in many hospitals and clinics in the last two decades. In the United States, the decision on using TCM continues to be a personal choice. Fortunately, consumers have easy access to data from trusted scientific sources. Knowing its potential dangers and benefits, TCM users can make informed decisions while others may take further precaution by discussing with their physicians.

In summary, the development of TCM in the United States is an ongoing and challenging process. Investing more research dollars in TCM to consolidate its true effect is a hotly debated topic. A practical concern for users is whether one should wait until TCM is fully validated before using it or if one should give it a try when other treatments fall short. If a person experiences therapeutic results, his or her story becomes another testimony toward the value of TCM as a healing approach in modern medicine.

References

Ahn, A. C., Q. Ngo-Metzger, A. T. R. Legedza, M. P. Massagli, B. R. Clarridge, and R. S. Phillips. 2006. "Complementary and Alternative Medical Therapy Use among Chinese and Vietnamese Americans: Prevalence, Associated Factors, and Effects of Patient–Clinician Communication." *American Journal of Public Health* 96(4): 647–653. doi:10.2105/AJPH.2004.048496

AHRQ. 2003. *Acupuncture for the Treatment of Fibromyalgia.* Rockville, Maryland: The Agency for Healthcare Research and Quality, Center for Practice and Technology Assessment. http://www.quackwatch.com/03HealthPromotion/fibromyalgia/ahrq.pdf

Braverman, C., C. Baker, and R. Harris. 2009. "Acupuncture and Oriental Medicine (AOM) in the United States" (*The American Acupuncturist* 47:22). http://www.aaaomonline.info/aom_in_us.pdf

Burke, A., T. Kuo, R. Harvey, and J. Wang. 2008. "An International Comparison of Attitudes toward Traditional and Modern Medicine in a Chinese and an American Clinic Setting." *Evidence-Based Complementary and Alternative Medicine: eCAM.* doi:10.1093/ecam/nen065

Burke, A., D. M. Upchurch, C. Dye, and L. Chyu. 2006. "Acupuncture Use in the United States: Findings from the National Health Interview Survey." *Journal of Alternative and Complementary Medicine* 12(7): 639–648. doi:10.1089/acm.2006.12.639

California Health Interview Survey. 2007. *CHIS 2009 Adult Public Use File. Release 1 [computer file].* Los Angeles, CA: UCLA Center for Health Policy Research.

Caring Connection. 2009. *Chinese Community Outreach Guide.* National Hospice and Palliative Care Organization. http://www.caringinfo.org/i4a/pages/index.cfm?pageid=3385

Cassidy, C. M. 1998. "Chinese Medicine Users in the United States. Part II: Preferred Aspects of Care." *Journal of Alternative and Complementary Medicine* 4(2): 189–202.

Chan, C. W., and J. K. Chang. 1976. "The Role of Chinese Medicine in New York City's Chinatown." *The American Journal of Chinese Medicine* 4(1): 31–45.

Chang, J. 1999. "Scientific Evaluation of Traditional Chinese Medicine under DSHEA: A Conundrum. Dietary Supplement Health and Education Act." *Journal of Alternative and Complementary Medicine* 5(2): 181–189.

Chen Jr., M. S. 1995. "Keynote Address of the Seventh International Conference on the Health of Chinese in North America: Health Status of Chinese Americans: Challenges and Opportunities." *Asian American and Pacific Islander Journal of Health* 3(1): 8–16.

Chen, X., H. Zhou, Y. B. Liu, J. F. Wang, H. Li, C. Y. Ung, L. Y. Han, et al. 2006. "Database of Traditional Chinese Medicine and Its Application to Studies of Mechanism and to Prescription Validation." *British Journal of Pharmacology* 149(8): 1092–1103. doi:10.1038/sj.bjp.0706945

Cheung, F., Y. Feng, N. Wang, M. F. Yuen, Y. Tong, and V. T. Wong. 2012. "Effectiveness of Chinese Herbal Medicine in Treating Liver Fibrosis: A Systematic Review and Meta-Analysis of Randomized Controlled Trials." *Chinese Medicine* 7 (1): 5. doi:10.1186/1749-8546-7-5

Chiu, J., T. Yau, and R. J. Epstein. 2008. "Complications of Traditional Chinese/Herbal Medicines (TCM)—A Guide for Perplexed Oncologists and Other Cancer Caregivers." *Supportive Care in Cancer* 17: 231–240. doi:10.1007/s00520-008-0526-x

The Cochrane Collaboration - Cochrane Reviews. 26 August 2012. http://www.cochrane.org/cochrane-reviews

Dong, X., E. S. Chang, E. Wong, B. Wong, K. A. Skarupski, and M. A. Simon. 2011. "Assessing the Health Needs of Chinese Older Adults: Findings from a Community-Based Participatory Research Study in Chicago's Chinatown." *Journal of Aging Research* doi:10.4061/2010/124246

Dower, C. 2003. "Acupuncture in California." *UCSF Center for the Health Professions.*

Eisenberg, D. M., M. H. Cohen, A. Hrbek, J. Grayzel, M. I. V. Rompay, and R. A. Cooper. 2002. "Credentialing Complementary and Alternative Medical Providers." *Annals of Internal Medicine* 137(12): 965–973.

Eisenberg, D. M., R. B. Davis, S. L. Ettner, S. Appel, S. Wilkey, M. Van Rompay, and R. C. Kessler. 1998. "Trends in Alternative Medicine Use in the United States, 1990–1997." *JAMA: The Journal of the American Medical Association* 280 (18): 1569–1575. doi:10.1001/jama.280.18.1569

Eisenberg, D. M., E. S. J. Harris, B. A. Littlefield, S. Cao, J. A. Craycroft, R. Scholten, P. Bayliss, et al. 2011. "Developing a Library of Authenticated Traditional Chinese Medicinal (TCM) Plants for Systematic Biological Evaluation—Rationale, Methods and Preliminary Results from a Sino-American Collaboration." *Fitoterapia* 82 (1): 17–33. doi:10.1016/j.fitote.2010.11.017

Ernst, E. 2004. "Are Herbal Medicines Effective?" *International Journal of Clinical Pharmacology and Therapeutics* 42(3): 157–159.

Ernst, E. and A. Fugh-Berman. 2002. "Complementary and Alternative Medicine: What is It All about?" *Occupational and Environmental Medicine* 59(2): 140–144. doi:10.1136/oem.59.2.140

Ernst, E., M. S. Lee, and T. Y. Choi. 2011. "Acupuncture: Does it Alleviate Pain and Are There Serious Risks? A Review of Reviews." *Pain* 152(4): 755–764. doi:10.1016/j.pain.2010.11.004

Ernst, Edzard. 2012. "Acupuncture: What Does the Most Reliable Evidence Tell Us? An Update." *Journal of Pain and Symptom Management* 43(2): e11–e13. doi:10.1016/j.jpainsymman.2011.11.001

FDA. 2012. "CFR - Code of Federal Regulations Title 21. Sec. 880.5580 Acupuncture Needle." http://www.accessdata.fda.gov/scripts/cdrh/cfdocs/cfCFR/CFRSearch.cfm?fr=880.5580

Food and Drug Administration. 2006. "Guidance for Industry on Complementary and Alternative Medicine Products and Their Regulation by the Food and Drug Administration." U.S Department of Health and Human Services.

Hanks, A. K. 2000. *Cancer and Traditional Chinese Medicine - Treating the Side Effects of Chemotherapy and Radiation with traditional Chinese Herbs.* Seattle, WA: Eastland Press. http://www.eastlandpress.com/resources/

Harris, E. S. J., S. D. Erickson, A. N. Tolopko, S. Cao, J. A. Craycroft, R. Scholten, Y. Fu, et al. 2011. "Traditional Medicine Collection Tracking System (TM-CTS): a Database for Ethnobotanically Driven Drug-Discovery Programs." *Journal of Ethnopharmacology* 135(2): 590–593. doi:10.1016/j.jep.2011.03.029

Henke, C. 2011. "Response to the Article of Ernst et al. 'Acupuncture: Does it Alleviate Pain and Are There Serious Risks? A Review of Reviews.'" *Pain* 152:755–764; *Pain* 152(9): 2183–2184; author reply 2184–2186. doi:10.1016/j.pain.2011.05.011

Hon, C. C., Y. C. Chow, F. Y. Zeng, and F. C. C. Leung. 2003. "Genetic Authentication of Ginseng and Other Traditional Chinese Medicine." *Acta Pharmacologica Sinica* 24(9): 841–846.

Hsiao, C.-F., H. H. Tsou, Y. J. Wu, C. H. Lin, and Y. J. Chang. 2008. "Translation in Different Diagnostic Procedures—Traditional Chinese Medicine and Western Medicine." *Journal of the Formosan Medical Association, Taiwan Yi Zhi,* 107(12 Suppl): 74–85.

Hsu, M. 2006. "Comparison of Asian Populations during the Exclusion Years." Summer Institute 2006, University of Delaware. http://www.udel.edu/readhistory/resources.html

Huff, R. M., and M. V. Kline. 1998. *Promoting Health in Multicultural Populations: A Handbook for Practitioners.* SAGE Publications.

Hui, K. K. 1999. "Harmonizing Traditional Chinese and Modern Western Medicine: A Perspective from the US." Traditional and Modern Medicine: Harmonizing the Two Approaches. WHO Consultation Meeting in Beijing: Regional Office for the Western Pacific. http://www.ceWestern Medicine.med.ucla.edu/research/publication.html

Hui, K. K., J. L. Yu, and L. Zylowska. 2002. "The Progress of Chinese Medicine in the USA." *The Way Forward for Chinese Medicine,* edited by K. Chan and H. Lee. CRC Press. Boca Raton, FL: CRC Press.

Hui, K.-K., E. K. Hui, and M. F. Johnston. 2006. "The Potential of a Person-Centered Approach in Caring for Patients with Cancer: A Perspective from the UCLA Center for East-West Medicine." *Integrative Cancer Therapies* 5(1): 56–62. doi:10.1177/1534735405286109

Institute of Community Health and Research. 2007. *Community Health Needs and Resource Assessment: An Exploratory Study of Chinese in NYC.* New York: NYU School of Medicine. http://asian-health.med.nyu.edu/dissemination/community -reports

Jabbour, M., M. Sapko, D. Miller, L. M. Weiss, and M. Gross. 2009. "Economic Evaluation in Acupuncture: Past and Future." *The American Acupuncturist* 49: 11–18.

Jang, M., E. Lee, and K. Woo. 1998. "Income, Language, and Citizenship Status: Factors Affecting the Health Care Access and Utilization of Chinese Americans." *Health and Social Work* 23(2): 136–145.

Kung, S. D., and K. W. K. Tsim. 2006. *Modernization of Traditional Chinese Medicine – A prospect from Western Medicine.* Hong Kong: Joint Publishing (HK) Co., Ltd.

Lam, C. N. 2010. *Use of Traditional Chinese Medicine among Chinese Americans in San Francisco.* San Diego State University, San Diego, CA. http://sdsu-dspace .calstate.edu/handle/10211.10/315

Lassiter, S. 1995. *Multicultural Clients: A Professional Handbook for Health Care Providers and Social Workers* (1st ed.). Westport, CT: Greenwood.

Lee, M. M., S. S. Lin, M. R. Wrensch, S. R., Adler, and D. Eisenberg. 2000. "Alternative Therapies Used by Women with Breast Cancer in Four Ethnic Populations." *Journal of the National Cancer Institute* 92(1): 42–47. doi:10.1093/jnci/92.1.42

Lee, M. M. and J. M. Shen. 2008. "Dietary Patterns Using Traditional Chinese Medicine Principles in Epidemiological Studies." *Asia Pacific Journal of Clinical Nutrition* 17 Suppl 1: 79–81.

Li, S. S. 2007. "Commentary—the Proteomics: A New Tool for Chinese Medicine Research." *The American Journal of Chinese Medicine* 35(6): 923–928.

Li, Y.-M. 2009. "Ten challenging issues in the clinical research of Chinese medicine." [Zhongguo Zhong xi yi jie he za zhi Zhongguo Zhongxiyi jiehe zazhi]. *Chinese Journal of Integrated Traditional and Western Medicine* [Zhongguo Zhong xi yi jie he xue hui, Zhongguo Zhong yi yan jiu yuan zhu ban] 29(5): 389–391.

Lin, F. 2005. "A Cross-Sectional Study of Socio-Cultural and Health Determinants of Complementary and Alternative Medicine Use by Chinese Patients with Mental Health Needs in an Urban Primary Care Setting." (Ph.D. Dissertation, Columbia University, New York.)

Liu, C., and R. M. Douglas. 1998. "Chinese Herbal Medicines in the Treatment of Acute Respiratory Infections: A Review of Randomised and Controlled Clinical Trials." *The Medical Journal of Australia* 169(11–12): 579–582.

Lu, A., M. Jiang, C. Zhang, and K. Chan. 2012. "An Integrative Approach of Linking Traditional Chinese Medicine Pattern Classification and Biomedicine Diagnosis." *Journal of Ethnopharmacology* 141(2): 549–556. doi:10.1016/j.jep.2011.08.045

Lum, O. n.d.. *Clinics of Geriatric Medicine: Ethnogeriatrics* 2(1): 53–67.

Ma, G. X. 1999. "Between Two Worlds: The Use of Traditional and Western Health Services by Chinese Immigrants." *Journal of Community Health* 24(6): 421–437.

Maciocia, G. 2005. *The Foundations of Chinese Medicine: A Comprehensive Text for Acupuncturists and Herbalists.* (2nd ed.). London: Churchill Livingstone.

Manheimer, E., and B. M. Berman. 2011. Letter to the Editor in response to: Ernst E, Lee MS, Choi TY. "Acupuncture: Does It Alleviate Pain and Are There Serious Risks? A Review of Reviews." *Pain* 152:755–764; *Pain 152*(9): 2179–2180; author reply 2184–2186. doi:10.1016/j.pain.2011.04.009

Manheimer, E., A. White, B. Berman, K. Forys, and E. Ernst. 2005. "Meta-Analysis: Acupuncture for Low Back Pain." *Annals of Internal Medicine 142*(8): 651–663.

Mayeno, L., and S. M. Hirota. 1994. "Access to Health Care." In *Confronting Critical Health Issues of Asian and Pacific Islander Americans,* edited by N. W. S. Zane, D. T. Takeuchi, K. N. Young, 347–375. Thousand Oaks, CA: Sage Publications.

Miltiades, H. B. and B. Wu. 2008. "Factors Affecting Physician Visits in Chinese and Chinese Immigrant Samples." *Social Science and Medicine 66*(3): 704–714. doi:10.1016/j.socscimed.2007.10.016

National Alliance on Mental Illness. 2011. *Mental Health Issues among Asian American and Pacific Islander Communities.* NAMI Multicultural Action Center. http://www.nami.org/Template.cfm?Section=ResourcesandTemplate=/ContentManagement/ContentDisplay.cfmandContentID=21026

National Center for Complementary and Alternative Medicine (NCCAM). 2010. *Traditional Chinese Medicine: An Introduction.* National Institutes of Health, U.S. Department of Health and Human Services.

NCCAM. 2010. *Acupuncture: An Introduction.* National Institutes of Health: National Center for Complementary and Alternative Medicine. http://nccam.nih.gov/health/acupuncture/introduction.htm

NCCAM. 2011. *Acupuncture for Pain.* National Institutes of Health: National Center for Complementary and Alternative Medicine. http://nccam.nih.gov/health/acupuncture/introduction.htm

NICOS. 2004. *Chinese Community Health Report Summary.* NICOS Chinese Health Coalition. http://www.nicoschc.org/projects.html

NIH. 1998. "NIH Consensus Conference. Acupuncture." *JAMA: The Journal of the American Medical Association 280*(17): 1518–1524.

Pagán, J. A., and M. V. Pauly. 2005. "Access to Conventional Medical Care and the Use of Complementary and Alternative Medicine." *Health Affairs (Project Hope)* 24(1): 255–262. doi:10.1377/hlthaff.24.1.255

Pang, E. C., M. Jordan-Marsh, M. Silverstein, and M. Cody. 2003. "Health-Seeking Behaviors of Elderly Chinese Americans: Shifts in Expectations." *The Gerontologist 43*(6): 864–874.

Parekh, H. S., G. Liu, and M. Q. Wei. 2009. "A New Dawn for the Use of Traditional Chinese Medicine in Cancer Therapy." *Molecular Cancer 8*(1): 21. doi:10.1186/1476-4598-8-21

Paterson, C., C. Baarts, L. Launsø, and M. J. Verhoef. 2009. "Evaluating Complex Health Interventions: A Critical Analysis of the 'Outcomes' Concept." *BMC*

Complementary and Alternative Medicine 9(1): 18. doi:10.1186/1472-6882 -9-18

Paterson, C. and P. Dieppe. 2005. "Characteristic and Incidental (Placebo) Effects in Complex Interventions Such as Acupuncture." *BMJ* (Clinical research ed.) 330(7501): 1202–1205. doi:10.1136/bmj.330.7501.1202

Pearl, W. S., P. Leo, and W. O. Tsang. 1995. "Use of Chinese Therapies among Chinese Patients Seeking Emergency Department Care." *Annals of Emergency Medicine* 26(6): 735–738.

Pittler, M., N. Abbot, E. Harkness, and E. Ernst. 2000. "Location Bias in Controlled Clinical Trials of Complementary/Alternative Therapies." *Journal of Clinical Epidemiology* 53(5): 485–489. doi:10.1016/S0895-4356(99)00220-6

Prensky, W. L. 1995. "Reston Helped Open a Door to Accupuncture." *The New York Times*. New York. http://www.nytimes.com/1995/12/14/opinion/l-reston -helped-open-a-door-to-acupuncture-011282.html

Sadler, G. R., K. Wang, M. Wang, and C. M. Ko. 2000. "Chinese Women: Behaviors and Attitudes toward Breast Cancer Education and Screening." *Women's Health Issues: Official Publication of the Jacobs Institute of Women's Health* 10(1): 20–26.

Shang, A., K. Huwiler, L. Nartey, P. Jüni, and M. Egger. 2007. "Placebo-Controlled Trials of Chinese Herbal Medicine and Conventional Medicine—Comparative Study." *International Journal of Epidemiology* 36(5): 1086–1092. doi:10.1093/ije/dym119

Srivastava, K. D., C. Qu, T. Zhang, J. Goldfarb, H. A. Sampson, and X. M. Li. 2009. "Food Allergy Herbal Formula-2 Silences Peanut-Induced Anaphylaxis for a Prolonged Posttreatment Period via IFN-γ–Producing CD8+ T Cells." *Journal of Allergy and Clinical Immunology* 123(2): 443–451. doi:10.1016/j.jaci.2008.12.1107

Su, D., and L. Li. 2011. "Trends in the Use of Complementary and Alternative Medicine in the United States: 2002–2007." *Journal of Health Care for the Poor and Underserved* 22(1): 296–310. doi:10.1353/hpu.2011.0002

Tabora, B. L., and J. H. Flaskerud. 1997. "Mental Health Beliefs, Practices, and Knowledge of Chinese American Immigrant Women." *Issues in Mental Health Nursing* 18(3): 173–189.

Tang, J. L., S.-Y. Zhan, and E. Ernst. 1998. "Review of Randomised Controlled Trials of Traditional Chinese Medicine." *BMJ* 319 (7203): 160–161. doi:10.1136/bmj.319.7203.160

Tom, L. A. S. H. n.d. *Health and Health Care for Chinese-American Elders*. University of Hawaii. http://www.stanford.edu/group/ethnoger/chinese.html

Ung, C. Y., H. Li, C. Y. Kong, J. F. Wang, and Y. Z. Chen. 2007. "Usefulness of Traditionally Defined Herbal Properties for Distinguishing Prescriptions of Traditional Chinese Medicine from Non-Prescription Recipes." *Journal of Ethnopharmacology* 109(1): 21–28. doi:10.1016/j.jep.2006.06.007

University of Maryland. 2001. *A New Profile of Chinese Americans in a New Century*. Asian American Studies Program, University of Maryland.

U.S. Census Bureau. 2012. "Facts for Features and Special Editions: Facts for Features: Asian/Pacific American Heritage Month: May 2012." http://www.census .gov/newsroom/releases/archives/facts_for_features_special_editions/cb12 -ff09.html

Uzuner, H., R. Bauer, T. P. Fan, D. A. Guo, A. Dias, H. El-Nezami, T. Efferth, et al. 2012. "Traditional Chinese Medicine Research in the Post-Genomic Era: Good Practice, Priorities, Challenges and Opportunities." *Journal of Ethnopharmacology* 140(3): 458–468. doi:10.1016/j.jep.2012.02.028

Wade, C., M. T. Chao, and F. Kronenberg. 2007. "Medical Pluralism of Chinese Women Living in the United States." *Journal of Immigrant and Minority Health / Center for Minority Public Health* 9(4): 255–267. doi:10.1007/s10903-007 -9038-x

Wei, H. F., G. Ji, P. Y. Zheng. 2009. "Study of Standardization of Syndrome Diagnosis: An Analysis of Current Status." *Journal of Chinese Integrative Medicine* 5(2): 115–121.

White, A. 2012. "Acupuncture: What does the Most Reliable Evidence Tell Us? A Correction." *Journal of Pain and Symptom Management* 43(5). doi:10.1016/j. jpainsymman.2012.02.002

Wong, L. K., P. Jue, A. Lam, W. Yeung, Y. Cham-Wah, and R. Birtwhistle. 1998. "Chinese Herbal Medicine and Acupuncture. How Do Patients Who Consult Family Physicians Use These Therapies?" *Canadian Family Physician (Médecin de Famille Canadien)* 44: 1009–1015.

Wong, R., C. M. Sagar, and S. M. Sagar. 2001. "Integration of Chinese Medicine into Supportive Cancer Care: A Modern Role for an Ancient Tradition." *Cancer Treatment Reviews* 27(4): 235–246. doi:10.1053/ctrv.2001.0227

Wong, W., L. K. C. Lam, R. Li, S. H. Ho, L. K. Fai, and Z. Li. 2011. "A Comparison of the Effectiveness between Western Medicine and Chinese Medicine Outpatient Consultations in Primary Care." *Complementary Therapies in Medicine* 19(5): 264–275. doi:10.1016/j.ctim.2011.07.001

Wu, A. P. W., A. Burke, and S. LeBaron. 2007. "Use of Traditional Medicine by Immigrant Chinese Patients." *Family Medicine* 39(3): 195–200.

Xue, X., T. Wang, Y. Zhang, J. Wang, G. Li, M. Zheng, Y. Zhao, et al. 2009. "Construction of Effectiveness Evaluation System for Traditional Chinese Medicine Interventions in Subhealth." *Zhong Xi Yi Jie He Xue Bao [Journal of Chinese Integrative Medicine]* 7(3): 201–204.

Yee, B., and G. Weaver. 1994. "Ethnic Minorities and Health Promotion: Developing a "Culturally Competent" Agenda" *Generations* 18 (1): 39–45.

Young, A. 1999. "A Study of Herbal Medicine Usage among Chinese Patients in Boston." *Between Heaven and Earth: An Introduction to Integrative Approaches to Health Care* (2nd ed., 18–20). American Medical Student Association. http:// www.amsa.org/AMSA/Libraries/Committee_Docs/heavenearth.sflb .ashx

Zhang, Y., L. Lao, H. Chen, and R. Ceballos. 2012. "Acupuncture Use among American Adults: What Acupuncture Practitioners Can Learn from National

Health Interview Survey 2007." *Evidence-Based Complementary and Alternative Medicine, vol. 2012:* 1–8. doi:10.1155/2012/710750

Zou, J., H. F. Shi, and Y. M Cai. 2008. "Epidemiologic Study on Basic TCM Syndrome in the Subhealth Population in the Zhengzhou Area." [Zhongguo Zhong Xi Yi Jie He Za Zhi Zhongguo Zhongxiyi Jiehe Zazhi]. *Chinese Journal of Integrated Traditional and Western Medicine* [Zhongguo Zhong Xi Yi Jie He Xue Hui, Zhongguo Zhong Yi Yan Jiu Yuan Zhu Ban] 28(7): 610–613.

CHAPTER TEN

Curanderismo: A Complementary and Alternative Approach to Mexican American Health Psychology

Jesse N. Valdez

The purpose of this chapter is to present *curanderismo* (a healing system) that incorporates the essence of its foundation with a parallel perspective from traditional folk medicine, health psychology, and the use of complementary and alternative medicine (CAM). *Curanderismo* belongs to a system of healing known by several names. Traditional, indigenous, or folk medicine are a few of the more well-known terms used. Traditional medicine includes knowledge and practices within different cultures in our current world and before the beginning of modern medicine.

The origin of *curanderismo* in the Americas can be traced back to the 15th and 16th centuries when Spain discovered and conquered the indigenous peoples of the New World. After liberation from Spain, newly formed countries of the Americas continued many of the Spanish traditions, including folk medicine. Mexican *curanderismo* is the precursor to the *curanderismo* that is practiced in the United States by Mexican immigrants and those who chose to become American citizens after the 1848 Treaty of Guadalupe Hidalgo (Griswold del Castillo 1990). Later Mexican immigration continued to keep *curanderismo* alive. *Curanderismo* as a system of traditional health care used by recent Mexican immigrants and Mexican Americans currently living in the United States will be examined.

Curanderismo and History

Folk and traditional medicine are well known and have been used in Europe and other parts of the world such as Africa, China, India, and Middle Eastern countries. Immigrants from different parts of the world bring their healing systems with them when they immigrate to America. Those who came as conquerors, *los conquistadores*, from Spain, for example, brought their own systems of medicine but also traditional healing systems (Foster 1953). Settlers from Western Europe such as the English also brought their own healing practices and medicine as practiced in old Europe during the 17th and 18th centuries (Hand 1980). These traditional medical practices were combined and integrated with New World American indigenous healing systems.

Spanish medical knowledge along with Spanish folk medical practices, were brought to America during the conquest (Foster 1953). When the Spanish arrived in Mexico, the Aztec civilization had developed theories about the etiology of illness, including physical and mental health. Health care providers specialized in diagnostics and treatment of disorders. Some of their treatment interventions had features that resemble modern techniques and interventions and their use of herbs and plants for medical purposes was advanced beyond Europe's (Padilla 1984). A blending of Spanish and indigenous medical practices began to occur when the indigenous healers borrowed what they believed to be superior medicine from the Spanish. The Spanish also developed an interest in indigenous healing practices and rituals (Foster 1953).

The then modern Spanish medicine consisted of the Greek Hippocratic humoral theory of four wet or dry, hot or cold humors. A disequilibrium in the humoral qualities caused illnesses. Spanish medicine also included the Arabic concept of health as a balance among all the individual's life domains in addition to Judeo-Christian beliefs and practices (Mulcahy 2010, Lucero and Velásquez, 1981).

Modern Curanderismo

The integrated traditional medicine practices have survived alongside modern medicine and are still used by current populations. Different ethnic groups will tend to use traditional practices based on their traditions and culture (Ortega-López 2006). These widespread healing systems, in some cases, are the only form of health care available in certain parts of the world (WHO 2008). *Curanderismo* is a way that *mejicanos* (Mexicans) and Mexican Americans communicate about illness and life problems. The Mexican culture, as influenced by indigenous and European healing systems, developed a system of health care for *la gente* (the people), *los mejicanos,* and the Mexican American community (Del Castillo 1998).

Mexicans and other Central and South American immigrants bring healing practices such as *curanderismo* to the United States. *Curanderismo* has been used extensively, especially by recent immigrants. As the immigrants socialize and acculturate into the American middle-class culture—Mexican Americans, for example—*curanderismo* may be used along with biomedical practices. Succeeding generations, especially as they move into the mainstream middle-class, move toward using modern alternative medical practices.

The well-educated, higher income level Mexican Americans, heavily socialized into the modern U.S. American culture, are unlikely to consider folk-practitioners. While there is little or no research to support this view, exceptions consist of anecdotal reports of urban healers (Avila 1999). One can examine this view from the perspective of early Americans with old-country traditional ties and with no access to medicine or medical practitioners, who were likely to have to resort to folk remedies (Hand 1980). Many used published sources from Europe since there was no medical service available (Hand 1980). Today's immigrants who come to America from traditional and rural regions, who begin their Americanization journey at the lower end of our economic ladder, still using their native language, adhering to their traditional religious practices, and those who have little formal education, find it necessary to use their traditions, including folk medical practices, in our modern industrialized country.

Thus, one must consider the factors that are necessary to support a rationale for the use of folk medicine and put such views in a proper context to understand the use of folk medicine in today's American society.

Description of the System: The Healing Model

Curanderismo, unlike modern biomedicine, does not separate the mind from the body. A spiritual dimension is acknowledged and addressed in the treatment of mental, emotional, and physical disorders in addition to the common life stressors and daily hassles. It also addresses the external environment and the individual within the natural world (Avila 1999). Nature is very much part of *curanderismo* and thus explains that treatment includes natural materials originating from or maintained by the earth such as plants, fruit, herbs, minerals, and animal products. In addition to those materials, other natural resources such as water, fire, and smoke, the natural cycles of the earth that include seasons, months, weeks, and days of the week, the sun (light of day), and moon (nocturnal darkness) are integrated into healing rituals.

Curanderismo has a collectivistic focus that does not separate the individual from his/her social and personal culture. The individual's family, community, society, and therefore culture, are included within the treatment and healing rituals. The individual is the focus of the treatment, but the family and the community are considered essential elements and are included whenever possible (Lucero and Velázquez 1981).

Holistic

A holistic approach that includes the physical, mental, spiritual, social, religious, cultural, and natural dimensions aims to achieve a balance among all the elements of the individual's life and experience with that of the natural and the supernatural. Thus, *curanderismo* encompasses entire dimensions that are not addressed by modern healing systems. It is this holistic approach that makes *curanderismo* attractive to different populations, especially those that are dissatisfied with the results of modern medicine and the brief and quick-paced for-profit practice of modern physicians. Other characteristics of modern medicine that makes it unattractive to *mejicanos* is that it is separated by specialties, at times requiring multiple appointments and referrals to different providers at different places. *Curanderismo* uses a holistic model that addresses the entire individual. Elena Avila stated, "In Western medicine the body goes to the hospital, the mind to the psychiatrist, and the soul and spirit to church. In *curanderismo,* the healing takes place under one roof" (Avila 1999, 29).

Religion

Other essential elements of the culture such as religion serve as a foundation and avenue to the spiritual and supernatural plane. Similar to the American indigenous tradition of accepting both the natural and spiritual world as one (Sanchez, Plawecki, and Plawecki 1996), it is common to imbed healing within the spiritual element. When religion, both Catholic and Protestant, is used as a base, it introduces religious faith and the metaphysical. Thus, there is no separation between the natural and the supernatural. The power of God and Christian saints are therefore seen as a central element in the healing process (Applewhite 1995, Treviño-Hernández 2005, Foster 1953). *Curanderismo* is a healing system that actively incorporates the individual's faith and belief systems that come from their religious and spiritual beliefs and traditional cultural practices (Trotter and Chavira 1981, Alegria, Guerra, Martinez, and Meyer 1977).

Factors Supporting Curanderisimo

Although *curanderismo* is considered to be folk medicine without substantial evidence that is it an effective healing system, its use has persisted for hundreds of years. Historical and sociocultural factors are among some of the factors that contribute to the continued use of folk medicine *curanderismo*.

New and recent immigrants, especially those from rural areas and lower socioeconomic status, continue to maintain their traditions. *Curanderismo* is one of those traditions.

There are objective indicators that American society's character is changing due to the continued influx of new immigrants (Carlson 1994, Kazarian and Evans 2001). This influx of new immigrants will be a factor that will continue to sustain the existence and use of traditional medicine including *curanderismo* (Garces, Scarinci, and Harrison 2006; Leclere and Lopez 2012).

Another factor that contributes to *curanderismo's* existence is its availability in many ethnic communities. Knowledge of home remedies contributes to availability of healing practices that does not involve having to expose oneself to the American bureaucratic system. The seriousness of an illness is another factor. If an illness is perceived to be within a *curandera/o's* treatment expertise, the folk healing system is used (Young and Garro 1982). The use of folk healers can also be influenced by a family's lower level of income (Higginbotham, Treviño, and Ray 1990).

When patients are dissatisfied with and refuse treatment by medical physicians, they seek the assistance of *curanderas* (female healers) *or curanderos* (male healers). This is more typical of low socioeconomic status recent immigrants. In this manner, *curanderismo* fills a void and serves as a backup system whereby the patient is at least being cared for by someone who may eventually encourage and convince them, perhaps with the help of the family, to seek western medical treatment. Dissatisfaction with health care provided by biomedicine, faith and trust, and perceived benefits of *curanderismo,* in addition to the spiritual and religious aspects are other important sustaining factors of *curanderismo* (Young and Garro 1982).

Dissatisfaction with mainstream medicine is polite way of accepting responsibility for not using such services. Underneath the dissatisfaction lies the unspoken reality uncovered by research. Researchers have identified determinants and barriers to health care services use by Mexican Americans and Latina/os (Anderson et al. 1981). Health disparities due to discrimination and repression leads to the avoidance of biomedicine and an increased reliance on *curanderismo* (MacLachlan 1997, Young and Garro 1982).

In other cases, when problems are not of a medical or psychological nature but more of a quality of life issue or due to common daily life hassles, individuals will also seek help from *curanderas/os* (curanderas and/or curanderos). When situations appear to be beyond the individual's control, *curanderismo* is used to help them deal with job loss, legal issues, government policy issues, and even threats to their identity (de la Portilla 2009). The Mexican culture thus guides individuals with life problems toward what is considered a source of relief, *curanderismo* (Ortega-López 2006).

Alternative and Comparative Curanderismo

From a multicultural health psychology perspective, in order to understand *curanderismo* the influence of socioeconomics, socioenvironment, and other community factors of health need to be applied. In many cases topics about multicultural issues are presented as if the topic has no connection to our society. Such topics are viewed as foreign and therefore strange and unknown. The result is a wide gap in our ability to understand. It is because the topic is viewed as coming from a foreign culture with no connection to our culture. This cognitive gap of understanding results in little or no understanding. The perspective is based on a cross-cultural model—two separate and distinct cultures with one assuming a dominant role and the other placed in an inferior position.

A multicultural perspective is one that is within the same place and the same shared environment. Multiple cultures interact with each other on a continuous basis. Cultures have a reciprocal effect on each other resulting in more complex social environments. The environment, context, and ecological systems are integrated into a traditional model of health psychology. Relevant multicultural factors, perspectives, and traditions are integrated. According to MacLachlan (1997), within coexisting cultures and subcultures, issues related to religion, gender, and theoretical, research, and practice exclusion, health disparities, and economical, oppression, discrimination, racism, and other factors that impact diverse and multicultural populations are integrated and expanded within multicultural health psychology. In addition, an attempt to understand *curanderismo* without understanding its patients and what they bring with them, may lead to significant misinterpretation and a confused understanding of its meaning. Molina, Zambrano, and Aguirre-Molina (1994) point out those moderator variables that impact health such as socioeconomic status, the patient's environment, and the community's culture which need to be considered.

It is also common for specific folk practices of certain regions and cultural groups to reciprocate and incorporate and borrow from one another (Clark, Bunik, and Johnson 2010). For example, one of *curanderismo's* goals is to have a person achieve a holistic balance among their physical, mental, spiritual, and natural life dimensions. The concept of wholeness and balance is common in other traditional healing systems such as those of American indigenous populations (Cervantes 2008) and other societies throughout history (Kazarian and Evans 2001). Balance is also a concept that is receiving some attention in western models of mental health. Lipworth, Hooker, and Carter (2011) state that "Balance is a powerful, culturally recognized concept related to living the best possible life, with profound effects on the ways in which people view, experience, and respond to their health-related circumstances" (15).

An American form of folk healing can also help clarify the meaning of *curanderismo*. *Curanderismo* can be understood from the perspective of Appalachian folk medicine (Cavender 2003), folk medicine of Europe and America (Hand 1980, Hatfield 2004), traditional medicine as practiced by African Americans (Mitchen 2007), and Native Americans (Campbell 1995, Sanchez et al 1996). Thus, *curanderismo* is not as uncommon or unusual as one would expect. Several American multicultural subgroups of our society have kept the traditions of folk medicine alive.

Curandersimo as Traditional Folk Medicine

The World Health Organization (WHO 2008) defines traditional medicine as health practices that use materials from multiple sources, spiritual interventions, along with manual exercises, to assess, treat, and prevent both physical and mental illnesses and to help individuals maintain physical and mental health.

Applewhite (1995) states that "folk healing is defined broadly as a set of health beliefs and practices derived from ethnic and historical traditions that have as their goal the amelioration or cure of psychological, spiritual, and physical problems" (28). Traditional medicine and folk healing systems have a long tradition in the United States and the world. These health care systems have been in use for hundreds of years and in some cases thousands of years. For example, it is well known that medicine derived from plants has always been an integral part of traditional medicine. Today's pharmaceuticals have developed medicine derived from plants to the degree that a significant percentage of current medications now derive from such sources. Traditional medicine has relied on nature and its practitioners have always known of its effectiveness in providing relief to their patients. Thus, today's biomedicine can claim that it has roots in traditional medicine as practiced by folk healers for ages in different parts of the world.

In addition to the use of natural plant ingredients to develop pharmaceuticals, many of the traditional medicine healing practices are now being integrated into modern medicine. Comparative and alternative medical practices such as acupuncture and herbal remedies are now part of mainstream medical treatments (Astin 1998, Johnson et al. 2012, Grzywacz et al. 2005). Traditional folk healing systems and traditional health care systems of medicine from around the world are being integrated into the health system of the World Health Organization (WHO). According to WHO (2008) traditional medicine and folk healing have spread beyond traditional cultural groups and are being called alternative or complementary medicine.

Curanderismo is both alternative and complementary medicine. *Curanderismo* is alternative medicine when a client is seen by a *curandera/o* who includes the person's energy, spirit, and religious beliefs in treatment without referral to or in conjunction with biomedicine. *Curanderismo* is complementary when a *curandera/o* treats a client with traditional *curanderismo* and also refers to and works in conjunction with biomedicine.

Prevalence of Curanderismo

Research that addresses the extent of usage of *curanderismo* is sparse. However, in the Mexican American communities, the practice of Mexican folk medicine continues to exist and is practiced by *curanderas* and *curanderos* not only in small rural communities but also in urban areas. However, it is difficult to guage the actual extent and use of *curanderismo* because *curandera/o's* presence is kept underground and undisclosed to the public (Applewhite 1995). A *curanderismo* researcher, de la Portilla (2009) indicated that although she communicated with healers and implemented the use of a survey, she could not estimate the number of *curanderas/os* in San Antonio, Texas (de la Portilla 2009). Research is inadequate due to poor research design. Accurate or at least useable documentation of rates of use are not available.

The Healers

Curanderismo literature usually provides a stereotypical portrayal of *curanderas/os* (Lucero and Velásquez 1981). There is a tendency to describe a *curandera/o* with simplistic and general terms that address only a limited range of values and characteristics (Lucero and Velazquez 1981). There are, however, more realistic portrayals. For example, Harris, Velásquez, White, and Renteria (2004) state that "*Curanderas/os* are considered very important and special persons within many Chicana/o communities throughout the United States. They are revered and respected for their role as healers, spiritual advisors, wise persons, and counselors" (115). Lucero and Velázquez (1981) present *curanderas* and *curanderos* as individualistic practitioners who have few unifying characteristics. There are regional differences. Backgrounds are diverse in terms of socioeconomic status, training, experience, treatment methods, and specialty areas.

Trotter and Chavira (1981) indicate that "*Curanderas/os* are the preeminent curers, analogous to physicians, who treat tradition folk illnesses and a variety of psychologically and socially disruptive complaints in the Mexican American community" (72). Others compare a *curandera/o* to a psychiatrist (Torrey 1986). Alegria, et al. (1977) see *curanderas/os* as general practitioners. On the other hand, these views of *curanderos* as professional medical providers move on a continuum to where just about anyone can participate in the profession of folk healers. Such a view is supported by Treviño-Hernández (2005), who claims that "A *curandero* can be anyone who prays and uses herbs to help others" (9).

Comparisons to biomedical professionals or common people in the street are inadequate. They compare a limited range of expertise that *curanderas/os* have, such as being able to establish a therapeutic counseling relationship (Avila 1999) or within a narrow range of physical treatment such as *sobadores* (bone setters). However, to accurately define Mexican/Mexican American *curanderas/os*, the range of *curanderismo's* specialties within the material and natural levels such as *curandera/o total* (professional or total *curandera/o*), *llerbera/o* (herbalist), *señora* (lady), etc., must be accurately understood.

Curanderas/os' expertise and ability extends beyond the material and the natural to the realm of the supernatural level. *Curanderas/os* who practice beyond the beginning levels are less apparent to the general public. For the more advanced folk healers, religion serves as a foundation for their healing (both Catholic and Protestant). God, saints, and holy individuals are considered the sole source of healing (Treviño-Hernández 2005). They are spiritual advisors able to address spiritual issues and some can make use of the supernatural for healing purposes (Harris et al. 2004). Skills and abilities of these healers are comparable to those who are clairvoyant and who have the ability and skills of mediums (Alegria et al. 1977). Thus, comparisons to physicians, psychiatrists, and community and family members, are inaccurate if the enormity of skills and expertise are not considered.

Abilities and range of practice descriptions identify large and extensive areas of expertise. Those who practice beyond the level of family members, *señoras* (ladies), *herbologists* (herbalists), and *sobadores* (massagers) include *curanderas/os* who work with serious physical ailments such as diabetes, asthma, and terminal cancer. *Curanderas/os* not only treat physical disorders, they are involved in addressing and resolving difficult social problems such as marital conflicts, family disruptions, issues about love, business, or home life, and conflicts in business partnerships. They can create supportive relationships similar to what is done in counseling relationships (Avila 1999).

Psychological disorders such as depression and anxiety and other major disorders such as conversion hysteria and thought disorders are part of their treatment areas (Arenas, Cross, and Willard 1980). *Curanderas/os* are also involved in helping people deal with *mal puestos* (hexes, curses) which from a psychological point of view can be considered different types of schizophrenia and related thought disorders (Roberts 1984,Trotter and Chavira 1981). It is apparent that these are wide-ranging, diverse, and different areas. While some *curanderas/os* employ a holistic perspective in their treatments and work at different levels of competency— not all disorders can be treated by a single *curandera/o.* There are specialties within *curanderismo* whereby different healers work and specialize in different disorders.

Curandersimo Specialty Types

Curanderismo is a healthcare system that includes *curanderas* and *curanderos,* but there are other specialists who operate within limited specialty areas only. Just as there are different types of medical specialties that are not practiced on a one size fits all modality, *curanderismo* also has different specialties that are used according to level of competence, specialty area, and client presenting problems.

Professional or Curandera/o Total

A *curandera/o total* (professional *curandera/o*) treats physical, social, psychological, and spiritual problems using curing techniques or a combination of techniques that are specific to their practice. Others can be distinguished by their specific practice of different levels of healing the material, spiritual, and mental (Del Castillo 1998, Trotter and Chavira 1981). A *curandera/o total* also works as an educator, advisor, consultant, and herbalist (Avila 1999).

The Specialists

Beyond the level of *curandera/o total,* there are different types of traditional practitioners divided according to specialty area. Although some of these specialty practitioners are identified as *curanaderas/os,* some may accept the title (some do not) but practice within mainly one or two specialty areas. They do not perform the total range of medicine or *curanderismo* healing systems and levels. These specialists are known for their skills and unique treatment techniques in treating certain disorders (Lucero and Velázquez 1981).

Consejera/o (advisor; counselor). All *curanderas/os* use *pláticas* (heart-to-heart talks) in their work; *consejeras* or *consejeros* specialize in counseling clients on a broad variety of issues.

Yerbero/a or **llerbero/a** (herbalist). *Yerberos* are herbalists and make extensive use of herbs and home remedies (Roberts 1984, Treviño-Hernández 2005). A *yerbero* may have competence in using herbs for medicinal practice but may not have the competence to work with a client dealing with other problems. Disorders of the gastrointestinal system may be treated by a *yerbero* since the focus of treatment may be on *empacho* (gastrointestinal problems) with the use of teas made of special herbs.

Partera (midwife). *Parteras* are lay midwives who usually have a fairly extensive knowledge of both mainstream and folk medicine. Some serve as adjuncts to obstetrical care in some areas. Some are professional and advertise their services; some are affiliated with physicians. The practice is regulated in some states and *parteras* are licensed as midwives (Roberts 1984, Alegria et al. 1977).

Sobador/a or **huesero/a** (person who massages; bone setter). *Sobadores* function as folk chiropractors who treat physical ailments using massage to relieve pain. A *huesero* is someone who does spinal adjustment and sets dislocated joints (Avila 1999). They administer *masajes* (massages) for generalized pain or nervous tension and *sobaditas* (little massages) for specific problems such as a sprains or cramps (Roberts 1984).

Señoras (ladies) are respected for their folk remedies. They are usually sought out by clients within their own neighborhood or community for curing mild ailments. *Señoras* have slightly higher status than the "women of the house" or family members who use home remedies. *Señoras* tend to be older women of a family (grandmothers, aunts) who are viewed as someone who can heal due to their knowledge of folk remedies and practices (Lucero and Velázquez 1981). Some *señoras* may also be professional readers of cards and use decks of cards to make predictions about the lives of clients in different area such as health, home life, social relations, and legal and business matters (Lucero and Velázquez).

Médica (medical healer). Lucero and Velásquez (1981) identify a *médica* as someone who practices medicine in their healing practices. These are usually individuals who have medical training such as nurses who can prescribe medicine in addition to home remedies (Alegria et al. 1977).

Espiritualista (spiritualist). A trance medium who works at the spiritual level. These healers are not very common now in the United States but common in other countries such as Mexico. Trotter and Chavira (1981) indicate that a *espiritualista* has the power to produce a link between this and the other world. The treatment revolves around spirit beings that inhabit another plane of existence. These healers enter a trance and act as a medium that establishes a line of communication between the client and the spiritual world (Trotter and Chavira 1981).

Urban Curanderas/os

Another category of healers is one that is now blended with modern medicine and to some extent the practice of modern psychological principles. This type of *curanderismo* is the one that is used in urban areas. There are *curanderas/os* that do not fit the profile of the older neighborhood *curandera* or *curandero* found in small communities and rural regions. Although a popular view maintains that most are middle aged women, modern *curanderas* are educated and middle class. Some may have backgrounds in related health fields such as nursing and have mental health training and degrees (Avila 1999). De la Portilla (2009) describes one *curandera* as "Aida, 31, successful business woman and mother" (69).

Secular Saints

Secular saints are not religious saints acknowledged by the Catholic Church but have a special place in *curanderismo* and are considered saints by the people and known as folk saints. They are individuals who have the power of God or other holy and supernatural entities to heal and cure. Two well-known folk saints are Don Pedrito Jaramillo and el Niño Fidencio. Originally from Mexico, Don Jaramillo had a large following during his lifetime of healing in Southwest Texas. *Fidencistas,* followers of el Niño

Fidencio, channel the healing power of el Niño Fidencio as part of their healing (Torres 2005).

Competence Levels

There are different levels of competence according to how the practitioner entered the practice, source of training, type of training, assessment skill level, treatment skill level, issues, problem, or type of disorder. There does not seem to be a division of practice according to type of population served. Categorization by interests, experience, training, and specialty practice can be used to organize *curanderas/os* within different levels of competence. Levels of competence are also determined by level of education, how much time is invested in the practice, how many clients are served per day, and sometimes by where they practice. Trotter and Chavira (1981) divide the practice of *curanderismo* into three levels.

Trotter and Chavira's levels are the material, the natural, and the supernatural. The level of competence increases with each level. At the material level, family members and *las señoras* (ladies) predominate. It is the primary level that is practiced by family members such as the mother, father, a relative, or someone who is well known in the community. Most of the specialists such as *yerberos* and *sobadores* work at the natural level. A *curandera/o total* can practice at all levels but unlike the other *curanderas/os*, they may have the skills of a medium who can work at the supernatural or spiritual level.

Profit or Non-Profit Services

There is also a division of *curanderas/os* by whether their practice is non-profit or if they charge for their services, or if they aim to make a profit by services provided. The genuineness of the *curanderas/os* is determined not by how much they charge but whether they charge at all. Clients appear to know that the "real" *curanderas/os* have a "sliding fee" scale and clients pay according to how much they can pay— from nothing to whatever they want to give.

The decision to charge may be determined according to the source of their power to heal. If their healing powers come directly from God, then the expectation is that they are to serve society without any self-interest at all. Other *curanderas/os* who have a more modern perspective believe that services should be provided for a fee since the *curandera/o* has expenses to maintain their practice (Avila 1999).

Practice Settings

Traditionally, *curanderas/os* have a special area in their homes where they practice, with an altar, candles, pictures of saints, and the Lady of Guadalupe (Alegria et al. 1977). Some of the more recent practitioners of *curanderismo* have what could be considered a physician's office—complete with a desk, massage table, medical books, and the model of a skeleton (Mull and Mull 1983, de la Portilla 2009). Other practice settings range from a temporally arranged space in a family's home to more elaborately decorated and designated private space in the home for healing purposes (Alegria et al. 1977). Most work at home and have convenient hours for people who work during the day and need flexibility in their hours to see a healer (Avila 1999). The flexibility in hours and convenience of the healer's setting is one reason why the services of folk healers are used more in comparison to the rigid schedules of professional physicians.

How They Become Healers

Family Tradition

Some individuals enter the practice due to the influence or encouragement of someone in their immediate or extended family, circle of acquaintances, friends, or community members. Their skill level and treatment areas are elementary and focus on minor illnesses according to well-known and very common cultural syndromes such as *empacho* (gastrointestinal disorder), and *mal de ojo* (bad or evil eye) (Treviño-Hernández 2005).

El "Don"—Gift from God

Divine power is accessed by a vision, a calling, or a dream. It is believed that divine power gives the needed therapeutic healing skills but only a minority of *curanderas/os* reported having acquired skills through divine vision (Del Castillo 1998). On the other hand, Treviño-Hernández (2005) indicates that "The belief that the power to heal comes from God is something that all *curanderos* believe" (9).

Avila (1999) challenges the popular belief, including that of Treviño-Hernández (2005), that all *curanderas/or* are born with a "don"—a gift from God. She considers a somewhat different view of the "gift from God." Individuals are indeed born with the ability to help others heal. However, this ability is very similar to a talent that individuals are born with, whether it is musical, athletic, or intelligence.

Self-Selection

Other individuals choose to become *curanderas/os* of their own desire. Their life goal is to give and serve others. These individuals "feel that it is their obligation and responsibility to help those who seek treatment and thus frequently extend their practice beyond the bounds of family, friends, and neighborhood" (Lucero and Velázquez 1981, 5).

Cultural Syndromes, Types of Disorders: What Curanderos Treat

Folk medicine refers to healing practices and ideas of the body and health maintenance that is known to members of a culture, spread informally as general knowledge, and practiced by members of the culture who have prior practice experience (WHO 2008). *Curanderismo* falls within the realm of traditional and folk medicine as practiced by traditional folk healers.

The most common type of conditions treated by practicing *curanderas/ os* include *empacho* (intestinal and stomach distress), *mal de ojo* (bad or evil eye), *and susto* (fright). These problems have a strong emotional component to them and some believe that they are caused by culturally associated situations (Harris et al. 2004).

Curanderas/os treat problems that can be categorized as emotional and somatic illness. For some patients it is natural to process emotional problems through somatization. *Curanderas/os* can be of help for such patients. The use of ritual prayer, massage, and reassurance can provide relief for what often turn out to be long-term complaints with a lot of psychosocial features (Harris et al. 2004).

Some of the specific cultural syndromes treated by *curnaderas/os* include the following:

Bilis. Bile; "gall, bitter secretion stored in the gall bladder" (McElroy and Grabb 2012, 24). Anger or suppressed anger is believed to be the cause of this illness and "symptoms are too much bile, gas, constipation, sour taste in mouth" (Campbell 1995, 68). Such a syndrome could be related to gallbladder problems—a physical disorder. Many *curanderas/os* interpret the *bilis* symptoms as a psychological disorder.

Caida de mollera. Defined as "*Hundamiento en la mollera o fontanela de la cabeza del bebé*" (sinked formation in a child's fontanel of its head) (Kemper, 1998, 79). While *curanderas/os* and the Mexican American public considered the cause to be dropping the baby, a swollen fontanel is viewed as possible symptoms of encephalitis and meningitis (Kemper 1998, 153). *Caida de mollera* is also considered to be a symptom of grave dehydration (79) or "baby dehydration" (Campbell 1995, 68).

Empacho. Defined as "blockage of the stomach, or the digestive track; also any kind of block to emotion or energy of the body" (Avila 1999,61). *Empacho* is considered to be "a type of indigestion or gastrointestinal infection that afflicts children and adults caused by an interaction between physiological and social factors. Stomach pains are attributed to intestinal blockage and fever that causes thirst and stomach bloating" (Falicov 1999, 107).

Mal de Ojo (commonly called the evil eye). The belief that social relationships contain inherent harm to the health of an individual, usually a child. "*Mal de ojo*" is not caused by a person who wants to hurt someone. It is done by one who admires a person, especially if it's an infant or child. If the admiring person does not touch or caress the admired child, the child becomes ill with *mal de ojo.* The antidote is physical contact, a touch, or hug (Treviño-Hernández 2005).

Mareo (dizziness). A form of dizziness, or simple anxiety or nervousness (Falicov 1999).

Nervios (nerves). A general state of distress connected to life's trials and tribulations; also describes a specific syndrome that includes headaches, sleep difficulties, trembling, tingling and *mareo,* a form of dizziness, or simple anxiety or nervousness (Falicov 1999).

Ataque de nervios (nervous attack). A sense of being out of control with dissociative experiences, seizure-like or fainting episodes, hyperventilation, crying spells, or shouting. Victims may experience amnesia. More common in women and people in lower SES (Falicov 1999).

Susto (fright; aka *Espanto*). The most universal trait of the belief is that *espanto* is thought to result from a magical fright through which the victim loses his soul. The soul thereafter remains captive or wanders aimlessly. "Suffering from traumatic encounter or shock. When the person *'se asusta'* suffers from shock—the good spirit leaves—the person is weak without protection—illness enters" (Treviño-Hernández 2005, 21). *Susto* is also regarded as a behavioral discord resulting from a combination of stressful events and the ineffective coping of the person in trying to meet social expectations.

Mal puesto (hex or witchcraft). A condition that does not fit with any other disorder and that is long lasting due in part to resistance to treatment (Falicov 1999).

Locura (psychotic disorder). A term used by Latina/os in the United States and Latin America. Although commonly used by Mexican Americans in the U.S. Southwest, it is very uncommon in the *curanderismo* literature.

Diagnoses and Etiology: Sources of Disorders and Problems Theory

Curanderismo does not follow a unified diagnostic system. One point of view is that there is an "immense variation in classification of illnesses and their symptoms, diagnosis, treatment techniques, and etiological explanations" (Lucero and Velázquez 1981, 5). Avila (1999) states that "*Curanderos* believe that it is not enough to heal the body, they must heal the wounded soul as well" (41). This holistic approach that includes working with a patient's soul puts some *curanderas/os* in a position where they are reluctant to label the disorder a mental illness (Arenas et al. 1980). While there is a diagnostic process in *curanderismo*, Avila (1999) claims that the use of a diagnosis will restrict a person's ability to heal.

Curanderas/os have a theoretical or philosophical perspective. For example, the following are statements made by *curanderas/os:* "Objects and materials contain energy; people can manipulate energy; the spiritual world and the physical are closely aligned and are in contact with each other; therefore, attitudes and state of mind can affect one's state of wellness" (de la Portilla 2009, 53).

Original theories of the causes of illness focused on God and religion. Illness was a result of having sinned or lack of faith (Arenas et al. 1980, Clark et al. 2010). These beliefs took root in sixteenth century Spain, when *sanadores* used their healing powers to provide medical help by patients thought to be ill due to supernatural causes (Tausilt 2009). Similar beliefs continue to influence people in today's society, especially among ethnic minorities but also in White individuals who still attribute the causes of illness to supernatural causes (Landrine and Klonoff 2001). The supernatural and religious aspects of the origin of health are congruent with the belief that health is the result of a balance between the spirit (*espíritu*), soul (*alma*), and body (*cuerpo*) (Zacharias 2006). The spiritual world is very much a part of a curanandera/o's diagnostic assessment of a person's illness. Clients are asked to talk about the spiritual system that they follow as part of the diagnostic phase (Avila 2009).

The original etiological theories have been impacted by biomedicine and psychology. Elena Avila (1999), a curandera and psychiatric nurse, states that "God does not make us sick. We get sick because we do not take care of ourselves, inherit an illness, or due to aging or atmospheric influence from an energy our body cannot resist (viruses, bacteria)" (21). Urban *curanderas/os* also use the theory of energy to explain problems. A San Antonio *curandera,* Lizzie, believes that illnesses are due to "negative energy, from bad luck; illness problems are passed among family members" (de la Portilla 2009, 86).

Disease is also attributed to stressful changes in the social world. It is believed that stress due to change disrupts the balance between the individual and environment. There are also changes in traditional norms and values, in addition to daily stresses in American urban life that affect the well-being of Mexican Americans especially. Although the family is seen as a source of support, there has been an increase in the absence of solid family support system, and general conflict between traditional and modern. Changes such as immigration to urban living are considered to be a cause of the breaking down of the family. The changing roles of women, changing standards of child socialization techniques, common social changes, are also all seen as factors in increasing susceptibility to illness (Arenas et al.1980, Kiev1968, Lucero and Velázquez 1981).

The World Health Organization's (2008) definition of traditional medicine includes the identification of and diagnoses of illnesses as cultural syndromes. Some believe that all societies, industrialized and nonindustrial ones, experience culture bound illness. For example, in the United States "going postal," and "Type A pattern behavior" could be considered American cultural bound syndromes (Clark, Bunik, and Johnson 2010).

Diagnostic Assessment

Curanderas/os conduct clinical assessments to help them determine and arrive at a diagnosis. Different diagnostic procedures are used. In the diagnostic phase of treatment, a healer may use divination (e.g., looking into a glass of clear water), or holding the patient's wrist to feel the pulse. The patient's pulse reveals more to the *curandera/o* than just the rate of heartbeat. Others may use clairvoyance abilities (Avila 1999). Mulcahy (2010), working with curandera Eva, stated that as her client described the multiple problems in his life, Eva "sees the multiple levels simultaneously: physical, mental, spiritual, and emotional" (38). *Curnaderas/os* can have insight into the ways a patient perceives their own illness within the context of their personal values. Treatment goals take these beliefs into consideration (Avila 1999).

The American Psychiatric Association's *Diagnostic and Statistical Manual of Mental Disorders* (DSM-IV-TR) (American Psychiatric Association 2000) is used to help clinicians arrive at a diagnosis in order to develop a treatment plan. The 2000 edition of the DSM-IV-TR includes "cultural syndromes" from different cultures throughout the world. The DSM format is criticized since the cultural syndromes are not used in any official diagnosis and are not included as part of the treatment. Although cultural syndromes are part of the DSM, they are in an appendix and are not used for anything significant (Harris et al. 2004). Others believe that the way the cultural syndromes are used implies that the conditions are not real or can be dismissed as exotic (Clark et al. 2010).

The Practice of Curanderismo

Although folk medicine and current biomedicine may have originated from similar healing roots thousands of years ago, within a set of health beliefs and practices derived from ethnic and historical traditions with the goal of easing the pain of psychological, spiritual, and physical problems (Applewhite 1995), the scientific practice of modern medicine is based on scientific investigation and research. Application and practice is governed by ethical and professional codes set up to protect the public from harm. The practice of *curanderismo* is in some minor aspects similar in its purpose, at least in its intent to heal individuals and restore them to health.

However, the practice of *curanderismo* is in many fundamental respects entirely different. It appears that *curanderismo* is difficult to place within modern models of medical treatment because it involves numerous different techniques, interventions, processes and different sources at many different levels. Although there may be some universal and fundamental aspects of healing that are used by folk healers, practitioners are independent, individualistic, and can create and borrow from whatever resources are available (Mulcahy 2010, de la Portilla 2009). Other than the moral, religious, and spiritual codes created by the more socially advanced societies, there are few legal or professional codes of ethics to guide treatment and protect the public. One important contribution from traditional folk medicine, however, can perhaps be considered as complementary and alternative healing avenues that can help attend to the illnesses and problems that biomedicine does not address or cannot reach.

Trotter and Chavira (1981) state that *curanderismos*, "...healing is an art that includes culturally appropriate methods of treatment delivered by recognized healers in the community who capitalize on a patient's faith and belief systems in the treatment process" (44). Avila (1999) states that "Treatment involves religion and spiritual belief of the *curandero*. It happens together with earth as the foundation and God as the source" (105).

Among the many treatments used by folk medicine and *curanderismo* are those that involve spiritual, symbolic, and sensory interventions. Treatments include healing rituals, applications of states of altered consciousness, therapeutic talk, sweat lodges, cleansing, and healing rituals (Clark et al. 2010). Confession, suggestion, prayer, and confrontation are additional treatments (Arenas et al. 1980). Massage, herbs, potions, and reassurance are used in the treatment of patients (Padilla et al. 2001). Practice involves using whatever is useful and available in treatment in an intuitive and creative way. The use of herbs, counseling, psychodrama, and spiritual cleansings, are acceptable treatment modalities. However, referral to medical doctors is always an option that healers consider when they assess that their treatments may not work (Avila 1999).

Mulcahy (2010) worked with Eva, a curandera, who said "I use the ninety-first psalm, the specialist for healing susto.The psalm: 'There shall no evil befall thee, neither shall any plague come nigh they dwelling/For he shall give his angels charge over thee, to keep thee in all my ways'" (39). According to Mulcahy, "Eva adds the native elements of using incense with little stones; you bring together the harmony of the four corners of the earth. Combining the biblical Word with indigenous beliefs in the earth's harmony highlights the syncretism that is central to the practice of a *curandera*" (40).

Curanderas Lizzie and Jo Ann teach people to pray. They "teach to pray to God out loud. . . . to talk openly and without fear of what is foremost on your mind and heart." . . . "The goal is for people to become self-reliant and self-sufficient. People need to acknowledge their own spirituality in order to move forward and to accomplish things in their lifetime." . . . "Not pay someone when they can do it themselves. . . . people can learn to heal themselves" (de la Portilla 2009, 86).

In some areas of practice, *curanderismo* is similar to modern-day practices. Folk healing practices within the realm of complementary and alternative medicine have been introduced and used within related health services. One type of *curandero* is the "*huesera/o*" (bone setter) or "*sobador/a*" who are *curanderas/os* who specialize in chiropractic and massage healing. They use a system of massage that is incorporated into the healing treatment. There are some *curanderas/os* that have their massage tables where they practice. Such equipment is now seen in *curanderas/os'* places of practice (Mull and Mull 1983).

Curanderismo and Empirical Research

Health psychology research has moved beyond descriptive models to a more direct approach toward including members of ethnic groups. However, including ethnic groups are used for group comparison purposes. Comparison of groups (e.g., African Americans and Asian Americans) results in assumptions that group membership can be used as a proxy for culture and ethnicity. All group participants are considered to be equal and homogeneous when only external group differences are considered. Within-group factors are ignored. This results in weak and perhaps even misleading research. More appropriate multicultural research needs to include psychological variables and variables that can be considered temporary measures at least.

Some researchers address questions regarding typical ethnic patient beliefs and behaviors only with ethnic research participants. Assumptions are made that if an illness or medical condition is included when collecting data from all participants, then some participants may endorse such illnesses more. Assumptions are also made that White individuals do not believe in or use spiritualism as part of their health beliefs or practices. Such questions or items are not included or addressed when collecting data from White research participants. However, when this is done, the research may be flawed. Research has indicated that research design is important. Participants will not endorse illness more if listed by researchers more because it was suggested by researchers. Research has also clearly indicated that Whites will endorse supernatural causes related to illness and health if such items are included in the data collection (Landrine and Klonoff 2001).

Most conceptual literature and research have examined *curanderismo* from anthropological, historical, and descriptive perspectives. The medical field has started to include some studies of *curanderismo* but again, it is descriptive in nature, reporting only frequencies and categories. Observation and the recording of what single individuals do and practice are descriptively recorded. There is little or no investigation with depth that allows a more revealing perspective that helps to understand the significant aspects of *curanderismo*.

Models used to investigate *curanderismo* are based on western models and pay no attention to sociocultural, historical, or stake holders' perspectives or input. Environmental and ecological factors are ignored. Issues related to oppression, discrimination, and racism are not considered. In any case, the minor attention paid to factors such as SES, gender, age, language spoken, composition of the samples used, and more significant variables such as acculturation is pointing the research in a more meaningful direction.

Landrine and Klonoff (1996) noticed a major weakness of their research: the lack of a measure of discrimination. Variables known to play a significant role in the health behaviors of all ethnic minority groups were not examined, namely, ethnic discrimination (Karlsen and Nazroo 2002, Landrine et al. 2006). These researchers pointed out that ethnic discrimination and segregation make up the larger social-structural context (Landrine and Klonoff 1996).

In order to understand *curanderismo,* the influence of socioeconomics, socioenvironment, and other community factors of health need to be applied. Direct effects of both SES and culture to avoid misinterpretation of the role of culture and class (poverty) on health need to be taken into account. There needs to be a search for cultural strengths that improve health and medical compliance of ethnic groups (Molina et al. 1994).

A significant factor that is missing in multicultural health psychology is *cultural validity.* Models used to investigate *curanderismo* are based on western models and pay no attention to stakeholders' perspectives or input. Environmental and ecological factors are ignored. Issues related to oppression, discrimination, and racism are disregarded. Minor attention paid to factors such as SES, gender, age, language spoken, and composition of the samples are not significantly integrated into data analysis and interpretation.

Functional equivalence, whether the values and behaviors have similar functions across cultures, is ignored. For example, assertiveness, showing pride, behaving for individualistic gain, are valued in mainstream White middle class America. However, these behaviors are frowned upon in more traditional Latina/o societies and communities. The behaviors' functions are dependent on the cultural setting (Quintana, Troyano, and Taylor 2001). Thus, rituals used in *curanderismo* have the function of providing a sense of wellbeing, but only in that cultural setting.

Conceptual equivalence is another factor that is disregarded in the study and understanding of *curanderismo.* Medicine and health are believed to mean something different than what modern biomedical treatment provides (Quintana et al. 2001). Many of the terms and concepts critical to understanding *curanderismo* have no conceptual equivalence in our modern middle-class American culture. The understanding of *curanderismo* may occur through the use of concepts relevant only to middle-class American culture through what is called *ethnocentrism. Ethnocentrism* results in a misunderstanding of what *curanderismo* means to people who depend on it for their healing.

CAM Research

Some recent research with complementary and alternative medicine (CAM) is including Latina/os and Mexican Americans as part of a diverse ethnic minority sample. Variables addressed include the use of *curanderos* (Hunt, Arar, and Akana 2000). Other CAM research focuses on the use of plants by Mexican Americans including the use of *aloe vera, nopal (prickly pear cactus)* for the treatment of diabetes and other conditions (Alarcon-Aguilara et al. 1998, Andrade-Cetto and Heinrich 2005).

Hunt et al. (2000) used a convenience sample of 43 low-income, low educated participants diagnosed with diabetes. Half of the sample chose to respond in Spanish. Using interviews, participants were asked questions such as "Have you ever used or heard of any other kinds of treatment for diabetes? Any home remedies or things like herbs or *curanderos*? Do you think that religion or your spiritual life can affect your health? Do you ever pray about your health or your diabetes?" (217). Sixty percent of the participants used herbs to treat their diabetes. Seventy-seven percent believed that God or prayer helped with diabetes. Only 15 percent (3 out of 20) ever used a *curandero*. Most of the participants, although they had heard about the use of herbs, did not use plants or herbs. The plant used most often by 39 percent of the sample was *nopal* (prickly pear); 31 percent used *aloe vera* and *nispero* (loquat leaves) and *ajo* (garlic) was used by fewer participants. Participants were more likely to use biomedicine rather than alternative methods. Results showed that if they were highly involved with alternative medicine, they were also highly involved with biomedical treatment. Regarding religion, rather than being fatalistic and abdicating care of their health to a higher power, many respondents said that God is important and they felt that God worked through the physicians and medications.

Curanderismo Research Recommendations

One psychological variable that is more appropriate is *ethnic identity* (Bernal and Knight 1993). An example of the use of ethnic identity is Gurung and Mehta's (2001) study of Asian physicians and their attitudes toward providing treatment to ethnic minority patients and toward alternative medicine. Their results indicated that a more pronounced ethnic identity was positively correlated to a favorable attitude toward providing treatment of ethnic patients and a favorable attitude toward alternative medicine. It is apparent that simply having a health provider with a similar ethnic background to the patients may not be effective. The more Westernized the healthcare provided, the less favorable were attitudes about treatment of ethnic patients and alternative treatments (Gurung and Mehta 2001).

Moderator Variables

While there are many psychological variables that can be used to increase the study of *curanderismo,* acculturation is presented here as an example of how different constructs can be used to explore other dimensions of *curanderismo.*

Research with acculturation has produced mixed and contradictory results. There is no consistent or standard way to assess and measure acculturation.

Most measures of acculturation do not measure the construct directly and are primarily proxy measures. There were disagreements about whether to include multiple factors of one-dimensional acculturation or whether to use single factors. For example, multiple factors included measurement of language, culturally relevant behaviors, and relationships with members of their ethnic group, and cultural values. Single factor proponents favored using generational level, preferred language usage, or place of birth. Some adhered to using demographic variables such as place of birth, preferred language use, and ethnic or racial group categories to measure acculturation.

Corral and Landrine (2008), in their study of health behavior with a sample of over 7,000 Mexican Americans used language and birth place as proxies for acculturation. They indicated that although such measures are the norm and are the sole measure of acculturation in population health surveys (e.g., CHIS, NHANES), they are limited in their capacity to capture the complexity of acculturation.

Effectiveness Research

Research has been conducted to determine if traditional medicinal herbs and plants have appropriate chemical ingredients that contribute to the plants' effectiveness. For the most part many of the current plants have not been found to have chemical properties that may contribute to the treatment's effectiveness. However, some empirical research has shown that traditional medicinal herbs can be effective and can provide relief of some clinical conditions. For example, research found that three traditional herbs used for many years by the Chinese have significant impact on the relief of depression (Xu, Luo, and Tan, 2004). Hunt, et al. (2000) reported that results of scientific laboratory research with humans and animals show that some plants such as *nopal* decrease serum glucose levels.

Beyond the Realm of Science: Magic and Witchcraft

Curanderismo is also viewed by some as something that involves magic and witchcraft (Falicov 1999). However, *curanderismo*, black magic, and doing harm appears to contradict the meaning of *curanderismo*—a healing system. *Curanderismo* is understood as a process to heal and to provide wellness and health and includes a religious aspect (Treviño-Hernández 2005). It is unlikely that religion, at least the Christian faith, is used to cause harm. Most of the rituals and the term *curanderismo* come from the Spanish word *curar* which means to cure or *sanar,* to heal. It is important to keep this definition in mind when learning about *curanderismo*. Therefore, there is little if any room in *curanderismo* for witchcraft with a harmful intention.

Not all *curanderismo* involves rituals and the supernatural. Many individuals are treated by some of the *curanderismo* specialties, such as a *sobador*, a healing procedure that does not involve any of the usual props such as prayers or eggs. *Sobadores* use massage and manipulate nerve points. The treatment is more like alternative medicine and not magic or witchcraft (Campbell 1995). Professional-style massage tables are usually part of medical equipment used for *sobadas* (massages) in semi-professional practice settings (Mull and Mull 1983).

Witchcraft and magic have remained part of *curanderismo* since a number of researchers and writers include such phenomena as a significant part of *curanderismo*. Trotter and Chavira, well-known anthropologists, who wrote *Curanderismo*, include magical problems as part of the *curandera/o's* role. They state that "For psychological, spiritual, or magical problems, the curanderos frequently combine the herbs, objects, and rituals into a special cure (*curación*) designed to eliminate a specific problem" (Trotter and Chavira 1981, 63). Concepts such as magic and witchcraft are difficult if not impossible to consider as part of modern and scientific medicine. Such concepts distance *curanderismo* from mainstream health care systems.

The perspective of having healers and witches intermingling with each other may come from the precursors of curanderos—the *saludadores*. In sixteenth century Spain, *saludadores* were known for, among a number of other powers, their healing powers. They were the ones who were called to help those who had been the target of a witch's evil eye. In this early period, *saludadores* and witches were separate and opposing sources of good versus evil (Tausilt 2009).

The separation of good and evil appears to have eroded the understanding of the healing purpose of *curanderismo*. Or perhaps it is because a minority of healers accept patients that believe they have been hexed. However, the majority have either not heard of *brujeria* (witchcraft) as being part of *curanderismo* (Avila 1999), or just flatly refuse to treat patients with witchcraft beliefs (Alegria et al. 1977).

Avila (1999), a well-known *curandera* and author, stated: "Personally, I have never had any experience, don't know any *brujos* (witches) who do things. Many academic people claim they do. I have never met anyone who used materials such as grave dirt and makes up evil spells to put in people" (27). Avila goes on to say that she knows from experience that "there are *curanderas/os* who take money from people, sometimes thousands of dollars and tell the clients they will do magic to remove the curse" (27). She also believes that "there are people who are as evil as the so-called *brujos* who supposedly caused the curse" (Avila 1999, 28).

Future of Curanderismo

Curanderismo is now included in CAM. If *curanderismo* continues to be viewed as traditional medicine and as an alternative healthcare system for Mexican Americans, then it can be predicted that *curanderismo* will continue to thrive—at least various components such as that of the *sobadores* (bone setters) and *yerberos* (herbalists). Surveys and descriptive research have also revealed that there is a segment of the American population that believes and practices holistic medicine including spiritualism. Thus, the mystical and spiritual part of *curanderismo* is bound to continue to be in demand if it is practiced in response to the demand of Americans.

Western medicine's and people's attention to complementary and alternative medicine (CAM) has lasted for a long time and has increased in recent times. There is now a process that appears to integrate traditional medicine and practices with CAM. There is a blending of practices that are now seen as outside of western scientific medicine but are used with healing practices to support health and wellness of society. Thus, *curanderismo,* as traditional medicine, especially the use of herbs, plants, and massage, can complement other healing practices.

Psychology, from a scientific point of view, does not help students or professionals fully comprehend the meaning or purpose of *curanderismo*. One of psychology's objectives, among other things, is to understand behavior in order to help people. The scientific method is used and an experimental model must be used. Results and outcomes must be measureable. Outcomes cannot be measured because they are not objective, e.g., subjective feelings. Psychological constructs are developed and theories are used to place these constructs within the reach of an experimental model. There needs to be something that can be measured. Scales are constructed based on the definition of the construct. The outcome of measurement is a quantitative number. These numbers can be analyzed using probability and inferential statistics. Experiments must be conducted according to specific procedures and standardized methodology. The intent is that the experiment must be conducted in a way that it can be replicated by others.

Healing systems such as *curanderismo* do not fit into the scientific method or experimental design because it includes a religious, spiritual, and supernatural perspective. Most of the literature also includes magic and witchcraft as a part of *curanderismo* and *curanderas/os* are seen as witches by some. The spiritual and supernatural are mystical and cannot be observed, much less measured. It cannot be quantified. Therefore, traditional healing systems such as *curanderismo* may be difficult to understand from a scientific point of view.

An even more difficult hurdle is the religious aspect that includes addressing and asking the power of God and saints to help heal a person. The popular literature, the media, and to some extent, our academic world have portrayed *curanderismo* as being "magic" and something that involves sorcery and witches. Therefore, psychology and *curanderismo,* as a whole, may be difficult if not impossible to connect and integrate. Some components of *curanderismo* such as the use of herbs and plants fit into what is already being used as part of healing systems.

Alegria et al. (1977) saw *curanderismo* as being difficult to integrate with modern medical practices due to the *curandero's* lack of education. They recommended the maintenance of the *curandero's* current practices along with training of curanderos to become knowledgeable about community resources and basic facts about symptoms related to major medical disorders (Alegria et al. 1977). While *curanderismo* may not be fully accepted by biomedicine and the modern medical establishment, its popular use will certainly continue due to the need of many of its multicultural consumers. Folk healing has endured for hundreds and thousands of years. It is likely that *curanderismo* will continue to thrive, in part because it is indispensible for many members of our society who lack access to mainstream health care due to health disparities. Multicultural health psychology and multicultural behavioral health can be a significant part of helping those Americans who believe in and use *curanderismo* in their daily lives.

Curandersimo and similar traditional healing systems need to be viewed from a multicultural health psychology perspective. Openness to what is similar and universal as opposed to what is different and foreign is necessary. Similarities and commonalities in healing systems can help ease the understanding and eventual acceptance of what may be beneficial to many within the broad expanse of several cultural systems.

References

Alarcon-Aguilara, F. J., R. Roman-Ramos, S. Perez-Gutierrez, A. Aguilar-Contreras, C. C. Contreras-Weber, and J. L. Flores-Saenz. 1998. "Study of Anti-Hyperglycemic Effect of Plants Used as Antidiabetics." *Journal of Ethnopharmacology* 61: 101–110.

Alegria, D., E. Guerra, C. Martinez Jr., and G. G. Meyer. 1977. "El Hospital Invisible: A Study of Curanderismo." *Archives of General Psychiatry* 34(11): 1354–1357.

American Psychiatric Association. 2000. *Diagnostic and Statistical Manual of Mental Disorders* (4th ed., text revised.). Washington, DC: Author.

Anderson, R., S. Lewis, A. L. Giachello, L. U. Aday, and G. Chiu. 1981. "Access to Medical Care Utilization among the Hispanic Population of the Southwestern United States." *Journal of Health and Social Behavior* 22: 7889–7905.

Andrade-Cetto, A. and M. Heinrich. 2005. "Mexican Plants with Hypoglycemic Effect Used in the Treatment of Diabetes." *Journal of Ethnopharmacology* 99: 325–348.

Applewhite, S. L. 1995. "Curanderismo: Demystifying the Health Beliefs and Practices of Elderly Mexican Americans." *Health and Social Work* 20(4): 247–253.

Arenas, S., H. Cross, and W. Willard. 1980. "Curanderos and Mental Health Professionals: A Comparative Study on Perceptions of Psychopathology." *Hispanic Journal of Behavioral Sciences* 2(4): 407–421.

Astin, J. A. 1998. "Why Patients Use Alternative Medicine: Results of a National Study." *JAMA* 279(19):1548–1553.

Avila, E. 1999. *Woman Who Glows in the Dark: A Curandera Reveals Traditional Aztec Secrets of Physical and Spiritual Health.* NY: Jeremy P. Tarcher/Putman.

Bernal, M. E., and G. P. Knight, eds. 1993. *Ethnic identity: Formation and Transmission among Hispanics and Other Minorities.* Albany, NY: State University of New York Press.

Campbell, R. C. 1995. *Two Eagles in the Sun.* Las Cruces, NM: EDITTS Publishing.

Carlson, A. W. 1994. "America's New Immigration: Characteristics, Destinations, and Impact, 1970–1989." *The Social Science Journal* 31(3): 213–236.

Cavender, A. 2003. *Folk Medicine in Southern Appalachia.* Chapel Hills, NC: The University of North Carolina Press.

Cervantes, J. M. 2008. "What is Indigenous about Being Indigenous: The Mestiza/o Experience." In *Latina/o Healing Practices,* edited by B. W. McNeill and J. M. Cervantes, 3–27. New York: Routledge.

Clark, L., M. Bunik, and S. Johnson. 2010. "Research Opportunities with Curanderos to Address Childhood Overweight in Latino Families." *Qualitative Health Research* 20(1): 4–14.

Clark, L., A. Colbert, J. H. Flaskerud, J. Glittenberg, P. Ludwig-Beymer, A. Omeri, and R. Zoucha. 2010. "Culturally Based Healing and Care Modalities." In *Core Curriculum in Transcultural Nursing and Health Care* [Supplement], edited by M. K. Douglas and D. F. Pacquiao. *Journal of Transcultural Nursing* 21(Suppl. 1): 236S–306S. doi:1177/1043659610382628

Corral, I. and H. Landrine. 2008. "Acculturation and Ethnic Minority Health Behavior: A Test of the Operant Model." *Health Psychology* 27(6): 737–745.

Davies, R. E., K. E. Peterson, S. K. Rothschild, and K. Resnicow. 2011. "Pushing the Envelope for Cultural Appropriateness." *The Diabetes Educator* 37(2): 227–238.

De la Portilla, E. 2009. *They All Want Magic: Curanderas and Folk Healing.* College Station, TX: Texas A&M University Press.

Del Castillo, R. 1998. "The Life History of Diana Velazquez: *La Curandera Total.*" In *La Gente: Hispano History and Life in Colorado,* edited by V. C. de Baca, 222–240. Denver, CO: Colorado Historical Society.

Falicov, C. J. 1999. "Religion and Spiritual Folk Traditions in Immigrant Families. Therapeutic Resources with Latinos." In *Spiritual Resources in Family Therapy,* edited by F. Walsh, 104–120. New York: The Guilford Press.

Foster, G. M. 1953. "Relationship with Spanish and Spanish-American Folk Medicine." *Journal of American Folklore 66*: 201–217.

Garces, I. C., I. C. Scarinci, and L. Harrison. 2006. "An Examination of Sociocultural Factors Associated with Health and Health Care Seeking among Latina Immigrants." *Journal of Immigrant Health 8*: 377–385. doi 10/1007/s 10903-006 -9008-8.

Griswold del Castillo, R. 1990. *The Treaty of Guadalupe Hidalgo: A Legacy of Conflict.* Norman: University of Oklahoma Press.

Grzywacz, J. G., W. Lang, C. Suerken, S. A. Quandt, R. A. Bell, and T. Arcury. 2005. "Age, Race, and Ethnicity in the Use of Complementary and Alternative Medicine for Health Self-Management: Evidence from the 2002 National Health Interview Survey." *Journal of Aging and Health 17*(5): 547–572.

Gurung, R. A. R., and V. Mehta. 2001. "Relating Ethnic Identity, Acculturation, and Attitudes toward Treating Minority Clients." *Cultural Diversity and Ethnic Minority Psychology* 7: 139–151.

Hand, W. D. 1980. *Magical Medicine. The Folkloric Component of Medicine in the Folk Belief, Custom, and Ritual of the Peoples of Europe and America.* Berkeley: University of California Press.

Harris, M., R. J. Velásquez, J. White, and T. Renteria. 2004. "Folk Healing and Curanderismo within the Contemporary Chicana/o Community: Current Status." In *The Handbook of Chicana/o Psychology,* edited by R. J. Velásquez, L. M. Arellano, and B. W. McNeill, 111–125. Mahwah, NJ: Lawrence Erlbaum Associates Publishers.

Hatfield, G. 2004. *Folk Medicine: Old World and New World Traditions.* Santa Barbara, CA: ABC-CLIO.

Higginbotham, J. C., F. M. Treviño, and L. A. Ray. 1990. "Utilization of *Curanderos* by Mexican Americans: Prevalence and Predictors. Findings from HANES 1982–1984." *American Journal of Public Health* 80, suppl.: 32–35.

Hunt, L. M., N. H. Arar, and L. L Akana. 2000. "Herbs, Prayer, and Insulin. Use of Medical and Alternative Treatments by a Group of Mexican American Diabetes Patients." *Journal of Family Practice* 49: 216–223.

Johnson, P. J., A. Ward, L. Knutson, and S. Sendelbach. 2012. "Personal Use of Complementary and Alternative Medicine (CAM) by U.S. Health Care Workers." *Health Services Research* 47(1): 211–227.

Karlsen, S. and J. Y. Nazroo. 2002. "Relation between Racial Discrimination, Social Class, and Health among Ethnic Minority Groups." *American Journal of Public Health* 92(4): 624–631.

Kazarian, S., and D. Evans. 2001. "Health Psychology and Culture: Embracing the 21st Century." In *Handbook of Cultural Health Psychology*, edited by S. S. Kazarian and D. R. Evans, 3–43. San Diego, CA: Academic Press.

Kemper, D. W. 1998. "Deshidratación." In *La salud en casa: Guía práctica de Healthwise* (Decimontercera edición), edited by T. Smith, 78–79. Boise, ID: Healthwise.

Kiev, A. 1968. *Curanderismo*. New York: The Free Press.

Landrine, H. and E. A. Klonoff. 1996. "The Schedule of Racial Discrimination and a Study of its Negative Physical and Mental Health Consequences." *Journal of Black Psychology* 22: 144–168. doi: 10.1177/00957984960222002

Landrine, H., and E. A. Klonoff. 2001. "Cultural Diversity and Health Psychology." In *Handbook of Health Psychology*, edited by A. Baum, J. Singer, and T. Revenson, 851–891. Mahway, NJ: Erlbaum.

Landrine, H., E. A. Klonoff, I. Corral, S. Fernandez, and S. Roesch. 2006. "Conceptualizing and Measuring Ethnic Discrimination in Health Research." *Journal of Behavioral Medicine* 29: 79–94. doi:10.1007/s10865–005-9029–0

Leclere, O. A., and R. A. Lopez. 2012. "The *Jornalero*: Perceptions of Health Care Resources of Immigrant Day Laborers." *Journal of Immigrant Health* 14: 691–697. doi: 10.1007/s10903.011–9516-z.

Lewis, M. K. 2002. *Multicultural Health Psychology. Special Topics Acknowledging Diversity*. Boston: Allyn and Bacon.

Lipworth, W. L., C. Hooker, and S. M. Carter. 2011. "Balance, Balancing, and Health." *Qualitative Health Research* 21(5): 714–725. doi:10.1177/10497323113199781.

Lucero, A., and D. Velásquez. 1981. "*Curanderismo: A Case Study of Etiology, Diagnosis, and Treatment Techniques of a Practicing Curandera.*" Monograph series. 2 (3). Washington State University.

MacLachlan, M. E. 1997. *Culture and Health*. New York, NY: Wiley and Sons.

McElroy, O. H., and L. L. Grabb. 2012. *Merriam-Webster's Spanish-English Medical Dictionary*. Springfield, MA: Merriam-Webster, Inc.

Mitchen, S. Y. 2007. *African American Folk Healing*. New York, NY: University Press.

Molina, C., R. E. Zambrano, and M. Aguirre-Molina. 1994. "Influence of Culture, Class and Environment on Health Care." In *Latino Health in the U.S.: A Growing Challenge*, edited by C. Molina and M. Aguirre-Molina, 23–43. Washington, DC: American Public Health Association.

Mulcahy, J. B. 2010. "Magical Thinking." *Anthropology and Humanism* 35(1): 38–46. doi:10, 1111/j.1549.2010.01051.x.

Mull, J. D., and D. S. Mull. 1983. "A Visit with a *Curandero.*" *The Western Journal of Medicine* 139: 730–736.

National Institute on Aging. 2002. *Información de salud para las personas de la tercera edad. Curanderos: Como conocer estafas en cuestionses de salud.* Gaithersburg, MD: Dept of Health and Human Services.

Ortega-López, R. M. 2006. "Cultural del dolor, salud y enfermedad: Percepción de enfermería, usuarios de salud y curanderos" [Culture of pain, health and sickness: Nursing, health users' and healers' perception.] *Cultural de los Cuidados* 10(19): 63–72.

Padilla, A. M. 1984. "Synopsis of the History of Chicano Psychology." In *Chicano Psychology* (2nd ed.), edited by J. L. Martinez, Jr. and R. H. Mendoza, 1–19. Orlando, FL: Academic Press, Inc.

Padilla, R., V. Gomez, S. L. Biggerstaff, and P. S. Mehler. 2001. "Use of Curanderismo in a Public Health Care System." *Archives of Internal Medicine* 161(10): 1336–1340. doi:10-1001/pubs.

Quintana, S. M., N. Troyano, and G. Taylor. 2001. "Cultural Validity and Inherent Challenges in Quantitative Methods in Multicultural Research." In *Handbook of Multicultural Counseling* (2nd ed.), edited by J. G. Ponterotto, J. M. Casas, L. A. Suzuki, and C. M. Alexander, 604–630. Thousand Oaks, CA: Sage Publications.

Roberts, R. E. 1984. *Ethnicity and Health: Mexican Americans. A Guide for Health Care Providers.* U.S. Dept. of Education National Institute of Education (ERIC). National Fund for Medical Education grant number MH 00047 NIMH.

Sanchez, T. R., J. A. Plawecki, and H. M. Plawecki. 1996. "The Delivery of Culturally Sensitive Health Care to Native Americans." *Journal of Holistic Nursing 14:* 295–307.

Sloan, R. P., E. Bagiella. and T. Powell. 1999. "Religion, Spirituality, and Medicine." *Lancet 353*: 664–667.

Tausilt, M. 2009 "Healing Virtue: Saludarores Versus Witches in Early Modern Spain." *Medical History Supplement 29*: 40–63.

Torres, E. 2005. *Curandero.* Albuquerque, NM: University of New Mexico Press.

Torrey, E. F. 1986. *Witchcraft and Psychiatrists: The Common Roots of Psychotherapy and its Future.* Northvale, NJ: Jason Aronson Inc.

Treviño-Hernández, A. 2005. *Curanderos. They Heal the Sick with Prayers and Herbs.* Tucson, AZ: Hats Off Books.

Trotter, II, R. T., and J. A. Chavira. 1981. *Curanderismo: Mexican American Folk Healing.* Athens, GA: The University of Georgia Press.

World Health Organization 2008. *Traditional Medicine.* Fact Sheet no. 134, December.

Xu, C., L. Luo,, and R. X. Tan. 2004. "Antidepressant Effect of Three Traditional Chinese Medicine in the Learned Helplessness Model." *Journal of Ethnopharmacology 91*: 345–349.

Young, J. C. and L. Y. Garro. 1982. "Variations in the Choice of Treatment of Two Mexican Communities." *Social Science and Medicine 16*: 1453–1465.

Zacharias, S. 2006. "Mexican Curanderismo as Ethnopsychotherapy: A Qualitative Study on Treatment Practices, Effectiveness, and Mechanisms of Change." *International Journal of Disability, Development, and Education* 53(4): 381–400. doi:10.1080/10349120601008522.

CHAPTER ELEVEN

Mexican American Medicine: History, Roots, and Key Maladies

Mario Tovar

There has been a recent increase of interest in traditional alternative approaches to medicine in Western societies. Nevertheless, the perception of these is still not as favorable as Western medical interventions (Van Der Riet 2011). This view may be influenced by a variety of factors such as level of acculturation (Barragan et al. 2011) and lack of research evidence showing the effectiveness of these healing strategies (Shekelle et al. 2005). In the United States, these types of alternative healing methods are frequently found in rural locations, and practiced by people of low socioeconomic status (Trotter II and Chavira, 1997). People that adhere to traditional medical practices such as those that address culture-bound syndromes are often viewed as ignorant as this approach to medicine is considered to be inferior and ineffective (Mysyk 1998, O'Nell 1975). The Mexican American population utilizes some alternative methods as cultural customs, several of which are implemented to treat culture-bound syndromes (Trotter II and Chavira 1997). To be able to provide services to people that utilize alternative folk medical practices, it is important to understand the interventions they may use as remedies, the types of conditions that are specific to their culture, and that these practices are not necessarily inferior, but simply different approaches to illness and discomfort, several of which have the same roots as contemporary Western medicine (Foster 1987).

The Mexican American Population

The term Mexican American is often used to describe people that reside in the United States and that are of Mexican descent. Nevertheless, this term can be used to describe very diverse populations. For examples, the term can be used to describe people that have some link or connection with Mexico, but the term Chicano can also describe people with these characteristics (Herrera 2010). Furthermore, the term Mexican American can be used to describe individuals that are of Mexican descent, but that do not have any connection or identity with Mexico. These individuals are also known as Pochos (Herrera 2010).

According to the U.S. census results from 2010, the Mexican American population had the largest growth amongst the Hispanic or Latino populations, reaching approximately 31.8 million (U.S. Census Bureau 2011). Furthermore, this number is distributed across the United States in the following manner: In the Northeast region, there are 918,188; in the Midwest, there are 3.5 million; there are 11 million in the South and 16.4 million in the West (U.S. Census Bureau 2011).

Even though the Mexican American population resides in different locations of the United States and therefore may differ in some socio-cultural characteristics, there are several commonalities of practices (Trotter II and Chavira 1997, Waldstein 2008). An example of this is the approach to medical interventions and cultural remedies, as well as well-identified culture-bound or folk medical syndromes (Waldstein 2008).

In the Mexican American population, there are four main folk medical syndromes: *Mal de ojo, caida de mollera, empacho,* and *susto* (Trotter II and Chavira 1997). Susto is possibly the most complex of these, due to its unique characteristics (e.g., the belief that it is caused as a result of the person suffering from it losing his/her soul), and similarities with more than one psychiatric condition known by Western medicine (American Psychiatric Association 2000).

The purpose of this chapter is to describe the nature to these types of conditions from a culturally relativistic perspective, including Emic/Etic approaches to the understanding of these ailments and their treatments. It contains information about the origins of Mexican American folk medicine, including influences from Ancient Greece, the Middle East, and Europe. In this chapter, I also describe in general terms the most common types of culture-bound syndromes found in contemporary Mexican American folk medicine, and finally, I provide a thorough description of the condition known as susto, including psychological, biological, and socio-cultural factors that may contribute to its presence and existence.

Western Origins of Mexican American Folk Medicine

Ancient Greek Medicine

Traces of ancient Greek medical practices can be found throughout Europe and in the Americas demonstrating its scientific nature. However, even within Greece, there was a transition from supernatural beliefs to a more systematic approach to medicine. Greek medicine originally considered ailments to be caused by supernatural forces. As such, the treatments needed to be supernatural and address mythological components (Fornaro, Clementi and Fornaro 2009).

The god of medicine was known as Asclepius. He was the son of the god Apollo and the nymph Coronis and was born shortly after Coronis was killed by the goddess Artemis (the twin sister of Apollo) because she was unfaithful to Apollo. Thus Asclepius was born in what was considered the first cesarean section from a dead mother. Asclepius was raised by the centaur Chiron, who was considered a master in herbal medicine and medical practices. From Chiron, Asclepius was able to obtain all the necessary information to heal the sick (Fornaro et al. 2009).

The medical system in ancient Greece was predominantly influenced by the Asclepius myth. Over 200 temples were erected in his name and served as centers to treat the ill (Vasiliadis, Grivas and Kaspiris 2009). These temples were known as Asclepions (Vasiliadis et al. 2009). The sick went to these temples to sleep and it was believed that while resting, they were to experience a prophetic dream in which they were going to be informed how to feel better. Some patients also claimed that Asclepius walked around them at night. This was possibly caused by wizard doctors dressed as gods who assisted in the healing process. It is believed that these doctors poisoned/drugged patients so they experienced prophetic dreams through drug-induced hallucinations (Fornaro et al. 2009). Furthermore, these witch doctors, also known as priest-physicians, were in charge of providing specific healing methods such as hydrotherapy, physiotherapy, hygienic rule, dieting, some therapies involving drugs and mildly intense surgeries (Vasiliadis et al. 2009).

The effects of herbs in Ancient Greek medicine were also an important concept that had its origins in mythology. Ancient Romans utilized the word *medicamentum* when referring to both poison and healing, demonstrating that it was crucial for the physicians to become familiar with the effects of medication which could help somebody get better or make an ill patient get worse (Chiappelli, Prolo and Cajulis 2005).

Humoral Medicine

Supernatural and magical elements of medicine could be seen in ancient Greek mythology and in applied practices. This approach to medicine was a constant variable across time and space throughout Europe (Cole 1993). These explanations for ailment became less frequent with the innovative interpretation and systematic approach to medicine by Hippocrates of Kos (460 BC-370 BC). Hippocrates is considered to be the father of medicine and one of the first to establish and use systematic observation to heal different medical and psychological conditions (Pikoulis et al. 1998; Vasiliadis et al. 2009).

Hippocrates followed the philosophical and empirical traditions and practices of Plato, Aristotle and Democritus. However, he added to ancient Greek medical traditions a systematic, empirical and scientific approach and discredited superstitious causes of illness (Pikoulis et al. 1998). Resulting from this new understanding of pathologies was the emergence of different theories such as the one of four humors. In it, Hippocrates suggested that the human body is composed of four humors (*Karsis*) or fluids that need to be in harmony for the body to be healthy. If there is an imbalance of these substances, the body suffers a physical or mental illness. The four substances are blood, phlegm, yellow bile, and black bile. (Pikoulis et al. 1998). A natural mechanism to reach homeostasis of the body was through the regular ways of expelling substances such as urine, sweat and excrement, a process that was known as *coction* (Pikoulis et al. 1998).

Each of these four humors had unique properties. Blood was considered to be hot and wet. Phlegm was cold and wet; black bile was thought to be cold and dry, and yellow bile was hot and dry (Androutsos et al. 2008). Additionally, these humors were linked to different parts of the body. Blood originated in the heart and phlegm was associated with the brain. Black bile was related to the spleen and yellow bile originated in the liver. Furthermore, the four properties were also related to the four ancient elements. Hot was associated with fire, cold with air, wet with water, and dry with earth (Hansotia 2003).

Hippocrates' approach to medicine included how to prevent any ailment in addition to the identification and treatment of conditions. To do so, moderation was emphasized in every aspect of life, including when consuming what were considered the six non-natural elements: air, sleep and waking, food and drink, resting and exercising, excretion and secretion, and passions or emotions (Androutsos et al. 2008). According to Hippocrates's humoral system of medicine, the ailments were treated by using remedies of opposite properties (e.g., a cold illness could be treated with a hot remedy). Additionally, the transference of illness from the person into an object was a legitimate method of treatment (Androutsos et al. 2008).

This theory of medicine changed the way ancient Greeks approached and treated illnesses. However, it was further developed by others such as Claudius Galen of Pergamon (130 AD-200 AD), who was a Greek physician that worked in Rome, first treating gladiators and eventually becoming personal physician of the emperor Marcus Aurelius (Vasiliadis et al. 2009). Even though several volumes of his work were destroyed in a fire in Rome, 118 treatises were saved. In his work, it is common to find references to Hippocrates (Vasiliadis et al. 2009).

Galen also made observations and assumed relationships between the different humors and the behavior and personality of individuals (Brown 2007, Capitanio 2008), something that Hippocrates had started with his humoral theory (Chiappelli et al. 2005). A person dominated by blood was believed to be warm and pleasant. A person with a dominant black bile humor was thought to be choleric and hot-tempered. An individual with a predominant yellow bile humor was considered to be melancholic, depressed and sad. Finally, a person with a dominant phlegm humor was thought to be phlegmatic or apathetic (Chiappelli et al. 2005).

From Greek Medicine to Arabic Influence

After the Greek and Roman Empires ended, the knowledge of philosophical and medical traditions expanded into other areas. Following the tradition of Hippocrates and Galen, advancements in medicine continued under the hands of Arab physicians (Editorial 2006).

During the 8th century, Islam was the most influential religion as it covered up to two-thirds of the known world at that time. Furthermore, Arabs were established in important Western locations such as Spain and Sicily (Saad, Azaizeh, and Said 2005). When they discovered the importance of obtaining information from Greek and Roman culture, they translated as much information as possible into Arabic. One of the most important and well-known translators in charge of this transition was Hunayn Ibn-Is'haq. He translated several works pertaining to Mathematics and science. Also, he was in charge of translating medical documents from Hippocrates and Galen (Saad et al. 2005). Because of access to this information, Arab physicians developed the most influential body of medicine at the time. One of the most recognized writers of medicine was Avicenna (980–1037) also known as Ibn Sina, denoting his Persian roots (Editorial 2006).

Avicenna wrote several books on philosophy, mathematics, astronomy and different areas of medicine such as gynecology and infections like tuberculosis (Editorial 2006). His work reflected several principles from Hippocrates and Galen like the humoral system of medicine (Pettman 2007). Although he was considered more of a philosopher than a physician, his major work was *The Canon of Medicine,* which was considered to be "the medical bible" during the 10th century, when it was written (Editorial 2006). In it, he explained and elaborated on humoral medicine and he added hot-cold properties to foods in addition to remedies for illnesses. For example, he explains barley to be cold and dry, whereas squash is considered cold and wet. Sesame seed was described as hot and wet and cloves hot and dry (Foster 1987).

From the 10th to the 12th centuries, Arab medicine continued to evolve thanks to several contributors and became such an important part of Western culture that the work of some physicians such as Avicenna were translated into Latin (Saad et al. 2005) and other Western languages such as German (Cole 1993). The understanding of Hippocratic medicine and the work of Galen and Avicenna led Europe to adopt a medical approach that combined traditional medicine and a systematic approach to investigating what could cure particular ailments (Cole 1993).

Traditional Folk Medicine in Europe

After Arab physicians' work was translated from Arabic to Latin, they continued to influence the teaching and practice of Medicine from the twelfth century until at least the seventeenth century. For example, Avicenna's work was published during this period, with the number of editions gradually increasing as the centuries passed (Saad et al. 2005).

Even though the 16th century European approach to medicine was primarily based on Avicenna and Hippocrates' works, there were some influences from traditional and folkloric practices. This was especially seen in places like Germany where physicians like Theophrastus Paracelsus von Hohenheim (1493–1541) incorporated both traditional and formal non-traditional medical practices to form a combination of folk medicine, alchemy principles, and occultism (Cole 1993). As part of his medical preparation, Paracelsus interviewed individuals from different parts of Europe. He focused on physicians as well as other common people that were aware of some healing practices that were often passed from generation to generation or that were considered common knowledge (Cole 1993).

Some traditional practices were established and developed because of the difficulty of accessing rural areas across Europe. Getting to these areas to treat ill people was especially difficult with the existence of contagious conditions/infections such as tuberculosis (Pettman 2007). Up to the 19th century, functionalism was the predominant theory of academic medicine. It suggests that an individual has to be treated as a whole and to help restore the organism's functioning, and therefore, it was required for the treating expert to be present at the time of the healing process, making it necessary for people that resided nearby, not necessarily trained physicians, to be familiar with some medical traditional knowledge (Androutsos et al. 2008).

Spain was no exception and also adapted these medical practices. Before the Moors were expelled from Spain, their influence was very significant, particularly in areas such as mathematics, philosophy and medicine. During the 15th and 16th century, the dominant medical approach taught in Spain was based on the teachings of Hippocrates, Galen, and Avicenna (Foster 1987).

Folk Medicine in the Americas

Anthropological work in Latin America suggests the principles of the humoral system of medicine were identifiable and constantly present in the New World. Traits of humoral medicine can be found in Haiti, Trinidad and Tobago, the American Southwest, and the Philippines (Foster 1987).

Furthermore, some researchers believed that people from non-European cultures developed a medical system characterized by utilizing a classification of illnesses and remedies with cold and hot properties, and such a system was designed to treat conditions by using the principle of opposition (Foster 1987). After several analyses, it has been mostly agreed that these medical practices originated in Ancient Greece, were translated by Arab scholars, and expanded across Europe. Medical books that were published pre and post-conquest in Spain show consistencies with European based content and therefore, demonstrate that what was being practiced in the New World after the conquest had the same elements as the information that was applied in Europe (Foster 1987).

It is possible that some elements of hot/cold properties existed in pre-Columbian times. For example, deities from the Aztec religious system were considered to have some of these properties. Tlaloc, who was the god of rain, was usually associated with cold properties (Foster 1987). Also, local foods were classified based on hot and cold properties (Artschwager Kay 1977, Foster 1987). This, however, does not mean that they utilized a medical system that included these properties and treated illnesses the way the humoral medical system suggests, that is by selecting and utilizing items with opposing characteristics (Foster 1987).

Even though there were some parts of Europe that incorporated the principles of the humoral system into folk and popular medicine such as Germany (Cole 1993), Spain only applied this medicinal system in formal and academic training and practice (Foster 1987). Once it arrived in New Spain, it was incorporated into popular practice by different means.

Initially, only some physicians and mainly religious leaders had knowledge of Hippocratic medicine. However, this changed as the Spanish conquistadores established hospitals in central locations such as Tenochtitlan, which was the economic, political, and religious center of the Aztec Empire. Later on, there were more hospitals created around this area, which led to medical staff being trained in this medical system (Foster 1987). Additionally, there were pharmacies established around New Spain's Empire. These were responsible for dispensing medicinal herbs and other minerals intended to treat the sick. These eventually incorporated and combined both Spanish and Native medical elements to treat both native and European illnesses (Foster 1987).

Finally, because the main political and religious goal of the Spanish government was to expand, exploit the resources, and evangelize and convert natives to Christianity, people started to travel and usually moved far from the center of the Empire's power, where all the hospitals and medical facilities were located. This led people to develop *recetarios*, which were home medical guides that described certain illnesses and ways to treat them. Remedies were based not only on herbs and minerals, but also on practices such as massages (Foster 1987). Common people eventually were able to have these *recetarios* and that is how some folk medicine practices developed in rural areas where there no physicians or other medicine staff (Foster 1987).

As people moved north of central Mexico, they carried and developed *recetarios*. One of the most complete and well-known was the one created by Juan de Esteyneffer, a Jesuit lay brother who traveled to Chihuahua. He titled this work *Florilegio Medicinal*, and in it, he described a wide variety of illnesses and herbs to treat them. He not only focused on European conditions, but incorporated local conditions and practices (Artschwager Kay 1977).

Esteyneffer's work is divided into three volumes that dealt with medicine, surgery, and pharmacology. He described the conditions that might be present and the remedies to treat them. Furthermore, he specified where people could find the medicinal herbs (Artschwager Kay 1977).

There are several accounts recorded that mention how priests, friars and other members of religious orders served as physicians due to the lack of medical staff. As these accounts express, such people were focused on dealing with the natives' souls as well as their health (Artschwager Kay 1977).

Some of the conditions found in the *Florilegio Medicinal* are easily identifiable and can be traced back to Europe and Greek medicine. However, there are other conditions that are of native origin and which have no equivalent in Western medicine. These illnesses and their remedies are believed to have existed since pre-Columbian times. One of these examples is known as *caida de mollera*, or fallen fontanelle (Artschwager Kay 1977). Conditions like this have survived and can still be identified in the northern part of Mexico and the south of the United States, particularly in Mexican American communities, and the remedies that were at one time recommended by recetarios are still being practiced today as folk medicine (Artschwager Kay 1977).

Mexican American Folk Medicine

Religious groups moved north of Mexico to evangelize native communities they found on their way. They took with them recetarios as they were moving away from major health centers such as hospitals and they needed to have some type of reference to deal with conditions. However, like Esteyneffer, the collection of additional conditions and remedies were added to what was already known (Artschwager Kay 1977). The religious orders in charge of evangelizing the natives established in the northern part of Mexico and the southern region of the United States medicinal practices and information about herbs and rituals that have survived until the present time (Artschwager Kay 1977).

After the addition of the northern states of Mexico, such as Texas, into the United States, the customs, traditions, and social characteristics remained constant features of the region. Among other customs, those involving healing practices can still be identified in today's society (Trotter II and Chavira 1997). Conditions and ways to treat them can be identified as those that were mentioned in the narratives of conquistadores and religious orders. In certain cases, these conditions have the same characteristics as illnesses found in Western medicine. However, there are several others that have no equivalent and, therefore, are unique in properties and treatments (Artschwager Kay 1977).

Some of these conditions deal with common physical symptoms such as a stomach ache or fever. However, there are others that might involve supernatural elements that are attributed to and explained by supernatural means in addition to physical discomfort (Trotter II 1991). The conditions that do not have an equal in Western medicine are considered traditional and to an extent folkloric and culture-bound. These conditions have identifiable symptoms and a traceable origin. The treatment of these conditions often involves medicinal herbs, supernatural practices and rituals and occurs only amongst the people of the region and culture (Trotter II 1991).

Even though these folk medical practices can be affected and influenced by the level of acculturation and assimilation of the practitioners and the community in general (Waldstein, 2008), there are several regions in the United States, particularly those with a high number of immigrants, where these healing methods can still be identified and recognized as legitimate (Baer and Bustillo 1993, Baer and Bustillo 1998, Baer et al. 2003, Trotter II and Chavira 1997).

Similar to mental disorders and Western medical conditions, culture bound syndromes in the Mexican and Mexican American cultures have symptoms that may overlap with each other. Because of this, the different conditions are identified according to other factors such as the length of time the symptoms are present or the cause of the syndrome (Baer et al. 2003).

Four Main Mexican American Folk Medical Syndromes

The most common culture-bound syndromes found in contemporary Mexican American society are those known as *caida de mollera, empacho, mal de ojo*, and *susto*. *Caida de Mollera* is literally translated as fallen fontanelle. This condition is only present in children and is identified when the upper part of the forming skull (fontanelle) of an infant sinks. Additionally, diarrhea, loss of appetite, fever and constant crying can occur (Baer and Bustillo 1998). This is believed to happen if the child hits his/her underdeveloped head, if the child is not cared for appropriately, or also if the nipple of the bottle or breast is removed too quickly from the infant's mouth (Baer and Bustillo 1998). This condition is believed to be treated by pushing up the palate, holding the infant upside down while shaking, putting soap on the submerged area, and holding the child upside down while placing the upper part of the head in water (Ortiz de Montellano 1987). There are records about this culture-bound condition that date to pre-Columbian times and reveal an origin prior to Spanish arrival in the New World (Ortiz de Montellano 1987).

Empacho is another folk medical syndrome that can be seen in contemporary Mexican and Mexican American cultures. Like Caida de Mollera, this syndrome has an organic origin. It is caused by the blockage of food in the intestines resulting from a bolus that was not properly digested. The bolus gets stuck to a wall of the intestines and can occur after swallowing an excessive amount of saliva. Sometimes the blockage is caused by other things besides food (Weller et al. 1993). The condition is also associated with inadequate eating habits such as eating too much, eating not well-cooked food or at an incorrect time of the day (Weller et al. 1993). The symptoms are constipation, diarrhea, indigestion, bloating of the stomach, vomiting, weakness, and lethargy (Weller et al. 1993). This condition can be treated utilizing several remedies. People suffering from empacho ingest teas and purgatives. Also, individuals can go to a specialist folk healer. In the Mexican American communities, this specialist is known as a *sobador* and provides a massage of the stomach (Trotter II 1991) or a massage of the back in which the skin is pulled back (Trotter II and Chavira 1997). This condition can be found in documents written during the colonization of New Spain such as recetarios (Artschwager Kay 1977).

A third common culture-bound syndrome that can be found in today's Mexican American society is known as *mal de ojo*, which literary means "evil eye." This condition can occur after an individual stares at something or someone with admiration. The person being observed can become sick or if the observation and admiration was directed toward a thing, then it can break or stop working (Trotter II 1991). One way to prevent this is by touching the thing or person admired shortly after the admiration (Holland and Courtney 1998). The population that is most vulnerable to this condition is young infants and older people. It is common to find amulets that can absorb the energy that can make a baby sick. These are called "deer's eye" and are usually bracelets that have a seed. It is believed that if they absorb the "evil," then break and prevent the baby from getting sick (Baer et al. 2006). Furthermore, if the person who admired the child does not touch him/her, then a ritual is performed as a healing method. It consists of brushing the child with herbs and a raw egg as the healer says prayers. Once this is done, the egg can be placed under the bed of the infant overnight (Trotter II 1991). On the following day, it can be determined if the "evil" was absorbed by cracking the egg. If the egg appears to be darker than usual, then it is said the egg has been "cooked" and therefore, absorbed the evil (Baer et al. 2006). Common symptoms of *mal de ojo* are similar to the common cold. The person might get fever, headaches and diarrhea (Trotter and Chavira 1997).

The folk medical syndrome known as *susto* is complex in interpretation and treatment. Even though the causes and explanation of this condition are usually supernatural in essence (i.e., the soul leaves the body), there are also elements that show a physiological reaction to the event such as hypoglycemia (Hatcher and Whittemore 2007). Additionally, because the treatment is based on the beliefs of the members of society and the expected positive outcome of the folk treatment, Western medicine is often ineffective in treating susto (Baer et al. 2003).

Susto as a Culture-Bound Syndrome

Susto, a Spanish word that is literally translated as "fright," and is often considered to be "magical fright" by some people that believe in folk medicine, is a syndrome that is caused by exposure to a shocking or traumatic event. Folk healers and members of the Mexican and Mexican American communities interpret the shock as the soul of the victim leaving the body (Trotter II 1991). It occurs in both children and adults and can eventually evolve into other folk syndromes such as *nervios* (Baer et al. 2003). Even though susto has symptoms that can be recognized and identified, they are diverse and sometimes vary depending on the victim, healer and culture. There can be both psychological and somatic symptoms. Major psychological symptoms are similar to depression such as insomnia or hypersomnia, loss of appetite, sadness and feelings of worthlessness. Somatic symptoms are fundamentally headaches, muscle aches, diarrhea and stomach aches (American Psychiatric Association 2000). Additionally, people suffering from susto experience severe anxiety and hypervigilance, nightmares and trembling and shaking (Rivera and Wanderer 1986).

When susto is not treated, the victim can have serious health complications. In extreme cases, people believe susto can be responsible for the death of the victim. If this does not occur, the victim can develop tuberculosis as a result of untreated susto. This is commonly known as *susto pasado* (Rivera and Wanderer 1986). Additionally, it is believed that susto can evolve and contribute to the development of diabetes (Hatcher and Whittemore 2007).

Even though there are some culture bound syndromes that might share similar symptoms with susto, there are substantial differences that make each diagnosis unique. For example, due to the symptoms of anxiety occurring in both of the diagnoses, people might misdiagnose susto with nervios. Nervios is a syndrome that results from several stressful and traumatic events. In contrast, susto is the result of experiencing only one single event. Also, nervios is usually not associated with death if left untreated; however, it can have severe repercussions on the victim's health.

These syndromes also differ in the treatment methods utilized to heal them. Nervios can be treated as a psychiatric disorder; susto is usually not as easily treatable by Western medicine. It requires a more complex treatment that involves rituals, prayers and other esoteric and natural methods (Baer et al. 2003). Another significant difference between susto and nervios is the age group each one of them affects. Susto is present in both children and adults. Nervios is only present in adults (Baer et al. 2003). Recent research has shown that both of these conditions are strongly related to depression and stress and suggests they are primarily the manifestation of mental health distress rather than anything exclusively physiological (Weller et al. 2008).

In addition to nervios, another commonly mistaken diagnosis with susto is known as *espanto,* which is also a type of fright as a result of a traumatic event. This syndrome, however, is usually attributed to the presence of a supernatural being such as a ghost or a demon. Nevertheless, an important similarity between susto and espanto is that it is believed they can both cause death in the victim if not treated properly. Regarding espanto, this extreme level of the syndrome is known as *espanto fulminante* (Rivera and Wanderer 1986, Tousignant 1979). Although there are some distinctions made between susto and espanto, the difference is not always clear as some people believe that susto can also be the result of supernatural causes. Therefore, the different diagnosis between these two syndromes is difficult and the possibility of this folk medical syndrome occurring in different locations characterized by the same symptoms but identified by different names is very likely (Landy 1985, Tousignant 1979).

Although some people from different locations have identified the soul leaving the body as a major explanation for what happens when a person suffers from susto, a research project revealed that this is not always the case. In the Rio Grande Valley, 951 individuals were asked about the nature of this condition. Most of the respondents were female and only 205 reported they had heard of soul loss being related to susto, even though all of them provided a description of this syndrome (Glazer et al. 2004).

Treatment for Susto

There are several methods to treat susto. Some of these approaches involve a single procedure and others require a combination of several healing strategies. The treatment usually depends on the healer. A considerable number of people view susto as a major spiritual problem because it is believed the victim loses his/her soul as a traumatic event is experienced or witnessed (American Psychiatric Association 2000). This might require a thorough ritualistic procedure that includes prayer. In contrast, other individuals believe that as a person experiences susto, the victim suffers from an episode of hypoglycemia, which requires an external materialistic intervention. The victim is provided with a spoonful of sugar to remedy the low glucose level in the body. This is often believed to be enough for the victim's body to find homeostasis and return to its normal level. Also, the victim may be given vinegar or water with salt (Weller et al. 2002). Often, susto is treated with herbal teas, particularly those made out of traditional folk medicine herbs such as *yerbaniz/Tageteslucida cav*. If this is not enough for the soul of the victim to return, a ritual consisting of sweeping the victim with medicinal herbs takes place. This is known as *barrida* (Trotter II 1991). The rituals may also involve laying the victim down on the floor in a cross-shaped position. The healer in turn begins to pray and often utilizes branches and ointments to conduct a barrida asking for the victim's soul to return to the person's body (Baca 1969).

A common herb that is used for the treatment of susto is *Adiantumtetraphyllum Humb. and Bonpl. Ex Willd* from the family *Adiantaceae*. This plant has properties to reduce, suppress and eliminate levels of anxiety and stress. This herb's use to treat susto demonstrates that this folk medical syndrome has a strong psychological component and that the term could be another way of interpreting psychological symptoms and possibly disorders (Bourbonnais-Spear et al. 2007). Even though people that reside in locations where susto is a well recognized and legitimate condition have access to different folk healers that can assist in the treatment, whether by providing the right type of substance such as a tea or by performing a supernatural ritual with the appropriate combination of the right herbs and prayers, most individuals prefer to deal with this condition in the home setting (Trotter II 1991).

Psychological Aspects of Susto

One of the most difficult aspects of attempting to adapt the diagnosis of *susto* to Western medicine standards is the fluctuation of its symptoms and the constant dependence on the culture to deal with the physical and psychological effects, including the understanding of the origin and type of treatment. Although susto could be considered a type of depressive disorder due to the symptoms the victims experience (e.g., loss of appetite, insomnia/hypersomnia, etc.), there are some characteristics that could fit susto into a different category of mental conditions such as anxiety or dissociative disorders (American Psychiatric Association 2000).

An important psychological distinction between susto and nervios is the nature of the origin of such conditions. Although the symptoms are similar, nervios is a condition that usually is longer lasting than susto. It could be proposed that the symptoms that accompany susto are not the representation of a Western analogy to the different types of depressive disorders. Instead, susto could be considered a type of panic attack and nervios can be an actual diagnosis of panic disorder (Baer et al. 2003, Cintrón, Carter and Sbrocco 2005).

Another similar psychiatric diagnosis that seems to overlap in symptoms with susto is Post-Traumatic Stress Disorder or PTSD. This disorder is characterized by the experiencing of a severely stressful and traumatic incident that causes the victim to avoid the possible stimulus that is related to the incident. Additionally, the victim experiences the traumatic incident recurrently in his/her mind, reacting with a physiological arousal in response to the incident (American Psychiatric Association 2000). It is possible that susto and nervios have some properties and similarities with PTSD, especially considering the social perception of individuals that reside in locations where the culture-bound syndromes are well known (Norris et al. 2001). Regarding the re-experiencing of the traumatic event or situation, it is important to clarify that susto is a culture-bound syndrome that can occur from hours to months and years after the traumatic incident happened (O'Nell 1975).

Susto also possesses some elements of what is known as dissociative disorder. Since one of the principal interpretations of susto involves the soul or spirit leaving the body, it has been stated that what the victims experience in susto is a dissociation that can affect the mind/body duality and have major consequences on the health and psychological well-being. (Trotter II 1991). People who suffer from susto can experience dissociation, as they believe their souls leave their bodies (Cintrón et al. 2005).

Physiological/Medical Aspects of Susto

As opposed to other folk medical syndromes, susto can occur in both children and adults. Therefore, the medical implications and analogies with Western society can occur across the lifespan. It is a complex culture-bound syndrome that has several descriptions of the symptoms resulting from it. Even though experiencing a traumatic and frightening event is the situational setting in which susto originates, the esoteric explanations together with the physical and psychological symptoms make it a broad condition.

Although the soul leaving the body is the most well known interpretation of the description of susto among the general population, there are also interpretations from a Western medicine perspective that suggest susto is the result of medical conditions. Because of its psychological components and due to the physiological symptoms, susto has a major impact on the victim's immune system (Trotter II 1991). Additionally, susto has several directly related medical symptoms such as diarrhea, headaches and different body aches (American Psychiatric Association 2000).

An important interpretation of susto in the medical setting is the sudden change of glucose levels in the blood. Hypoglycemia, sometimes as a result of diabetes, appears to have a significant effect on the victim's change of behavior and the onset of psychological symptoms in addition to physiological ones (Flaskerud and Ruiz Calvillo 2007). Since diabetes is a common condition within the Hispanic population in the United States, there are popular beliefs that express a relationship between Type II diabetes and susto. Even though most people that suffer from this medical condition are aware of the causes for diabetes and the treatment according to Western medicine, there are some interpretations incorporating susto as the cause of Type II diabetes. People know that major risk factors for acquiring and developing diabetes are poor eating habits, lack of exercise and heredity; however, they also attribute the frightening and traumatic event that made them experience susto as a major contributor (Flaskerud and Ruiz Calvillo 2007, Hatcher and Whittemore 2007).

The treatment for diabetes is also influenced by the folk remedies that treat susto. In addition to expressing an unpleasant and negative attitude toward insulin, people tend to seek out alternative methods of treatment for diabetes. Two of the major approaches to treat this condition are prayer (sometimes involved in rituals) and herbal remedies such as teas (Hatcher and Whittemore 2007).

Another association between susto and Western medicine is the occurrence and correlation with epilepsy. It is often believed that epilepsy can result after experiencing a severe traumatic event, such as what triggers susto. Children suffering from epilepsy are specially affected by this condition (Baca 1969, Rivera and Wanderer 1986). Also, when susto affects pregnant women, the fetus can be impacted (Rivera and Wanderer 1986).

When susto is left untreated, it can develop into a more severe variant of the same culture-bound syndrome known as *susto pasado*. This condition can lead to the death of the victim, especially if the victim is a child

(Rivera and Wanderer 1986). The major characteristics of susto pasado are exhaustion and coughing. Because of this, it is believed that susto pasado can also evolve into tuberculosis (Rivera and Wanderer 1986). According to Mexican American folk healers, if susto pasado is treated even after it has evolved into tuberculosis, Western medicine can be utilized and is effective in the treatment for tuberculosis (Baca 1969).

Social Aspects of Susto

Susto is greatly influenced by the culture that legitimizes and considers it a real condition that can be suffered by the members of a particular group or society. It incorporates the knowledge and the practices of a specific culture and the different components that surround this folk medical syndrome. It also relies and depends on the values and several factors found in society.

Susto is known in Mexico, Guatemala, Puerto Rico and other countries of Latin America. Additionally, it is also known in some social sectors of the United States. This is likely the result of immigration and the transmission of knowledge from generation to generation. Although this culture-bound syndrome is not always recognized as susto, there are different names that describe conditions with the same characteristics (Landy 1985).

Even though it is possible for this syndrome to be experienced by children and adults and equally by males and females, there is a greater rate of women experiencing or admitting suffering from susto than males (Baer et al. 2003). It is also usually experienced by people with low socio-economic status and with low standardized and academic/formal education (O'Nell 1975). Even though some members of society do not receive formal education through the school system, knowledge is transmitted by other members of their family such as parents (Waldstein 2008)

Another social aspect that appears to be relevant to the diagnosis, treatment and recognition of susto involves the level/lack of acculturation of individuals residing in the United States. People that have resided in the United States and away from their countries for a longer time tend to lose the knowledge and belief in folk medical syndromes, diagnosis, and treatment via traditional methods (Baer and Bustillo 1993).

Individuals that have knowledge of these syndromes often witness a major rejection of culture-bound syndromes from the Western medicine perspective. Because of this, it is likely that individuals that suffer from them do not go to a physician. Instead, they opt to go to a healer to receive the treatment the victim requires (Baer and Bustillo 1993). Another possible reason why this occurs is related to economic situations. Whenever a member of the family is ill, the condition is first treated within the family. If this does not work, then a friend or acquaintance is consulted. If this is also ineffective, then a professional folk healer is consulted (Villasenor and Waitzkin 1999).

Susto could be the result of psychosocial stressors. If some people do not meet with the socially expected requirements, then they might start feeling pressured and, as a result, develop susto. The roles that the individual is unable to meet can vary and be from different social settings such as work, home, etc. Due to the stress and anxiety that this causes, the person gets into a very intense state of anxiety and starts to experience the symptoms that characterize susto (O'Nell 1975). This theory is consistent with the definition of a culture-bound syndrome because the social roles and expectations solely depend on the culture and the society of the individual. Additionally, this also helps explain why susto is more common in females than males as they might be unable to meet major social expectations in some cultures like the Zapotec in Mexico, such as giving birth and rearing children (O'Nell 1975).

This theory, however, would not help explain the reason why children also suffer and are diagnosed with susto. Even though they also need to fulfill certain roles within society (e.g., going to school, follow rules set by parents), the social impact of these roles may not be as socially significant as those that have to be met by adults. Additionally, an alternative explanation for why women report suffering from susto more often than men is that one characteristic of victims of this condition is passivity. This type of behavior is usually not common in males from societies where susto is recognized. As a result, women might simply more often admit suffering from susto than men. However, this does not mean that women are actually suffering more from this condition than males. Another important social characteristic of susto is the relatively easy and simple way in which it is treated and cured. Even though susto is recognized as causing severe symptoms in the victim and even the possibility of dying if it is left untreated, the way of curing it is simple, inexpensive and usually can be done by a member of the family or a known folk healer (Uzell 1974).

Further Considerations

There is no evidence to demonstrate an equivalent condition in the Western medicine realm to the folk medical syndrome known as susto.

According to Western medicine, culture bound syndromes are not as legitimate and often are seen as a set of symptoms resulting from a medical/psychological condition (Weller et al. 2002).

The need for multicultural competence in the medical/psychological field is necessary, especially when treating individuals that have certain beliefs that are not the same as the health professional. The lack of this understanding can greatly harm people if they lose confidence in going to the doctor when they really need to (Baer and Bustillo 1993).

The healing process that incorporates rituals, prayer and the administration of certain medicinal components such as teas made from specific herbs appears to be similar to the practices found in Western medicine. There are some stereotypes that influence the social perception of *curanderos* or folk healers. They usually receive training in folk medicine and are widely known among the members of their community. They are given several classifications depending on the perception of the person. However, if there is skepticism and the person classifying the curandero has never attempted to receive help from him/her, then it is likely that the classification will be more negative, such as the one found in witches or evil persons working with evil elements (Press 1971).

In American society, although there is not one single medical/psychological condition that might resemble the exact symptoms of susto, there are some authors that believe this syndrome is equivalent to what is known as grief. Even though grief is not necessarily a pathological diagnosis, it has some commonalities with the symptoms experienced in susto. For example, there can be a combination of symptoms of anxiety and depression (Houghton and Boersma 1988).

One of the major obstacles in finding and defining susto in terms of Western medicine is the prevalence of several symptoms that could fit the description of diverse conditions such as anxiety disorders and mood disorders from a psychological perspective and stomach conditions that can result in diarrhea from the medical perspective. Attempting to continue to look for an equivalent condition in Western medicine might be useless as susto is experienced only by certain groups, cultures or societies (American Psychiatric Association 2000). A sociocultural approach needs to be included whenever conducting medical/psychological assessments and the understanding of the healing process from a broad perspective in addition to psychological, physiological, and spiritual aspects. These components are necessary to be able to provide accurate and appropriate services for people across cultures and ethnic backgrounds.

References

American Psychiatric Association. 2000. *Diagnostic and Statistical Manual of Mental Disorders* (4th ed., text rev.). Washington, DC: Author.

Androutsos, G., A. Diamantis, L. Vladimiros, and E. Magiorkinis. 2008. "Health and Disease in Ancient Greek Medicine." *International Journal of Health Science* 1(2): 32–36.

Applewhite, S. 1995. "Curanderismo: Demystifying the Health Beliefs and Practices of Elderly Mexican Americans." *Health and Social Work* 20(4): 247–253. http://www.naswpress.org/publications/journals/hsw.html

Artschwager Kay, M. 1977. "The *Florilegio Medicinal:* Source of Southwest Ethnomedicine." *Ethnohistory* 24(3): 251–259. http://www.ethnohistory.org/sections/journal/index.html

Baca, J. E. 1969. "Some Health Beliefs of the Spanish Speaking." *The American Journal of Nursing* 69(10): 2172–2176.

Baer, R. D., and M. Bustillo. 1993. "Susto and Mal de Ojo among Florida Farmworkers: Emic and Etic Perspectives." *Medical Anthropology Quarterly, New Series* 7(1): 90–100.

Baer, R. D. and M. Bustillo. 1998. "Caida de Mollera among Children of Mexican Migrant Workers: Implications for the Study of Folk Illnesses." *Medical Anthropology Quarterly, New Series* 12(2): 241–249.

Baer, R. D., S.C. Weller, J. G. De Alba Garcia, M. Glazer, R. Trotter, L. Patcher, and R. Klein. 2003. "A Cross-Cultural Approach to the Study of the Folk Illness *Nervios.*" *Culture, Medicine, and Psychiatry* 27: 315–337.

Baer, R. D., S. C. Weller, J. C. González Faraco, and, J. Feria Martín. 2006. "Las Enfermedades Populares en la Cultura Española Actual: Un Estudio Comparado Sobre el Mal de Ojo." *Revista de Dialectología y Tradiciones Populares* 61(1): 139–156.

Barragan, D. I., K. E. Ormond, M. N. Strecker, and J. Weil. 2011. "Concurrent Use of Cultural Health Practices and Western Medicine During Pregnancy: Exploring the Mexican Experience in the United States." *Journal of Genetic Counseling* 20: 609–624. doi:10.1007/s10897-011-9387-4

Boozang, K. M. 1998. "Western Medicine Opens the Door to Alternative Medicine." *American Journal of Law and Medicine* 24(2–3): 185–212. http://www.bu.edu/law/central/jd/organizations/journals/ajlm/index.html

Bourbonnais-Spear, N., R. Awad, Z. Merali, P. Maquin, V. Cal, and J. T. Arnason. 2007. "Ethnopharmacological Investigation of Plants Used to Treat Susto, a Folk Illness." *Journal of Ethnopharmacology* 109: 380–387. doi:10.1016/j.jep.2006.0 8.004

Brown, R.T. 2007. "Galen: Developer of the Reversal Design?" *The Behavior Analyst* 30(1): 31–35.

Capitanio, J. P. 2008. "Personality and Disease." *Brain Behavior and Immunity* 22(5): 647–650.

Chiappelli, F., P. Prolo, and O. S. Cajulis. 2005. "Evidence-Based Research in Complementary and Alternative Medicine I: History." *Advanced Access Publication* 2(4): 453–458.

Cintrón, J. A., M. M. Carter, and T. Sbrocco. 2005. "Ataques de Nervios in Relation to Anxiety Sensitivity among Island Puerto Ricans" [Electronic version]. *Culture, Medicine, and Psychiatry 29*: 415–431. doi: 10.1007/s11013-006-9001-7

Cole, R. G. 1993. "In Search of a New Mentality: The interface of Academic and Popular Medicine in the Sixteenth Century." *Journal of Popular Culture 26*(4): 155–172.

Editorial: 2006. "Time for the Renaissance of Medicine in the Middle East." *Lancet* 367, 959. doi: 10.1016/S0140-6736(06)68398-0

Flaskerud, J. H. and E. Ruiz Calvillo. 2007. "Cultural Competence Column. Psyche and Soma: Susto and Diabetes." *Issues in Mental Health Nursing 28*: 821–823. doi: 10.1080/01612840701415991

Fornaro, M., N. Clementi, and P. Fornaro. 2009. "Medicine and Psychiatry in Western Culture: Ancient Greek Myths and Modern Prejudices." *Annals of General Psychiatry* 8 (21): 21–28.

Foster, G. M. 1987. "On the Origin of Humoral Medicine in Latin America." *Medical Anthropology Quarterly New Series 1*(4): 355–393.

Glazer, M., R. D. Baer, S. C. Weller, J. E. Garcia de Alba, and S. W. Liebowitz. 2004. "Susto and Soul Loss in Mexicans and Mexican Americans." *Cross-Cultural Research 38*(3): 270–288.

Hansotia, P. 2003. "A Neurologist Looks at Mind and Brain: 'The Enchanted Loom.'" *Clinical Medicine and Research 1*(4): 327–332.

Hatcher, E. and R. Whittemore. 2007. "Hispanic Adults' Beliefs about Type 2 Diabetes: Clinical Implications." *Journal of American Academy of Nurse Practitioners 19*(10): 536–545. doi:10.1111/j.1745-7599.2007.00255.x

Herrera, S. R. 2010. "The Pocho Palimpsest in Early 20th Century Chicano Literature from Daniel Venegas to Américo Paredes." *Confluencia 26*(1): 21–33.

Holland, L, and R. Courtney. 1998. "Increasing Cultural Competence with the Latino Community." *Journal of Community Health Nursing 15*(1): 45–53. doi:10.1207/s1 5327655jchn1501_5

Houghton, A. A., and F. J. Boersma. 1988. "The Loss-Grief Connection in Susto." *Ethnology 27*(2): 145–154.

Landy, D. 1985. "Review: A Syndrome and its Meaning." *Science, New Series* 228(4701): 850–851.

Mysyk, A. 1998. "Susto: An Illness of the Poor." *Dialectical Anthropology 23*(2): 187–202.

Norris, F. H., D. L. Weisshaar, M. L. Conrad, E. M. Diaz, A. D. Murphy, and G. E. Ibañez. 2001. "A Qualitative Analysis of Posttraumatic Stress among Mexican Victims of Disaster." *Journal of Traumatic Stress 14*(4): 741–756. doi:10 .1023/A:10130422222084

O'Nell, C. W. 1975. "An Investigation of Reported 'Fright' as a Factor in the Etiology of Susto. 'MagicalFright.'" *Ethos 3*(1): 41–63.

Ortiz de Montellano, B. 1987. "Caida de Mollera: Aztec Sources for Mesoamerican Disease of Alleged Spanish Origin." *Ethnohistory 34*(4): 381–399.

Pettman, E. 2007. "A History of Manipulative Therapy." *The Journal of Manual and Manipulative Therapy* 15(3): 165–174.

Pikoulis, E., C. Waasdorp, A. Leppaniemi, and D. Burris. 1998. "Hippocrates: The True Father of Medicine." *American Surgeon* 64(3): 274.

Press, I. 1971. "The Urban Curandero." *American Anthropologist, New Series* 73(3): 741–756.

Rivera, G. and J. J. Wanderer. 1986. "Curanderismo and Childhood Illnesses." *The Social Science Journal* 23(3): 361–372.

Saad, B., H. Azaizeh, and O. Said. 2005. "Tradition and Perspectives of Arab Herbal Medicine: A Review." *Advance Access Publication* 2(4): 475–479.

Shekelle, P. G., S. C. Morton, M. J. Suttorp, N. Buscemi, and C. Friesen. 2005. "Challenges in Systematic Reviews of Contemporary and Alternative Medicine Topics." *Annals of Internal Medicine* 142(12): 1042–1047.

Tousignant, M. 1979. "Espanto: A Dialogue with the Gods." *Culture, Medicine, and Psychiatry* 3(4): 347–361.

Trotter II, R. T. 1991. "A Survey of Four Illnesses and Their Relationship to Intracultural Variation in a Mexican American Community." *American Anthropologist* 93(1): 115–125.

Trotter II, R.T. and J. A. Chavira. 1997. *Curanderismo: Mexican American Folk Healing* (2nd ed). Athens, GA: University of Georgia Press.

U.S. Census Bureau. 2011. "The Hispanic Population: 2010 Census Briefs." http://www.census.gov/prod/cen2010/briefs/c2010br-04.pdf

Uzzell, D. 1974. "'Susto' Revisited: Illness as Strategic Role." *American Ethnologist* 1(2): 369–378.

Van Der Riet, P. 2011. "Complementary Therapies in Health Care." *Nursing and Health Sciences* 13: 4–8. doi:10.1111/j.1442-2018.2011.00587.x

Vasiliadis, E. S., T. B. Grivas, and A. Kaspiris. 2009. "Historical Overview of Spinal Deformities in Ancient Greece." *Scoliosis* 4(6): 1–13.

Villasenor, Y., and H. Waitzkin. 1999. "Limitations of a Structured Psychiatric Diagnostic Instrument in Assessing Somatization among Latino Patients in Primary Care." *Medical Care* 37(7): 637–646. doi:10.1907/0000565-199907000-00003

Waldstein, A. 2008. "Diaspora and Health? Traditional Medicine and Culture in a Mexican Migrant Community." *International Migration* 46 (5): 95–117. doi: 10.1111/j.1468-2435.2008.00490.x

Weller, S. C., R. D. Baer, J. G. De Alba Garcia, M. Glazer, R. Trotter, L. Pachter, and R. Klein. 2002. "Regional Variation in Latino Descriptions of Susto." *Culture, Medicine and Psychiatry* 26: 449–472.

Weller, S. C., R. D. Baer, J. G. De Alba Garcia, and A. L. Salcedo Rocha. 2008. "Susto and Nervios: Expressions of Stress and Depression." *Culture, Medicine, and Psychiatry* 32: 406–420.

Weller, S. C., L. M. Pachter, R. T. Trotter II, and R. D. Baer. 1993. "Empacho in Four Latino Groups: A Study of Intra-and Inter-Cultural Variation in Beliefs." *Medical Anthropology* 15: 109–136.

CHAPTER TWELVE

Mediator between Man and the Gods: Shamanism and Health

Kimberly L. Howell

How the clouds pass silently overhead!
How the earth darts on and on!
And how the sun, moon, stars, dart on and on!
How the water sports and sings!
(Surely it is alive!)
How the trees rise and stand up – with strong trunks –
With branches and leaves!
(Surely there is something more in each of the trees –
Some living Soul!)
O amazement of things!
Even the least particle!
O spirituality of things!

Walt Whitman, *Song of Sunset*

When posing the question, "What is a shaman?" the answers are wide-ranging and varyingly interpreted. To some there is an indigenous heritage and bloodline associated with the title. For others, it is simply having the gift to heal or perhaps travel to other worlds by way of altered states of consciousness (ASC). Shamanism is one of humankind's most ancient spiritual and healing traditions that appears to have been common to hunter-gatherer societies worldwide (Eliade 1964, Winkelman 2010). Many authors have made identifications of shamanic work as being synonymous with the work of soul (Wolfe 1998). While shamanism has also been defined as "the ability to journey beyond this world and into the supernatural otherworld" (Williams 2010, 2), Wolfe in particular states, "The shaman taps into the purest forms of Nature's energy" (Wolfe 1998, xiii) perhaps identifying one sizeable incongruence between indigenous and post-modern, traditional practices of health and healing—that being, nature and the ability to communicate with nature. I would add to these definitions that the shaman is primarily the mediator between god and man, an individual divinely gifted to travel to other worlds for the purpose of communicating with god and nature with the ultimate outcome of healing. The sacred call to become the mediator between man and the gods is a notion somewhat foreign in many psychotherapeutic and biomedical environs.

The journey of the shaman is a most powerful one and in the shamanic world—much like Whitman's *Song of Sunset*—a spiritual essence connecting man with nature and the spirit worlds. Jung viewed shamanism as the earliest precursor to analytical psychology and construed Franz Mesmer's work with hypnosis and animal magnetism as more shamanic than scientific (Smith 2007, 145). On the surface, the shamanic journey is a transformative process used for healing of the body and soul, as well as for soul retrieval. However, within these practices lies the gift of speaking deeply to the soul.

Arguably, shamanic journeying provides a divination and parting of the veils between worlds of the seen and unseen and enacts a force that can help awaken and restore one to physical and psychical wholeness (Ingerman 2004), working alongside traditional psychotherapeutic and Western biomedical treatments. Regarding physical and psychical healing and therapies, there continues to be a substantial disconnect between the tribal ways of healing and finding that pure and sacred connection between the gods and man, between the known and unknown, between the depths of the soul and heights of consciousness. The prerequisite pathologizing found in the Western biomedical model is often an incongruent fit with shamanic treatments.

This chapter will pursue ideologies surrounding shamanism and indigenous practices including altered states of consciousness, including how these methods can possibly work in conjunction with traditional, psychotherapeutic approaches. Following a description of the different types of shamans and shamanic practices in America, I review different cultural groups using shamanism and focus on one specific aspect of shamanism, journeying, utilized in shamanic practices. I then review the notion of tribe, family, and community in addition to the treatments, philosophies, and approaches used in shamanic practice. I conclude with a discussion of health-related findings within shamanic and alternative medicine and briefly touch on the Westernization of practices such as yoga. For the purposes of this work, *alternative medicine* is defined by White as a medical system based on alternative paradigms for understanding healing and illness outside of the Western realm and model (White 2000, 671). General mention of the terms *shamanism* and *shamanic practice* fall synonymously within the overarching designation of *neo-shamanism* and *core shamanism* (Harner 1980) and for the purposes of this chapter are intended to either amalgamate the entirety of shamanism or imply non-denominationalism.

The Origins and Cultures of Shamanism

> In other traditions demons are expelled externally. But in my tradition demons
> are accepted with compassion.

Machik Labdron

Origins of Shamanism

The title *shaman* or *saman* originated amongst the Eastern Siberian Tungus-speakers but what is more widely known as shaman or shamanism has gone by many other designations including *page*, *anagkkut*, seer, medicine man, and *arendiouannens* (Narby and Huxley 2001, Walsh 2007). These terms should not be confused with other titles by which shaman have been mistaken including that of the sorcerer or occultist. In the case of the former, there are aspects which fit solidly within the sphere of shamanism including altered states of consciousness and the ability to act as proxy with unknown forces through communicating with the spirit world.

According to Van Gennep, "There can be no shamanic belief or cults, and therefore no shamanic religion, for the simple reason that the word does not designate a set of beliefs that manifest themselves through a set of customs. It merely affirms the existence of a certain kind of person who plays a religious and social role." (Van Gennep 1903, 51). However, I would argue that this expansive characterization of Van Gennep does not fit the sharp foci of shamanism, principally that of altered states of consciousness. The compartmentalization of "a person who plays a religious and social role," undoubtedly fits deftly in the borders of organized religion, but debatably, not shamanism. Systematized religions do indeed have spiritual conduits who can commune with the spirit world on behalf of parishioners, such as with the Roman Catholic priesthood, but the dissimilarity lies with said healing, response to a physical disease, psychic or physical malady being delivered solely by the shaman. Intercessory or individual prayer for healing is a component of many organized religious structures, but such is not generally the case with shamanic practices in which the channel or intermediary for healing is exclusively held by the shaman who receives said powers through communication with the spirit world.

Identifying North American Sects

Narby and Huxley (2001) refer to the shift in documented shaman in areas such as Siberia, the Canadian Arctic, and British Guiana when anthropologists began to observe the activities of these groups in the second half of the nineteenth century with the commonality again being the ability to communicate with the spirit world on behalf of the healing of others.

In the early 1800s, anthropologist Boas engaged in ethnographic research among the Inuit medicine men referred to as "angakoq." This group of medicine men was more widely viewed as priests who possessed the capacity to intervene in matters of sickness or to even obstruct death (Boas 1887, 47).

The challenge in identifying shamanic sects in North American culture is in differentiating religious practice, medical professions stemming from the Western biomedical model, practitioners of witchcraft, and healers who do not associate with shamanism in its indigenous manifestation. In some groups, the shamans are those who have experienced the benefit of shamanic practice, thereby becoming wounded healers as is the case with the Zuni Pueblo. However, it is argued that the Zuni Pueblo do not fall within the definition of shaman versus being that of a society of wounded healers due to the characterization of North American shamanic cultures focusing on communion with spirit and central focus on the healing and soul retrieval within their own communities (Smith 2007, 36). There are many practicing shamanic communities in North America and the following section focuses on a few such communities but is by no means an exhaustive catalogue of shamanic designations.

Tungus Shaman

The Siberian indigenous groups, Tungus shamans, credited with being the origin of shamanism, were largely spiritual in nature and comprised of both men and women. It was not until the 18th Century that the term *shaman* made its way into Western realms (Znamenski 2007). In the 1920s, what Znamenski calls "indigenous primitives" (2007, 52) initiated the sharing of their tribal knowledge with the inhabitants of the Southwestern United States. The Jungian notion of the hero fantasy began to grow in the United States along with the archetypal conceptualization of cowboys and Indians. The cultural divide, coupled with increasing interest in what was becoming shamanic practice in the United States, would be a mere ripple in the East-West, Traditional-Non-Traditional approaches to health and wellness.

Aboriginal Canadians

Among Aboriginal Canadians, there is a divide between those who are entrenched in more modernized, Western practices and those who have remained true to aboriginal practices including the hunter-gatherer who remains solidly connected to nature and natural engagements with shamanic practice. Studies by Polimeni and Reiss provide clinical evidence that there is a perceptible propensity toward hallucinations and delusions among the Aboriginal Canadians who are more entrenched with natural shamanic practices than among those who are adapted to post-modern society (2002, 246).

Hmong Shaman

Hmong Americans have a storied history with shamanic practice. The Hmong shamanic lineage embraces the concept of the body as the container of all souls and that disease occurs when there is a disruption with one or more of these souls. Conquergood addresses one of the most crucial means for healing these disruptions in body and soul—the *Hu Plig,* or Soul Calling—a ritual which calls the disrupted soul back to the "bodily community" (Conquergood 1991, 5). In the Hmong shamanic tradition, the shaman is the only individual who has the capacity to intervene with the wayward soul(s). Similarly to the *curanderismo* tradition, discussed previously, Hmong-American shaman are supportive of Western biomedical practices, including prescription medications. Hmong shamans also engage with medical facilities to work collaboratively toward healing those in the Hmong community, with the Hmong-American shaman having the ability to tend to both the somatic and psychical needs of the patient.

Curanderismo

Among Mexican-Americans there remain the traditions of the practice of curanderismo—from the Spanish verb *curar* meaning to heal (see chapter 10 in volume 1 of this series). This tradition of healers follows practices falling within three approaches: 1) material healing, 2) spiritual healing, and 3) psychic healing (Trotter 2001, 130). This rich tradition of healers, much like the Hmong, also practice modern biomedical approaches to health and healing including the use of prescription medication and body work such as massage and reflexology. The practice of curanderismo also involves the entering into of altered states of consciousness in some instances, but also borrows richly upon other practices including magic and traditional prayer as a means of channeling healing.

Arendiouannens

Arendiouannens are Huron and Iroquois lineages of shaman who participate in acts of divination including the analysis of dreams and predicting future events (Lafitau cited in Narby and Huxley 2001, 24). This divination of the Arendiouannens is notable in large part due to the diversity of abilities exhibited by shaman across time such as the ability to heal, communicate with plant and animal life, and in some cases, the ability to take life.

Overarching Cultures of Shamanism

The practice of shamanism is often generational, thereby dictating a communal following. Initially the equivalent of a village healer, the shaman led the community in not only medicinal, physical acts of healing, but also in soul retrieval and healing of the psyche. It is the latter that has caused the greatest gap in cultural sensibilities most notably among Western culture as a collective. Williams posits, "In traditional societies, shamanism is sometimes considered only a short step from madness" (2010, 22). And by all accounts and purposes, there remains a pall of judgment in the field and tradition of shamanism as a legitimate method of therapy or healing.

Becoming a shaman is often through lineage or from a spiritual or otherworldly call. In many Rocky Mountain shamanic sects, the shamanic authority always occurs through "ecstatic experience" (Eliade 1987, 21) which is in tune with communication directly with God or the gods in an effort to bring healing to the individuals who are in need or the community as a whole. It is this facet that differentiates Western shamans from those in other cultures. Asian shamans often fall more solidly into the category of being solely religious (versus borrowing from nature or the underworlds) as is the case with those who engage in what is called "Yellow Shamanism," which blends aspects of Buddhism with shamanic practice.

Journeying: Otherworld, Upperworld, Underworld

> We are always in both worlds, because there aren't really two.
>
> Gary Snyder

Although there is extensive discussion of the role of altered states of consciousness in shamanism (see Winkelman 2010), not as much has been

Table 12.1   Comparison of Shamanism and Jungian Practices

	Shamanic View	Jungian View
Health	Living in accord with the will of the sacred.	Result of wholeness, living in accord with the promptings of the archetypal self.
Pathology	Imbalance caused by violating the will of the sacred.	Imbalance (one-sidedness) caused by violating the wholeness and integration demanded by the archetypal self.

written about the more Jungian elements of shamanism. It is the notion of the upperworld and underworld that link shamanism to fields such as analytical (Jungian) psychology as well as religious traditions such as the ideology of heaven (above) and hell (below). This is a discernible difference in comparison to the Western biomedical representation where there is rarely, if ever, any comparison to above and below, upperworlds or underworlds. It is debatable whether Austrian psychologist C.G. Jung was a shaman, however his fascination and practice of active imagination—in which he would drop into the under-world and engage in active imagination with the images encouraged—have been well documented.

Eliade's work frequently reflects upon the linking of the upper and underworlds (Eliade 1987) and there are North American examples of shamanic engagements stemming from this link, such as the Ojibway where practices often include symbolic representations of the axis linking the upper and underworlds (Smith 2007, 17) and interactions with a "therapeutic field" during underworld journeys which could yield answers to the cause of disease and varied disorders (Porterfield 1987, 734).

Jung possessed a vast kinship with nature and connection with the ideology of the presence of soul in all forms including plant and animal forms. Jungian practices also share similar views to that of shamanism as can be seen in comparison in Table 12.1 made by Smith (2007, 124):

It is in the underworld where the notion of time becomes a factor. Western biomedical constructs dictate set structures as pertaining to time, chronologically speaking. Medical doctor appointments are often set within specific time parameters with static appointment times. Conversely, the shaman operates on *kairos* or divine time. A drop into the underworld as reported in some cases can last for several days while the "patient" waits for the diagnosis from the shaman upon their return. Eliade writes, "by its very nature, sacred time is reversible" (Eliade 1968, 68) and furthers this by differentiating how time is viewed also from the religious perspective. Current religious models also have a sense of *chronos* or numeric, tangible time versus *kairos.* The heads of many Western religious practices may have a head or leader similar to a communal shaman, but the journey to the underworld is atypical as is the notion that sacred time is "reversible."

This journeying to the otherworlds is well documented. Harner references the practice among the Coast of Salish Indians of Washington State who would as a group of shaman travel to the spirit world as a collective. The practice among this sect of shaman to travel as a group is not common. Also an uncommon practice among the Coast of Salish was the inclusion of the community in joining them in chanting as they began their journey to the underworld (Harner 1980, 70).

There is a considerable level of importance to be given to the transformation of the shaman. Going through the hero's journey into the depths only to again arise, is paralleled in the journey of the shaman and the shamanic transformation process. In *Jung and Shamanism in Dialogue,* the author speaks of how Jung would allow himself to "drop" into the underworld (Smith 2007, 84). This dropping can be viewed as parallel to the experience of the shaman when entering the trance state; both are an experience of entering and journeying through the underworld and communicating between the gods and man. Jung's method of journey into the unconscious world and encountering spirit presences was by way of active imagination.

When Jung discusses interactions during altered states of consciousness with a character by the name of "Philemon," it is reflective of the fantasy images that provide the insight deep into the psyche. For Jung, Philemon acted as a type of shamanic guide into the psyche and bridged the communication with the gods, much as psychotropic plants can serve the shaman (Jung 1989, 183). In *Memories, Dreams, Reflections,* Jung further states that everything in the unconscious seeks outward manifestation (Jung 1989, 3). The shaman enters ecstatic trance in order to see the soul of the other/patient. In line with Jung's thought, there is substantial force in images and these images can help unlock the doors to the underworld, providing fundamental healing and restoration.

The shaman possesses the gift of entering into the trance state, at times with the help of psychotropic plant life, in order to gain unity with nature and to heighten the numinosity of the spiritual transformation (Smith 2007, 141), a viewing of these soul images, if you will. Shamanic ritual provides a container for transformation. Jung's thoughts on ritual were that it effects a transformation, including the death of the old self and rebirth; a transformation from a lower to a higher level of consciousness (Smith, 2007, p. 162). It is this transformation that serves not only the objectives of the shaman, but those the shaman is called by the gods to serve.

Notion of the Tribe, Family, and Community

*Nature, psyche, and life appear to me like divinity unfolded—what more could
I ask for?*

C.G. Jung

A further separation between shamanic and traditional Western approaches toward health includes the notion of tribe or family. Biomedical practices often include a variety of practitioners and specialists (e.g., General Practice, Obstetrics, and Oncology). However, core shamanic practices (Harner 1980) embrace the notion of the tribe, family, and community. Often, in shamanic communities there is a lineage of shamans who have imbedded themselves and their work among their people and communal collective.

It is this separation from the notion of tribe that is lacking in Western medical models with rare and reaching exceptions being that of a practice among family members. However, the sense of tribe is the fiber of the shamanic culture. Westernized shamanic approaches do embrace cross-indigenous approaches, particularly among those who are schooled in shamanism by watered-down instructional methods, such as through a line of shamans who have at no point had contact or instruction with an indigenous teacher. This includes practitioners who are readily found via internet searches. An internet search for "San Francisco Bay Area Shaman" yielded results for a host of options from lay-shaman, including journeying trips and soul retrieval training. These types of practices could be viewed as a diluted form of shamanism as it eliminates the indigenous lineage of the practice. These modern approaches allow the general population to embark upon practices which in many societies have been closely protected and deemed sacred. Additionally, the reasonableness of such activities could be questioned for those who are engaged in the rigors of daily life.

The introduction of economic systems may be a driving force in traditional versus non-traditional shamanistic practices including that of yoga. Kim et al. (citing Henry) argues that this shift in economic patterns not only influences the cultural shift as a whole but also the dominance of religion (Kim et al. 2006, 88) in Western cultures. With this infusion of economic and religious focus came a pulling away from native practices and a more broad focus on the gods and nature. With this cultural shift came uprooting of various specific religious factions versus the concept of god in nature or the shaman as a conduit for the gods as an alternate to the universal, omnipotent, omnipresent God encapsulated in oneness.

Treatments, Philosophies, and Approaches

> *If one way be better than another, that you may be sure is nature's way.*
>
> Aristotle

The following will address some of the main treatments and philosophies of shamanism including the importance and impact of nature on shamanic practices and the value of animals and animal totems.

Nature and Plant Life

Plant life is an integral part of shamanic practice, primarily as a means of entering altered states of consciousness. In many instances, these plants are a part of sacred rituals above and beyond those that are engaged in by the shaman as a part of the healing and divining process. The processing of plants, such as those that will be discussed, is also a sacred activity. Many of these plants require that the preparation process be monitored and observed only by those with the purest of intent and with the power and knowledge to handle the spirit of the plant in a way that will end up being most helpful to the shaman in transporting between the gods and man and for the essential journeys to the underworld. At times, these plants are handled with such devotion of their sacredness that the shaman may engage in singing (known as *icaros*) to the plant life in preparation for ceremony (Heaven and Charing 2006, 89).

One very important point to make with regard to the topic of psychotropic plant use for shamanic purposes is the occasional misconception that surrounds this practice. The use of this type of plant life, or any method to enter trance, it not with the intention to "get high" or numb oneself from present consciousness – it is, like the title of this paper, a means for humans to reach the depths, speak with the gods, and bring soul healing. Some shaman claim that the powerful dreams, visions, and psychedelic effects come not from the plant, but from the spirits which created the plants.

The power of medicinal plants has indeed created an unfortunate opportunity for abuse. This includes what de Rios calls "charlatan psychiatry" (cited in Winkelman 2005, 209) in which groups of individuals take spiritual retreats led by people who are nothing less than imposters posing as shamanic healers who use those seeking a spiritual experience to defraud them of money and in some cases to prey upon tourists sexually.

While there are a host of plants that are used in shamanic ritual, the following is an overview of those most prominent in shamanic ritual and ceremony – San Pedro Cactus, the Seguro, and Ayahuasca. The following is an account of a post-hallucinogenic drink experience in Harner's "The Sound of Rushing Water."

> He had drunk, and now he softly sang. Gradually, faint lines and forms began to appear in the darkness, and the shrill music of the *tsentsak,* the spirit helpers, arose around him. The power of the drink fed them. He called, and they came. First, *pangi,* the anaconda, coiled about his head, transmuted into a crown of gold. Then *wampung,* the giant butterfly, hovered above his shoulder and sang to him with its wings. Snakes, spiders, birds, and bats danced in the air above him. On his arms appeared a thousand eyes as his demon helpers emerged to search the night for enemies (1968).

This account demonstrates not only the images that can appear during ingestion of medicinal plants during shamanic ritual, but also the essentiality of power animals and the messages they can provide to the shaman, in the above account, within the Jivaro shamanic community. Following is an overview of a sampling of medicinal plants used in shamanic practice and the groups among whom these practices are used. With these plants, a common side effect is the muddling of sensory modalities and in some cases, a heightening of all sensory modalities (de Rios 2003).

San Pedro Cactus

With the establishment of the importance of the transportation of the shaman, I will now address various methods of shamanic healing through plant life. Admittedly, what most captured my attention about the plant life of the shaman is the shamanic journeying experienced by the ingestion of the San Pedro cactus. As noted in *The Gift of Life,* "San Pedro" is known as the "Keeper of Keys" . . . [and] guardian of the doors of Heaven, so the San Pedro plant is called "guardian of the doors of remedy" (Glass-Coffin 1998, 64).

San Pedro cactus is most often cut, boiled and the remaining liquid ingested by the shaman and at times participants of the shamanic ritual ceremony. Like many other entheogenic substances used in the aboriginal religions of the Americas, the use of the hallucinogenic San Pedro cactus is ancient and its use has been a continuous tradition in Peru for over 3,000 years (Rudgley 1998).

In Glass-Coffin's, work, the author speaks of a time when attending a healing with curanderas Olinda and Isabel upon ingesting San Pedro. The author notes that Olinda felt as if San Pedro himself had possessed Isabel as demonstrated during the ceremony that she began speaking with the voice of a very old man (1998, 64). The powerful transformation that San Pedro provides is thought to bring the shaman to a more heightened connection and communication between the upper, middle, and underworlds.

With the demonstrated powers of the San Pedro cactus, there were, and continues to be, varying schools of thought on its potency, value, and legitimacy. Rudgley (1998) notes that early European missionaries had very negative views of the use of this particular cactus. However, another Spanish missionary, cited by Rätsch, admitted the medicinal value while reviling it:

> It is a plant with whose aid the devil is able to strengthen the Indians in their idolatry; those who drink its juice lose their senses and are as if dead; they are almost carried away by the drink and dream a thousand unusual things and believe that they are true. The juice is good against burning of the kidneys and, in small amounts, is also good against high fever, hepatitis, and burning in the bladder.

Rudgley (1998) notes that the experiences noted by the shaman are vastly different from those who have perhaps experienced San Pedro outside of the shamanic setting or through word of mouth. He notes that most shamanic input states that the San Pedro cactus provides the shaman with a great level of vision and a detachment from the body accompanied by a great level of tranquility. Additionally, he notes that some shamans add that it heightens the senses and provides a celestial transformation and ability to tap into the telepathic sense.

Seguro

Another shamanic potion is that of the seguro which is a ritually prepared jar of herbs thought to provide protection against daños. The jar is also filled with water from sacred lagoons as well as other fragrant substances spoken to the shaman and thought to be most powerful and appropriate for the need at hand. The powers within these mystical substances are called upon by the shaman (Glass-Coffin 1998, 23). According to San Pedro maestro, Juan Navarro, a *seguro* is a friend or ally (Heaven and Charing 2006, 101) since, as can be imagined, the journey of the shaman can at times be filled with solitude and devoid of allies. The seguro is also used as a spray during the ceremony by the shaman. During this time, the shaman may elect to spray the mesa altar or recipient of the services of the shaman as part of providing protection.

Ayahuasca

Ayahuasca is used in the shamanic work of various clans. This is the shamanic medicine of the Upper Amazon which originates from the ayahuasca vine and leaf of the chacruna plant. This plant is also grown and used in Mastizo healing sessions in certain parts of Peru. An element of beauty surrounding ayahuasca is the very meaning of its name which is Quechuan for "the vine of souls." Ayahuasca is typically boiled into a tea, and when ingested is said to cause the appearance of astonishing visual images. In interviews with individuals who have had the experience of ayahuasca during shamanic ceremony, there is mention of experiences as far ranging as "seeing demons" to "visions of regressed life forms." Some reported an intense nausea from the ingestion of this plant, but all state that the images revealed were signs from the upper and underworlds.

Research is currently being developed surrounding the possible medicinal properties of ayahuasca for conditions such as cancer and drug addiction, hopefully highlighting the importance of using naturopathic means to become more unified with mother earth and natural healing.

As the Western world in particular pulls further away from tribal ideologies and increases dependency on manufactured pharmaceuticals, we distance ourselves as a global collective from the sacredness of nature. While there are other methods of shamanic trance that are indeed sacred and viable such as meditation and drumming, the life that plants provide to the shamanic experience is imperatively important. It increases the criticality of studying this plant life, increasing knowledge of psychotropic plants, and working to restore the habitats that house these tools of the shaman.

The future of shamanic plant life vary depending on the geographic stance. For example, certain psychotropic plants, such as San Pedro cactus, can be purchased in the United States with relative ease. There are hosts of "botanical" sites offering cacti, seeds, and essences, with most sites offering a disclaimer that the items on the website(s) are not for human consumption, have not been approved by the Food and Drug Administration (FDA), and there is no culpability on the part of the vendor in the event a customer chooses to ingest the products.

As has been discussed in this chapter, among the differences between indigenous and tribal societies with those of modern, Western societies, a substantial discrepancy lies in the area of nature and community. This issue is not only one that lies solely within the modernized United States. In Northern Peru, the knowledge of medicinal plants is still taught orally, leaving a possibility that the many benefits of plant life may continue to be passed down to other generations. The most serious threat to this ancient tradition is the destruction of the lands on which shamanic plant life flourish. This is being experienced primarily in the Peruvian coastal plains. In addition, the Andean ecosystems and sacred lagoons are also in danger of extinction due to the increase in large-scale mining activities (Bussmann and Sharon 2006).

There are marked differences between alternative or shamanic methods of medicine and that of traditional practices:

- The Limitations of Resources
  Particularly in Peru where there is a considerable focus on shamanic plant life and harvesting, resources are limited, unlike the pharmaceutical industry which is able to create and produce products to heal in laboratories and on manufacturing lines.

- Driven By Nature
  Nature itself drives the output of shamanic plant life. Seasonality and elevation are merely two factors that can drive how a plant grows and how much of any given plant can be produced in certain climates. These plant species are also impacted by global issues such as urbanization and global climate shifting.
- Community Network
  The production of shamanic medicinals is often a community undertaking and a delicately interwoven tapestry of family and villagers who not only understand the land, but understand the intricacies of shamanism and how the plants they as a community work to grow will be used not only to help heal, but to transport the shaman on a journey to the underworld where the answers and souls are located.
- Scalability of Consumerist Production
  The production of these indigenous plants is frequently produced by lesser-known and smaller scale producers. In many cases, the plant growers are women who lack the financial backing to increase crops or to ship the products.

The shamanic plant life mentioned in this section represent only a fraction of the medicinal plant life located on this expansive planet, but represents that touch of earth that works as the vital vehicle of shamanic trance, revelation, healing and restoration. The overall value of these plants is over $1.2 million U.S. per year in Peru alone (Bussmann et. al 2008).

Power Animals

With roots in the natural environment, there is a logical leap to the presence of animal presentation or images in shamanic practices. The Southeastern Cherokee tribe would often diagnose disease or eruptions of the psyche as retribution by animal spirits or one's animal totem (a spirit guide in animal form). Offerings would often be made specifically to the offended animal by the shaman by dressing like and communicating with the animal during a state of trance and during underworld journeys. According to Smith, "Cherokee therapeutics presupposes a kind of sympathetic magic" (2007, 22) often projected toward or on the offended animal causing the disharmony in body, psyche, or both aspects. Harner (1980) refers to the synchronicities that often manifest with power or spirit animals and the significance of unexpected encounters with animals, most notably when the shaman assigns a power animal to the afflicted person.

Another important differentiating factor between shamanic and Western biomedical practices is that of treatments that are scientific and those that are not. It is widely apparent that shamanic traditions and rituals do not adopt standard scientific approaches. Western biomedical practices do not typically include actions such as trance, dreams, otherworld journeying, and shape shifting in an effort to heal and retrieve souls—the latter of which is certainly outside the scope of most medical practice within the United States. These approaches, which are generally not tested by clinical trials or within the limits of scientific measures, will be addressed with additional information being provided as to how they are enacted by the shaman and the standard results and outcomes of such approaches.

Trance

The origination of sacred chants and drumming which lead the shaman into trance belongs concretely to the Native American population in North America. Walsh notes that the beats of a drum at a tempo of 200 to 220 beats per minute will allow even a novice to enter into an altered state (Walsh 1989). Entering the trance state is a key, initial step toward communion between man and the gods. The entrance of the trance is often brought on by chanting or drumming. It is through these vehicles that the shaman is able to transport himself to the underworld in an effort to diagnose the presenting illness or disease. Often during the journey, the shaman is able to gather images or messages from other worlds to take back and act upon in order to bring healing. In the case of the Central Eskimo shaman, there is no drum utilized to enter into ASC and it is done simply through concentration.

Noll (citing Richardson) states, "contemporary psychologists do not regard mental imagery as an interesting empirical phenomenon, but as a hypothetical entity whose existence must be proved in the course of experimental investigation" (Noll et al. 1985, 443). Throughout time, including within holy scriptures, dreams and visions have been documented. I would contend that in primitive times as well as modern times, the visions and journeys that have been experienced by shaman do not have to be proven "real" in order to present healing to the afflicted.

Dreams

Shaman, Medicine Grizzlybear Lake (in Grasse) states, "The calling [to be a Native healer] comes in the form of a dream, accident, sickness, injury, disease, near-death experience, or even actual death" and that such events are all a vital segment of how shamanic wisdom is obtained (Grasse 1996, 134). In keeping with Jungian thought, what is likely the most valuable aspect to the shaman's dream is the images obtained and how those images can be used to heal as well as communicate with the gods and animal spirits believed to be the cause of the presenting disorder(s). Jung stated,

Nobody doubts the importance of conscious experience; why then should we doubt the significance of unconscious happenings? They also are part of our life, and sometimes more truly a part of it for weal or woe than any happenings of the day (Jung 1974, 99).

It is the notion that the solitary value of shamanic healing occurs in conscious awareness that can be viewed as misguided. The images, messages, and gifts from the gods during the shamanic journey should be viewed as equally valuable as conscious communication.

Health-Related Findings

> *May all sentient beings enjoy happiness and the root of all happiness.*
> *May we all be free from suffering and the root of suffering.*
> *May we not be separated from the great happiness devoid of suffering.*
> *May we dwell in the great equanimity free from passion, aggression, and prejudice.*
>
> The Four Limitless Ones Chant

Woodman states, "Crucial to the healing process, therefore is working creatively with the rejected body" (Woodman 1982, 56). Many shamanic practices provide the opportunity for those afflicted with physical or psychical wounding to work through this "rejection." This is often accomplished through creative and spiritual means such as travel such as underworld journeying and communication with animal spirits. The Western biomedical model is an industry versus ritual or indigenous process and it can be viewed as a consumerist-driven mechanism that often does not help or heal in the process. However, the detail of the non-commercialized focus of shamanism provides yet another means for individuals seeking health and healing; it allows a deeper communion with nature and with someone gifted with the ability to travel to the underworld and communicate with nature and the gods on their behalf. In the section, "America at Risk," Sabini quotes Jung,

> We are awakening a little to the feeling that something is wrong in the world, that our modern prejudice of overestimating the importance of the intellect and the conscious mind might be false. We want simplicity. We are suffering, in our cities, from a need of simple things (Sabini 2002, 8).

Jung's words ring true today. There is an inherent trust that the biomedical approach and those that are science-based are the lone means of health and healing and if not lone, still largely considered to be the best means. There is a prejudice against healing methods that are not steeped in science and proven time and again.

There are other benefits of shamanism from the standpoint of the efficacy of shamanic treatments of physical and psychical health. Smith (citing Eliade) claims the particular province and power of the shaman lies in the disorder of psyche (2007, 64). By grasping Jungian traditions of psyche/soul fissure and recovery correlations can be made with shamanic traditions and therapeutic applications. For example, were a community member of an indigenous shamanic practice to present symptoms of dissociative identity disorder (multiple personality disorder), the shaman might conduct the diagnosis as well as therapeutic, prescriptive measures by way of trance, drumming, and a visit to the underworld to retrieve the "whole" soul that has dissociated from the conscious realm.

It is the cultural beliefs rooted in the afterlife and the supernatural that bind the healing gifts of the shaman to the community (Singh 1999, 132) where diseases and disorders are typically considered an issue of an unbalanced life versus an unbalanced diet or lack of routine exercise as is often the case in most Western medical and scientific health approaches. According to Singh (1999, 133),

> Healing implies wholeness or a state of equilibrium. For the shaman, good physical and mental health imply not only that the individual is free from suffering, but also that the individual…is in a harmonious relationship with all things…biological, social, psychological, physical and cosmic…

There are drastic shifts in the paradigm of the Western approach to health, healing and wellness not only among practitioners but also within health organizations with a palpable modification of the medical model to that which is more holistic. This includes not only tending to the manifesting bodily ailments and diagnosing of symptoms but to treatment of the "biological, social, psychological, physical" of which Singh wrote. However, not included in this treatment is that of the "cosmic," also again referring to Singh. While models are being modified to embrace more shamanic or holistic practices, this often does not include the aspects of the cosmic which so deeply permeate shamanic culture and treatment.

Other studies have been conducted demonstrating the possible efficacy of shamanic practices such as drumming and chanting including alterations in the central nervous system stimulated by shamanic drumming or chanting resulting in marked effects upon neurochemistry (Money 2001, 129).

Klein compares the effect to that attained in beta-endorphin states:

> The same psychotropic effects as shown in clinical trials with beta-endorphin can also be observed the North American Indian ceremonials...We may further propose that the release of these substances could be triggered by the same conditions known to induce altered states of consciousness in the rituals under discussion; notably pain, acoustic and kinetic stimulation, hypoglycemia, and dehydration, in combination with physical exertion (340).

Studies also document the value and equivalencies between shamanism and schizophrenia. According to Polimeni and Reiss the origins of schizophrenia are as ancient as shamanism (2002, 244). The authors further this by claiming the similarities between schizophrenia and shamanism could lead to increased insight into the origins of psychosis (p. 245). Returning to the concept of the religious aspects of shamanism and the connection between the gods and man, there are common threads between the religious models of shamanism and that of schizophrenia with delusions among schizophrenics often exhibiting as not only bizarre behaviors but adopting the persona of religious characters such as Jesus Christ or believing that they are being spoken through by the gods. In the Western biomedical model, this behavior is analyzed and diagnosed as a disorder. In shamanic practices, these behaviors are standard and within the realms of orthodoxy.

Winkleman (2001) broaches the subject of alternative approaches to substance abuse treatment including shamanic practice and the effects of these approaches on those suffering from such abuse. Non-traditional, indigenous methods as seen in the shamanic tradition tend to be marginalized in Western culture, thus making some of these treatments challenging in conventional settings. In the case of substance abuse, many seeking treatment use the chemicals which they are abusing as a means of escape or expanded awareness. Treatment of addiction in non-traditional approaches often utilizes rites and rituals for both the purification of body as has been noted within the Malaysian and Thai Buddhist treatments (Winkleman 2001, 342). In another study, researchers sought to compare the effects of a spiritual retreat on depression and post-acute coronary syndrome (ACS). This study conducted by Warber et al. resulted in data showing that among 41 participants, those who participated in the spiritual retreat had significantly lower scores at all post-intervention measurement times (P.002) (Warber et al. 2011).

One notable issue with measuring the prospective efficacy of shamanic therapeutic treatments is that most conducted research has been done by anthropologists and not necessarily those skilled in biomedical traditions.

Walsh presses this even further by suggesting that while shamanic practices do not sit solidly within the branches of traditional medicine and healing methods, there can be a tendency to consolidate the work of the shaman with that of other healing practitioners including Buddhism or yoga (Walsh 1994).

Traditional, biomedical treatments have a large number of journals recording the statistics of the efficacy of treatments and pharmaceutics. Historically, there has been documentation of the work of the shaman but this work has been done without the necessity of cataloguing whether or not the journey of a shaman and the shaman's medicinal treatments have or have not been effective in their treatment. A further component could quite possibly be the lack of technology in most indigenous settings. Walsh aptly refers to the "technology of the sacred" (1999, 34) and how the realm of shamanic tradition creates generational knowledge through the sharing of the shaman's wisdom. But there could be room for future in-depth studies of the efficacies of shamanic treatments. Winkleman addresses this from the standpoint of the lower brain structures which are affected when in ASC and the change in function of the body's neurotransmitter systems (Winkleman 2002) as well as the efficacy of alternative healing approaches based in ASC in comparison with formalized substance abuse treatment programs (Winkleman 2001).

In ethnographic research I conducted in 2009 collecting the stories of self-identified women healers in the United States, there were many exchanges of information of how patients or clients had been transformed through the process of working with them. One particular woman who identified as a shaman stated that "It's a rarity if one finds this road (that of a shaman) by grace." The women I interviewed commented that they are outsiders who feel that their work is invalid as it does not fit neatly within the compartmentalized notions of traditional health and well-being or because they do not possess the training or licenses to practice medicine. As one such recipient of multiple "healings" throughout this work, I can attest when one is in need of physical or psychical repair, few questions are asked after the healing is conducted.

Yoga and Shamanism: Commonalities with Western-Adopted Practices

Sacred space is an integral part of living yogically.

Christy Turlington

A recent internet search for shamanic healers in the greater Los Angeles area yielded many results. While legitimate practitioners certainly fall within this number, this volume raises the issue of ethical standards and practices when an indigenous field enters the mainstream, particularly when unregulated. This includes the practice of yoga, which is an indigenous, ritualistic engagement. Yoga has burst onto the U.S. scene to the point of becoming mainstream, and it appears shamanism may be following suit, with some researched shamans even offering their services via Skype or over the telephone.

With the treatment of what can be called spiritual ailments, resulting traditions may draw practitioners using the mantle of indigenous shaman in order to lure those desperate for treatments offered in non-traditional mediums. In the postmodern Western world, there are countless practices stemming from primitive, indigenous, cultural practices that do not necessarily maintain the original connotations. Ethically speaking, the emergence of indigenous healing functions into einstream practice can prove problematic. When factoring in issues of medical confidentiality and considerations of legal dictates, there can be a blurred line between indigenous practices and those of modern, traditional practices including the question of whether or not indigenous practices should be held to the same standards of confidentiality of patient health. Granted, when elbow to elbow in a yoga studio, there is an implied openness, but this does not negate the necessity of ethics nor should it be an open gateway to remove oneself from the original significance and importance of indigenous practices.

Many spend every second filling time and space with cell phone calls, texting on their smart phones, or shuffling to the next tune on their iPod. Postmodern minds are moving non-stop. It is no small wonder the Western capitalist world found a way to turn that chatter of the mind into profit. Enter the commercialized yoga studio and the shaman for hire.

The Yogasutra 1.17 identifies four supportive factors: reasoning (vitarka), "refined" reflection (vicāra), sublime happiness (ānanda), and sense of "egoity" (asmitā) (Sacrini and Ferraz 2009, 250). There is a distancing from the true heart of indigenous practices within the Western geographic sphere where many are engaged in a quest for these supportive factors such as reflection and happiness mentioned in the Yogasutra. This quest is investigated largely, but not solely, through the lens of analytical psychology in an effort to illuminate the psyche and gain clarity on how the healing of the soul can be incorporated into the individual as well as collective. This is evidenced not only in yogic practice but also in the uptick in "drive-thru" or convenience shamanism.

The idea of yoga being a vehicle toward clearing the mind through controlled breathing should be an indicator of why this practice has been bastardized in many ways in Western culture. The yoga "market" in the United States consists largely of Hatha Yoga practice. This practice involves breathing and meditative exercises which are thought to have positive physical benefits such as improved health, stress reduction, and as touted in some studios, weight loss. It is these factors that make this practice enticing to the U.S. population as many clamor to be as physically fit and attractive as possible. Conversely, shamanism as well, with the advent of technological interfaces such as Skype, has also opened the door to the potential bastardization of indigenous practices such as shamanic healing.

Perhaps it is the mindset of open-access which causes the commoditization of yoga as well as shamanism. What makes luxury most desirable is that it is often viewed as unattainable to the masses. If yoga is free and available to all, then it can be argued that it could not be remotely glamorous and far outside of the scope of celebrity and if you can find a shaman easily in your own community who is willing to be paid with natural resources or not paid at all, it is likely less desired in this day and age. This contemporary re-versioning of an indigenous practice has played into the hands of capitalists in that it has become a tremendously lucrative segment. More than $30 billion was generated by the commercialized yoga industry in 2004 as the number of Americans engaging in this practice rose to over 20 million people (Fish 2006, 191). There was a 43 percent increase in American adults practicing yoga from 2002 to 2005 (Berger et al. 2009, 36) and there are growing numbers of train-the-trainer courses for the shaman.

There has been an influx of anti-yuppie yoga blogs and websites cropping up on the World Wide Web. The following is from an anti-yuppie treatise posted on the Yoga Dawg website (www.yogadawg.com) posted on the door of a New York City yoga studio:

> The yuppie yogi is a slacker; a pretty girl/boy, shaved, sexed, and clothed in high-end yoga togs whose soul is void of the yogic spirit. The yuppie yogi is the devil; scraping and bowing before the cesspool of the Industrial-Yoga-Complex while spouting regurgitated propaganda of unity, happiness and harmony that they found in pop-yoga magazines. These semi-educated yuppies espouse the simulated experience of yoga "stuff" while their brains are filled with fluff and the repugnant rambling of the scores of clueless yuppie yoga teachers.
>
> The true yogi is not a nice man or woman, concerned only with yoga's popularity and trendiness. The true yogi shouts unpleasant truths from the mats of countless yoga studios and forces upon the yuppie yogi the ghastly consequences of surrounding their bodies and souls with a narrow minded and timid yoga elite who too long has perverted the concept of yoga.
>
> The true yogi does not stand in tadasana in famous yoga studios; nor chant Om among the mindless yuppie yogis participating in pop-kirtans, nor pranam before a pimp-celebrity, bobo yoga star. Stop Yuppie Yoga NOW!!

While there may be exaggerated overtones in the above-quoted edict, there is an evident movement which finds the Western polishing of yogic practice a far cry from its spiritual foundations and it can be anticipated that the shaman—at least the Westernized version—may stand the same fate. One factor driving this divide is that of the commoditization of yogic practices. Fish (2006) addresses the issue of intellectual property rights issues recently surfacing as the practices of developing countries become more popular stateside. The capitalistic drive within the United States has seen a marked increase in the patenting of yoga studios, clothing, accessories, and the like. Most notable of the intellectual property issues is the Bikram Yoga College of India founded by Bikram Choudhury when in 2002, Choudhury attempted to impose copyright and trademark cease and desist orders to competing studios and practitioners engaging in similar yogic practices. This action sparked heated debate as to whether or not yogic practices and knowledge were private or public in proprietary nature and begs the question of whether or not primitive practices such as shamanism have an "owner."

It can be argued that this consumerism has a vice grip on the allowance of soul and that it has driven us to the point that indigenous practices such as yoga and shamanism that are deeply rooted in spirituality cannot escape the opportunity to yield a profit. Clearing the mind is no longer important. Happiness is overrated. There is no time for reflection, reasoning, or any of the factors in the Yogasutra.

In an effort to nurture and develop the individual and collective soul of Western culture, one must first strip away the mask of the glamorous persona which lurks within so many and find the sacred space. The desire to be loved and wanted based on the external must be obliterated in order to expose what lies in the depths, such as the capitalist drive and lure of commercialism that attempts to fill an insatiable abyss. The quiet sanctity of space can be a launching pad for the silence essential to calming the mind. It is during this still quiet, that psyche often speaks.

Arguably, the manner in which this therapeutic work can begin is to turn back toward the spirit of indigenous practices such as yoga, shamanism, and meditation and repair the incongruence between the capitalist drive and original tenets of soul imbedded in many of these indigenous practices. By creating and revering sacred space, steps can be made toward acknowledging one another as individuals with the forward motion of that action being recognizing the wounding of souls.

Conclusion

East and West can no longer be kept apart.

                                                                    Goethe

It has been questioned whether or not the traditional practice of sha-manism can exist in postmodern, Westernized culture. What should be considered is what contributory factors these practices can have not only on psychotherapeutic work but also on Western biomedical therapies. Quoting Winkleman, "Shamanism reflects the primordial spiritual prac-tices of humanity" (2001, 348) and it is this thread of humanity which could lead to a joining together of the Western biomedical and indigenous shamanic models. Additionally, there is a divide in many of these engage-ments between the practice at hand and communion with the gods and nature in order to mend ailments in body as well as soul.

In an attempt to address how changes could be broached with regard to shifting Western views of shamanism, Jilek addresses how past practice has included demonizing and pathologizing the role of shaman, but how strides can be made toward accrediting the work of the shaman as a "time-honored ritual through which practitioners heal sick people or divine the future" (Jilek 2005, 13). I am encouraged by the author's call-ing out for a "revival of shamanic healing and ceremonialism" (14). These rich traditions have worked for countless generations of indigenous peo-ples and continue to work today even through often stigmatizing eyes of those revering only traditional approaches to health, healing, and well-being.

Levi-Strauss, in addressing the parallels of shamanism and psychother-apeutics, states, "Actually the shamanic cure seems to be the exact coun-terpart to the psychoanalytic cure, but with an inversion of all the ele-ments. Both cures aim at inducing an experience, and both succeed by recreating a myth which the patient has to live or relive" (Levi-Strauss 1949, 110). It is this view which can assist in the facilitation of bridging both indigenous and traditional approaches—the view that both ap-proaches to healing engage with the mythic notion of treatment and equate to the opportunity for new life.

This bridging is exhibited in the modern-day practices of the Hmong shaman. In Merced, California's Mercy Medical Center, Hmong-American shamans have been integrated into the practice of health and healing. This medical center has implemented a first of its kind program to recognize indigenous healers and also train them in biomedical practices so they are able to practice their craft within the confines of a modern medical center.

This integration is not without obstructions including the necessity to ensure that Hmong shaman are abiding by certain biomedical standards of disease prevention such as prohibiting the use of animals used in certain shamanic healing ceremonies.

While there remains a substantial amount of work to be done to determine if these practices can be therapeutically beneficial to biomedical issues, there remain many options that may include at a minimum augmenting the traditional biomedical structures as well as other non-traditional therapies such as yoga and herbal therapy that may have some similitude of efficacy. A barrier to marrying traditional and indigenous practices lies in the consumerist forces for the Western environs which habitually dictate the mindset that healing comes at a monetary cost and must be legally and medically standardized and regulated.

According to Mokelke, "The shamanic way teaches us that each of us can have our own autonomous relationship with the helping spirits—loving, wise, and transcendent spiritual beings. We can find answers for ourselves, not as a matter of belief, but through direct experience" (Mokelke 2012, 24). The direct contact with the highest power or the ability to act as spiritual conduit in an effort to return the gift of healing to the afflicted is noble as is the concept of healing one's community—all underpinnings of overarching, or what could be called, non-denominational shamanic practice.

Jung expressed that when indigenous societies are exposed to modern evolution there can be a loss of the meaning of their lives and their ancestry (Sabini 2002) and I would further this thought by reflecting on the layers of core shamanic practices that have been addressed in this chapter. They offer a vast benefit not only from the standpoint of cultural value, but also from the position of supplementing the traditional, biomedical model with native traditions. This approach allows for a unification of cultures and beliefs outside of the jurisdiction of structured religious or medical practice.

Core shamanism and shamanic practices have no official manuscript or decreed dogma, but are an inventive collective of those called to heal and who are divinely gifted to communicate with the gods and spirit world on behalf of others in their communities. Jung is quoted, "The Western idea—particularly late Christianity—is of course to cure your neighbor, to help him, with no consideration of the question, *Who* is the helpers?" (Sabini 2002, 214) and this bolsters the concept of how central the shamanic principle of communing with the underworld, spirit, nature, god can be and how this is a Western disconnect in many instances with the "healers" themselves and begs the question, With whom is my physician consulting?

Perhaps there can be room for a healing community in which one communes with the gods and spirits working in conjunction with another who communes with the traditional medical community.

It is the return to the sacred and communion with the gods that lies firmly within the scope of shamanism (as well as religious functions that do not focus on a single religious conduit such as a shaman) to communicate on behalf of the afflicted and to connect with god and nature in an effort to heal and restore to wholeness. A paradigmatic shift is necessary to bridge the gap between Western and traditional healing approaches to those indigenous practices that may be considered unorthodox or perhaps antiquated. This bridging of cultural mindsets could serve to not only help and heal but to also keep primitive and indigenous practices true to their originations and continue the work of the shaman as the mediator between man and the gods.

References

Achterberg, J. 1985. *Imagery and Healing: Shamanism and Modern Medicine.* New York, NY: Shambala.

Berger, D., E. Silver, and R. Stein. 2009. "Effects of Yoga on Inner-City Children's Well-Being: A Pilot Study." *Alternative Therapies in Health and Medicine* 15(5): 36–42.

Boas, F. 2001. "The Angakoq Uses a Peculiar Language and Defines Taboos." (1887)." In *Shamans through Time,* edited by J. Narby, and F. Huxley. New York, NY: Putnam.

Bussmann, R. and D. Sharon. 2006. "Traditional Medicinal Plant Use in Northern Peru: Tracking Two Thousand Years of Healing Culture." *Journal of Ethnobiology and Ethnomedicine* 2: 47.

Bussmann, R.W., D. Sharon, and J. Ly. 2008. "From Garden to Market? The Cultivation of Native and Introduced Medicinal Plant Species in Cajamarca, Peru, and Implications for Habit Conservation." *Journal of Ethnobotany Research and Application* 6: 351–361.

Campbell, J. 2004. *Pathways to Bliss.* Novato, CA: New World Library.

Cicchetti, J. 2003. *Dreams, Symbols, and Homeopathy Archetypal Dimensions of Healing.* New York, NY: North Atlantic Books.

City of Los Angeles Public Affairs. 2009. *Cities within the County of Los Angeles.* http://lacounty.gov.

Conquergood, D. 1991. "Establishing the World: Hmong Shamans." *CURA Reporter* 19(2): 5–10.

De Rios, M. D. 2003. "The Role of Music in Healing with Hallucinogens: Tribal and Western Studies." *Music Therapy Today* 4: 3.

Eliade, M. 1964. *Shamanism: Archaic Techniques of Ecstasy.* New York: Pantheon Books.

Eliade, M. 1968. *The Sacred and the Profane: The Nature of Religion.* New York, NY: Harvest Books.

Eliade, M. 1987. "Shamanism: An Overview." *Encyclopedia of Religion* 13.

Fish, A. 2006. "The Commodification and Exchange of Knowledge in the Case of Transnational Commercial Yoga." *International Journal of Cultural Property* 13(2): 189–206.

Glass-Coffin, B. 1998. *The Gift of Life: Female Spirituality and Healing in Northern Peru.* Albuquerque, NM: University of New Mexico Press.

Grasse, R. 1996. *The Waking Dream: Unlocking the Symbolic Language of Our Lives."* Wheaton, IL: Theosophical Publishing.

Hall, C. S. and V. Nordby. 1999. *A Primer of Jungian Psychology.* New York, NY: Penguin Group.

Harner, M. J. 1968. "The Sound of Rushing Water." *Natural History* 77(6): 28–33, 60–61.

Harner, M. J. 1982. *The Way of the Shaman.* New York: Bantam Books.

Harris, J. P. 2001. *Jung and Yoga the Psyche-Body Connection.* Toronto, ON: Inner City Books.

Heaven, R., and H. G. Charing. 2006. *Plant Spirit Shamanism Traditional Techniques for Healing the Soul.* New York: Destiny Books.

Ingerman, S. 2004. *Shamanic Journeying: A Beginner's Guide.* Boulder, CO. Sounds True Publishing.

James, W. 1901/1958. *Varieties of Religious Experience.* New York, NY: New American Library.

Jilek, W. G. 2005. "Transforming the Shaman: Changing Western Views of Shamanism and Altered States of Consciousness." *Investigación en Salud* 7: 8–15.

Jung, C. G. 1974. *Dreams.* Princeton, NJ: Princeton University Press.

Jung, C.G. 1989. *Memories, Dreams, Reflections.* New York, NY: Vintage.

Jung, C.G. 1999. *The Essential Jung.* New York, NY: Princeton University Press.

Kim, U., Yang, K-S., and Hwang, K. K. 2006. *Indigenous and Cultural Psychology: Understanding People in Context.* New York, NY: Springer Science and Business Media LLC.

Klein, N. S. 1981. "The Endorphins Revisited." *Psychiatric Annals* 11: 137–142.

Leonard, L. S. 1998. *The Wounded Woman.* Boston, MA: Shambala.

Levi-Strauss, C. 1949. "Shamans as Psychoanalysts." Republished in J. Narby and F. Huxley, eds., 2001, *Shamans through Time: 500 Years on the Path of Knowledge.* New York, NY: Tarcher/Putnam.

Mokelke, S. 2012. "Core Shamanism and Daily Life." *Shamanism Annual* 22: 23–25.

Money, M. 2001. "Shamanism as a Healing Paradigm for Complementary Therapy." *Complementary Therapies in Nursing and Midwifery* 7: 126–131.

Noll, R., J. Achterberg, E. Bourguignon, L. George, M. Harner, L. Honko, and M. Winkelman. 1985. "Mental Imagery Cultivation as a Cultural Phenomenon: The Role of Visions in Shamanism [and Comments and Reply]." *Current Anthropology.* 26(4): 443–461.

Polimeni, J. and J. P. Reiss. 2002. "How Shamanism and Group Selection May Reveal the Origins of Schizophrenia." *Medical Hypotheses* 58(3): 244–248.

Porterfield, A. 1987. "Shamanism: A Psychosocial Definition." *Journal of the American Academy of Religion.* 55(4): 721–739.

Reilly, D. 1995. "Research Homeopathy and Therapeutic Consultation." *Alternative Therapies in Health and Medicine.* 1(4): 65–73

Rudgley, R. 1998. *The Encyclopedia of Psychoactive Substances.* Little, Brown, and Company.

Sabini, M. 2002. *The Earth Has a Soul: The Nature Writings of C. G. Jung.* Berkeley, CA: North Atlantic Books.

Sacrini, M. and A. Ferraz. 2009. "Some Remarks on the Yogasutra." *Philosophy East and West* 59(3): 249–262.

Singh, A. 1999. "Shamans, Healing, and Mental Health." *Journal of Child and Family Studies* 8(2) 131–134.

Smith, C. M. 2007. *Jung and Shamanism in Dialogue.* Victoria, BC: Trafford Publishing.

Stein, M. 1998. *Jung's Map of the Soul: An Introduction.* Chicago, IL: Open Court.

Trotter, R. T. 2001. "Curanderismo: A Picture of Mexican-American Folk Healing." *The Journal of Alternative and Complementary Medicine* 7(2): 129–131.

Turlington, C. 2003. *Living Yoga Creating a Life Practice.* New York, NY: Hyperion.

Turner, V. W. 1995. *Ritual Process Structure and Anti-Structure.* New York, NY: Aldine de Gruyter.

U.S. Census Bureau. 2000. *City of Los Angeles Statewide Statistics.* http://factfinder.census.gov.

Van Gennep, A. [1903] 2001. "Shamanism Is a Dangerously Vague Word." In *Shamans through Time,* edited by J. Narby, and F. Huxley. New York, NY: Putnam.

Walsh, R. 1989. "Shamanism and Early Human Technology: The Technology of Transcendence." *Revision* 12(1): 34–40.

Walsh, R. 1994. "The Making of a Shaman: Calling, Training, and Culmination." *Journal of Humanistic Psychology* 34(3): 7–30.

Warber, S. L., S. Ingerman, V. L. Moura, J. Wunder, A. Northrop, B. W. Gillespie, and M. Rubenfire. 2011. "Healing the Heart: A Randomized Pilot Study of a Spiritual Retreat for Depression in Acute Coronary Syndrome Patients." *EXPLORE: The Journal of Science and Healing* 7(4): 222–233.

Williams, M. 2010. *Follow the Shaman's Call: An Ancient Path for Modern Life.* Woodbury, MN: Llewellyn Publications.

Winkelman, M. 2001. "Alternative and Traditional Medicine Approaches for Substance Abuse Programs: a Shamanic Perspective." *International Journal of Drug Policy* 12(4): 337–351.

Winkelman, M. 2002. "Shamanism as Neurotheology and Evolutionary Psychology." *American Behavioral Scientist* 45(12): 1875–1887.

Winkelman, M. 2005. "Drug Tourism or Spiritual Healing? Ayahuasca Seekers in Amazonia." *Journal of Psychoactive Drugs* 37(2): 209–218.

Wolfe, A. 1998. *In the Shadow of Shaman*. Woodbury, MN: Llewellyn Publications.

Woodman, M. 1982. *Addiction to Perfection: The Still Unravished Bride : A Psychological Study*. Toronto, Canada: Inner City Books.

Woodman, M. 1984. "Psyche/Soma Awareness." *Quadrant* 17(2): 25–37. New York, NY.

Yoga Dawg. http://www.yogadawg.com/news11.htm

Young-Eisendrath, P. 1985. "Reconsidering Jung's Psychology." *Psychotherapy* 22(3): 501–515.

Znamenski, A. 2007. *The Beauty of the Primitive: Shamanism and the Western Imagination*. New York, NY. Oxford Press.

CHAPTER THIRTEEN

Vodou in North America: Healing One Person, Healing the Universe

*Benjamin Wendorf
and Patrick Bellegarde-Smith*

Haitian Vodou, a neo-African religion, is rooted in ancient theology, tracing back to principles found throughout West and Central Africa. It is a spiritual and philosophical system, pervasive and vital for followers and their society. Additionally, Vodou (as we refer to it below) provides health and wellness for its followers, via a holistic health care system that addresses sickness as an ailment of the body and the spirit. This health care was born from a number of factors including a complex history of oppression, colonization, and neglect, as well as perseverance, ingenuity, and innovation on the part of Haitian people. In this chapter, we will look at the ancient origins of Vodou and its mischaracterizations before presenting its core principles and approaches to health and wellness. By the end, readers will see that Vodou is indeed more than a religion; rather, it is an all-encompassing explanation of the universe, past, present and future.

Vodou has a very real presence in North America, thanks to frequent emigrations of Haitian citizens and refugees over the centuries. By 2010, the Haitian Diaspora numbered nearly 1.1 million citizens in the United States and Canada (U.S. Census Bureau 2010, Statistics Canada 2007); in the United States alone the Haitian-descent population grew from 290,000 in 1990 to 845,000 in 2010 (U.S. Census Bureau 2010). These data are focused primarily on respondents who identified their ancestry as "Haitian."

Due to illegal immigration and a failure to report Haitian ancestry, the number of persons of Haitian descent (Haitian Americans, Haitian Canadians) is much larger, possibly one of the largest national diasporas in the world (Bellegarde-Smith 2011). Most of the self-identifying Haitians are located in New York and Florida in the United States (U.S. Census Bureau 2010) and in Quebec in Canada (Statistics Canada, 2007).

There is also a contingent of Haitian descendants in New Orleans, who combined with other Caribbean migrants and enslaved Africans to create "Voodoo;" though not to be confused with Vodou, there are many similarities between the two. Both trace back to West African roots (most prominently, the *Vodun* religion) and the herbal remedies described below are nearly identical. Their divergence is largely in voodoo's use of *gris gris*, or charms and amulets that carry spiritual powers and symbolism (and actually seemed to have more Central African roots) (Desch-Obi 2005), and the "Voodoo Queens," or priestesses, who attained a sort of celebrity in the 19th century U.S. press that gave them individual power and influence in the community (Fandrich 2005). It was this form of African religion that became mythologized by the American press and Hollywood, and the use of charms (including dolls) came to be considered by the non-practicing American public as synonymous with the bulk of African religions conceptualized under an umbrella term "voodoo." Disaffected with the negative (at times oppressive) attention and misrepresentations of their practices, Voodoo practitioners have historically hidden the authentic ceremonies (Fandrich 2005), making it hard to assess the current impact and population of the religion outside of a proportion of African Americans in the bayous of Louisiana.

In terms of Vodou, it is wrong to assume that all Haitians or those with Haitian Creole ancestry practice the religion, though determining the number of Vodou practitioners in the population is difficult due to the influence of Christianity as a dominant system, the tendency of Haitians to use Christian symbolism and constructs to conceal Vodou practices, and the stigmatization of Vodou in North America more generally (beyond Christian denunciation) (Michel 2007). It is also wrong to assume that all Vodou practitioners are Haitian; Vodou has a growing population of African Americans and persons of European descent in many large cities of North America (including New York, Miami, Atlanta), the former group retracing African religious roots and the latter attracted to humanistic principles.

More tangible evidence of Vodou's influence is the demand for Vodou priestesses and priests, called *manbos* and *houngans* respectively. Two renowned Vodou leaders, Alourdes Margeaux (known popularly as Mama

Lola) and Jacqueline Epingle, are both located in North America, Lola in Brooklyn and Epingle in Montreal (Bellegarde-Smith and Michel 2007). KOSANBA (an acronym for the Congress of Santa Barbara, first convened in 1997), an association formed by scholars of Vodou in Haïti, has devoted itself to the preservation and study of Vodou all over the world, including areas of North America where some of the scholars are located.

Population aside, Vodou carries greater significance as a theology transported intact across the Atlantic. As Bellegarde-Smith argued in his introduction to *Fragments of Bone,* the core theology of neo-African religions, which the enslaved Africans carried with them to the numerous ports of the Americas, survived a variety of environments and manifested themselves in the forms of new religions such as Vodou, Brazilian *Candomblé,* and Cuban *Santería* (Bellegarde-Smith 2005) (see chapter 14 this volume for more on the latter). As we will discuss below, these principles are quite clearly tied to theologies in Western and Central Africa, and in fact carry similar names, expressions, and rituals (Aborampah, 2005; Bellegarde-Smith, 2005). This mirrors a larger body of scholarship that draws attention to the transmittance of numerous cultural characteristics—planting methods, architecture, burial practices—across the Atlantic (Mitchell 2005, Ogundiran and Falola 2007).

History

Any understanding of Vodou is inextricably tied to understanding its history; Vodou is defined by its connections to ancestry, the Haitian Revolution, and other important events in Haitian history. For example, the earthquake of 2010 has assumed an important place in Vodou folklore; called the "Goudougoudou," it was a terrible reminder of the power of nature. It was also a reminder of the persistence of foreign oppression; lost in the devastation of the earthquake itself was Canadian and American profiteering, the kidnapping of Haitian children (though this was briefly publicized in the United States), and the renewed presence of American military forces on Haitian ground (Bellegarde-Smith 2011).

Vodou's origins are traced primarily back to present-day Benin, where the African religion *Vodun* is so prevalent it is one of the official religions of the country. Though popular among the Fon people there, Vodun is also practiced in present-day Ghana, Togo, and Nigeria, and shows influences stretching from the Ewe in eastern Ghana, through the Yoruba in Nigeria, and all the way to the Bakongo in central Africa (Fennell 2007, Montilus 2007). In addition, Vodou demonstrates some influence from the small population of Taíno and Arawak that survived Spanish colonization (Bellande-Robertson 2007), and has incorporated some of the iconography and expressions of Christianity. On the one hand, this incorporation has been used as a means of preserving Vodou in the face of persecution, though it should also be viewed as the recognition of the divinity in these symbols and philosophies (Christophe 2007, Sager 2012). Like Hinduism, Unitarian Universalism, and other religious systems, Vodou is not exclusive of concepts from other religions, provided they are agreeable to Vodou philosophy.

The Atlantic Slave Trade brought an extraordinary amount of violence to enslaved African peoples, but one of their powerful expressions of humanity was their efforts to come together in the spirit of resistance and survival, and create new communities in the Americas. These new communities coalesced around organizational principles of the African continent, resulting in a variety of African-derived religions and ideas about forming a society. In the case of Vodou, society is guided by a series of principles or body of knowledge called *konesans* (Bellegarde-Smith 2005). The *konesans* were heavily influenced by the oppression experienced by many Haitians in the colonial system; one of the more brutal plantation colonies, Haïti (called Saint Domingue by the French) was a vital source of sugar for the world, and the French made incredible fortunes from it which they used to industrialize their homeland. While France prospered, the harvesting of sugar cane involved long hours in insufferable heat and humidity for the enslaved laborers. Their lives were made considerably worse by the treatment and neglect of slavemasters, who took advantage of a slave market flush with "commodities" by routinely working the enslaved to death. A grim detail told the tale: despite centuries of influx of enslaved Africans, at the beginning of the Haitian Revolution in 1791, well over a majority of the enslaved laborers had been born in Africa (James 1963).

Vodou became synonymous with resistance and survival in this environment; Vodou provided the organization for enslaved African society, the treatments for its members that fell ill in mind and spirit, and the *konesans* for the maroon societies that developed when the enslaved peoples fled (Price-Mars 1928). When rebel leaders began to form resistance and revolutionary movements, they found ready support among enslaved Africans, poor planters, and half-European, half-African (some free, most enslaved), who were discriminated against by a wealthy group of French planters and colonial officials. Vodou and leaders such as Toussaint Louverture and Jean-Jacques Dessalines proved to be the talismans for the large enslaved population; Louverture's presence was so tireless and ubiquitous that many Vodou followers saw him as manifestations of Vodou deities (James 1963). Centuries later, populist priest Jean-Bertrand Aristide would receive the same honor, both due to his populist messages and his survival through over a dozen assassination attempts (Bellegarde-Smith 2011).

Louverture's reaction to Vodou was a premonition of things to come; over the centuries, like Louverture, most Haitian governments *publicly* demonstrated a negative view of Vodou, as did the American government in its occupation of Haïti from 1915 to 1934, and some governments (most prominently, the Duvalier dictatorships from 1957 to 1986) would actually distort Vodou into a tool of oppression. Ironically, many if not most of these same leaders practiced Vodou in "secret," including Louverture (Montilus 2007). The primary reason for this was that Christianity was considered by the leadership (and the Haitian upper class) to be more presentable in the international community; Vodou was also viewed as being in direct competition with Christianity. Haitian scholar Jean-Price Mars would call this rejection of Vodou "collective Bovarism," in reference to Gustave Flaubert's fictional Madame Bovary, who presents herself as an upper-class aristocrat but, at her own peril, uses remedies and "potions" in secret (Price-Mars 1953).

The confluence of general unrest and willful neglect has left the rural Haitian population to its own devices for health care continuously since the first enslaved Africans landed on the island. Even in the contemporary era, there is one physician for every ten thousand Haitians (Beauvoir 2007), and the recent earthquake damaged some of the health care infrastructure in Port-au-Prince and surrounding towns. Thus, most Haitians who have come to North America likely have very little experience with Western medicine (Beauvoir 2007). Instead, they have lived in a society with its own definitions of sickness and health, malady and remedy, developed over the centuries by the observations and experimentation of manbos and houngans. Their holistic health care system, as we shall see below, carries strong connections to methods from the African continent, though it is also influenced by the local Caribbean environment.

Finally, Vodou has for centuries been characterized by (mostly European Christian) outsiders in regards to its differences and perceived inferiority to dominant European cultures. The U.S. government and Hollywood took to these characterizations readily, the former to stigmatize a powerful religion that had a history of revolution, the latter to generate revenue from its caricature (Bellegarde-Smith and Michel 2007). They created an entire mythological practice ("voodoo") presided over by "witch doctors" wielding "voodoo dolls" and vexing spells. None of these depictions were true to Vodou theology, but they had social weight; the caricatures were at times comical (*Major League*), belittling (the song "Witch Doctor" written by Ross Bogdasarian, Sr.), or sinister (Pat Robertson's claims that Haïti's earthquake and poverty was due to a "pact with the devil") (Bellegarde-Smith 2011). These distortions and fabrications have led to stigmatization of Vodou in North America.

Vodou Theology: A Focus on Person

The first step to explaining the theology of Vodou and its approach to health and wellness is focused on determining "personhood." By recognizing the place of a person within Vodou, we can start to understand some of the reasons that a person might be ill in body and spirit.

As Guérin Montilus writes, a "person" is one who has "consciousness of the relationship of oneself to oneself and an awareness of the existence of the external world of beings, objects, events, and facts—all of which intersect" (2007, 1). A person is the center of their universe; a powerful Haitian phrase is "When you look into the cosmic mirror, the image that beams back at you is the image of God" (Bellegarde-Smith 2005, 60), but as he/she is inextricable from the universe, he/she should be aware of his/her impact upon it. This agency is also expressed in the Vodou, "There are no messiahs: only you stand at the center," which also alludes to the humanistic nature of African religions. That universe extends into the past, to the ancestors, whom you will join when the time comes, to the unborn of the future, and to the deities; both your ancestors and the deities are a strong presence in your life, reminding you of vital lessons and occasionally there for communication through trance possession (Bellegarde-Smith 2005).

Scientifically speaking, a human is energy, and this concept is integral for Vodou. That energy can make you happy or sad, healthy or sick, and one of the most important roles for manbos and houngans is to bring balance to that energy (Beauvoir 2007). This balance is reflected in a number of Vodou sayings, including idioms concerning "God" ("God is neutral, neither good or bad, but 'cool'"), "poison" ("Everything is poison; nothing is poison"), and "good and evil" ("The objective for each life is to master both the forces of good and the forces of evil") (Bellegarde-Smith 2005, 59–60). In each case, the expressions seek to dismantle hardened dichotomies; the one for poison is most interesting, as the lesson is that, in trace amounts, very few things cause death, and in large amounts even good things can cause death. All of these expressions are a challenge to the person to maintain balance in their lives.

Health and Sickness

Having established personhood, to really understand health in Vodou you must understand how healthy and sick persons are designated and diagnosed. Max-G. Beauvoir, one of the most-respected houngans in Vodou, notes that "a body is not a simple machine that is designed to become ill. On the contrary, the machine is intelligent and heals itself in most instances" (2007, 122). Therefore, health is constantly being reaffirmed as the body endures a multitude of challenges (heat, cold, cuts, bruises, colds and other minor illnesses, and negativity). The manbos and houngans are trained in the process of maintaining the body (which, in turn, maintains the community, then the universe) by assuring the sound functioning of all the primary functions of the body. They also examine and help with maintaining equilibrium, and a general feeling of well-being (Beauvoir 2007). At the base level, Vodou is preventative, ensuring the best possibility for members of the community to avoid maladies but also to be strong, in this case, balanced, enough to recover from most illnesses.

As a future ancestor, everyone has a role in Vodou societies as a teacher, a listener, a helper, even if they are not manbos or houngans. Even children can teach the elderly, particularly if a Lwa speaks through them; as children are viewed as the ancestors reborn, they carry with them *konesans* that they could express. The point is that, without a clear hierarchy in Vodou, position and power gives way to a communal sense of being, wherein power is reestablished as something accessible to all and most prevalent in the community (Michel 2007). This can also provide an indicator of a sort of sickness; those who do violence to the community, or purposefully separate themselves from it, are unhealthy as well. It is more of a behavioral sickness, and those who are ill either address their problem themselves with the help of a manbo or houngan, or their illness is addressed by spirits in ceremony. In serious cases of violence done to the community, particularly in the event of a repeat offender, manbos and houngan have the power to turn the person into a "zombie," essentially using a combination of herbs that will render the person incapacitated. Regardless of the severity, a Vodou follower should not be surprised if their neglect emerges in the form of messages from Lwa during possession (Michel 1996, Beauvoir 2007).

Of course, there are also much more serious situations that call for specialized medical help, and because of this there are additional Vodou experts. For instance, *dokté zo* are bone-setters for broken limbs, *dokté féy* are "leaf doctors" or herbalists that help with more complicated remedies, and *fanm chaj* are midwives (Kail 2008, Beauvoir 2007). Inflictions like diabetes and hookworms also receive special treatment (Beauvoir 2007, Colon 1976, Wolpert et al. 2008). In contemporary Haïti, and among members of the Haitian Diaspora, it is not uncommon to consult Western medicine for some very serious illnesses, provided the facility and medicine are accessible and affordable.

Constructs

Frequently, Vodou is misinterpreted as a polytheistic religion; as Michel notes, Vodou is monotheistic, though not in the same ways that Christianity, Islam, or Judaism are monotheistic. The Creator in Vodou, known as *Bondye,* is not involved in the daily existence of followers, nor is Bondye consulted to do so (Michel 2007). Michel notes that, rather than hinging on Bondye, Vodou "is based on a conception of reality that includes life's goals, forces that determine the fate of living things, proper social organization, balanced interpersonal relations, and practices that promote the welfare of the community"(2007, 34). Most importantly, this is a flexible system, capable of adapting, being applied where needed, hiding when necessary, and bringing its followers together again to remember the ancestors and share communications with the spiritual world. This flexibility is historically tied to the persecution of Vodou during the colonial era, as well as subsequent persecution and distortion under Haitian and American occupation governments.

Vodou is dictated by the universe constructed on two planes: the spiritual or metaphysical plane—called *ye gaga*—and the physical plane—called *ye gli* (Montilus 2007). These planes are not separate in any sense of the word; Vodou depicts them as intersecting, forming what is called a "crossroads" where the two planes meet. The crossroads is a vital element of Vodou when one intends to communicate with the deities. In fact, every ceremony is conducted within the crossroads, either symbolized using the intersection of trees or poles with the ground or elaborate designs drawn on the ground including a crossroads within the figure (Ogundiran and Falola 2007). The indication is that the spiritual and the physical are always connected, and in ceremony the participants emphasize the intersection to bring the spiritual deities forward.

The deities themselves, called *Lwa,* are not viewed as equals with Bondye; nevertheless, they are considered much more active in affecting the everyday lives of followers (Michel 2007). Each Lwa is attributed particular characteristics of life, be they love, fertility, war, justice, etc., and they are consulted accordingly. Some of the most "common" Lwa referenced are:

- *Legba,* the keeper of the crossroads or "gates" to the spiritual world; if the other Lwa communicate in a ceremony, it is because Legba has been appealed to and chooses to allow it
- *Dambala,* one of the "oldest" deities, and thus most frequently consulted for general advice
- *Ayida Wedo,* "wife" of Dambala

- *Ogou,* who brings justice and confers power; Ogou makes alloys of justice and power
- *Azaka,* the archetypal peasant and worker who dispenses money and is seen as the patron of agriculture
- *Ezili Freda,* love, sensuality, and beauty
- *Ezili Danto,* mother, she is also a warrior
- *Gran Brigit* and *Bawon,* death and cemeteries, ancestors and reborn children
- *Gédé,* the spirit of death and sexuality (Daniels 2007, Appendix)

Each of these Lwa are represented by particular offerings (Ogou, for instance, likes cigars and rum) and symbols. In the eras that Vodou was viciously persecuted, followers used Catholic saints' names to represent Vodou Lwa, which proved to be so effective in protecting and hiding Vodou that Catholic décor is still commonly used among Vodou followers. It is important to emphasize that there are many variations on the names of the Lwa, though they frequently sound the same, and there are similar deities found in West African *Vodun* (though sometimes carrying out different functions).

The topic of possession is where one should tread carefully. Possession as a concept has been particularly misrepresented by the Western world as a diabolical or damaging possession and one that is difficult to remove. This is definitely not the case in Vodou, as possession is a regular process during ceremonies, and an outcome that is desired by the participants. This is because the possession is neither malicious nor nonsensical, but the bringer of important *konesans,* and in some cases balance to a person's "energy" (Beauvoir 2007). Just as importantly, it takes specific or personal challenges and situations and moves the person into the realm of universal truths, applicable beyond the person and even the community, though in no way compromising the ability to instruct either one (Boddy 1994, Crosley 2007).

Actual possession itself occurs typically in Vodou ceremonies after Legba has been appealed to and allows the participants and the Lwa access to one another—possession can also occur in rare cases outside of ceremony, usually in times of great stress (Beauvoir 2007). At that point in time, any person in the group could be possessed by Lwa, typically Lwa that have been summoned by gifts or are frequently present on that day of the week. The possession is a mounting of one's spirit by the Lwa, and the person who is mounted will exhibit the mannerisms and the outward characteristics of the Lwa. For example, you will remember that Ogou likes cigars and rum; a person mounted by Ogou will take up a cigar that had been brought as an offering and drink the rum as well.

Though the Lwa have some characteristics of gender identity, they can mount a person of any gender.

There are "rough" and "controlled" possessions; the former are very expressive and active, though no less of a communication that needs to be discussed and interpreted. The controlled possessions are more focused on achieving harmony and balance within the person who is mounted. They are conducted by a "trained" individual who has been initiated as a spiritual healer. Rough possessions are those carried out by the uninitiated (Beauvoir 2007). In both types, the possession could take minutes, hours, or in rarer cases days. Each possession involves messages that need to be received and understood, and those who have been possessed are no more stigmatized nor revered than any other within the community. Thus, possession becomes a matter of course, something that happens, experienced with the community, discussed within the community.

Vodou followers also have more personal means for spiritual and physical health. Most of these followers have shrines that can be used for individual prayer and recognition of ancestors. Rarely do these shrines outwardly look like areas of Vodou worship, and sometimes it is almost impossible to distinguish them as shrines at all. As mentioned above, many have Catholic or Christian relics and symbols and other objects not visibly associated with Vodou; once again, this is part of the legacy of the oppression Vodou followers experienced (Michel 2007).

A final effective structure in place for health is a preliminary channel to manbo or houngan consultation, a series of idioms and quick remedies that are passed via interpersonal relationships. Beauvoir refers to this as the "Phytotherapeutic Social Systems" all the offered advice is considered a suggestion, and the remedies are simple in their application. With the frequent challenges to balance that life poses, these communal remedies reinforced beliefs in common wisdom and involved interpersonal relationship in maintaining health (Beauvoir 2007).

Remedies

As mentioned above, Vodou remedies are the results of centuries, if not millennia, of experimentation and herbal knowledge. The transference of this knowledge, especially across the Atlantic, has been aided by the similar climates and plant life of West and Central Africa to the Caribbean. An overwhelming majority of these healing methods are focused on preventive health and holistic healing, combining physical medicine with the maintenance of spiritual balance. There is a method to each one of these diagnoses and treatments, beginning with the consultation.

The consultation with the manbo or houngan oftentimes involves possession as a way for communicating the patient's problems; interestingly, it is the manbo or houngan that will be possessed and identify the illness. The patient can either agree that the healer has correctly identified the problem or seek the advice of a different healer (Beauvoir 2007).

When a satisfactory diagnosis is made, the healer will determine whether to engage the healing process using the primordial elements earth, fire, or water, all of them pertaining to restoring the patient's metaphysical balance in an attempt to prepare him/her for the subsequent use of herbs via aromatherapy, baths, or consumption. The use of songs and dances are not uncommon to influence the energy of the patient, and the knowledge gained from some of the treatments can inform home remedies used in such a way as mentioned above, when a healer is not available (Beauvoir 2007, Weniger 1991).

The remedies run the gamut of local plants and their utilization, including the use of ground roots, barks, leaves, and extracts. They also involve activities such as sitting over sacrificed animals or being in the presence of the blood of a sacrificed animal, as the offer is believed to influence a change in the person's inner spirituality. Blood is considered the essence of life, and its use in treatment is viewed as a powerfully positive energy, in the same ways that other religions might use olive oil or anointed water (Solomon 2002, Beauvoir 2007). One example is *Nepeta caria,* more commonly known as "catnip," which is used for its calming properties, though it can also be used as an all-purpose pain reliever and balancer for energy. Closely related mints such as peppermint, spearmint, and lemon mint are also frequently used to this end (Jordan 1975, Laguerre 1987).

Women also have particular remedies in regards to easing menstrual pain, abortion-inducing remedies, and for helping with labor pain. Red sage and vervain are believed to help with menstrual flow, and both could be potentially used for abortions, while verbena is used for labor pain issues. Oak bark douches are also used for general hygiene and are believe to ease menstrual flows (Jordan 1975,Kloss 1987).

In some cases, there is a strong suggestion that what is regarded by Western medicine as the "placebo effect" is primarily what drives the effectiveness of the remedies (Bootzin and Bailey 2005). For Vodou healers, this placebo effect is inseparable from the holistic healing process, a psychological benefit that comes with other elements of the remedies that physiologically improve the quality of life. We would argue that the confluence of pain relief, stress relief, and the confidence of the patient in the healer's (and the Lwa) abilities to help—all tangible, "real" benefits—can enhance the placebo effect and lend to an overall satisfactory healing experience. It is for this reason that Beauvoir refers to this "holistic" medical system as the one that has been the best fit for a majority of Haitians and (per our argument) a large number of the Haitian Diaspora (Beauvoir 2007).

Efficacy

The matter of efficacy of Vodou medicine, while historically complex and hard to verify, has become easier with the growth of multicultural approaches to psychology, advances in understanding life scientifically, and more recent studies looking at the effectiveness of herbal medicines. A number of scholarly organizations have also been formed for the study of the use and effectiveness of Vodou medicines and practices, including Traditional Medicine in the Islands (or TRAMIL, formed in 1983) and the previously-mentioned Congress of Santa Barbara (or KOSANBA; Weniger 1991, Bellegarde-Smith 2005). To a degree, the success of some medicines and practices from East and South Asian cultures have aided the interest in the work of these organizations, and have also provided useful templates for testing and research of these multicultural health approaches.

Since the earnest efforts of groups like TRAMIL to research remedies in the 1980s, a number of herbs and plants have been shown to provide substantial health benefits. The plants *Simarouba excelsa* (called *quassia* by healers) and *senna* have been commonly used for expelling worms and for general digestive disturbances, both common problems in Haïti (Kloss 1987, Laguerre 1987, Santillo 1987). In fact, over eighteen additional remedies exist in Haïti for similar afflictions, all of which have demonstrated some effectiveness scientifically against the worms (Neptune-Rozier 1997, Beauvoir et al. 2001). Wolpert et al found in more rigorous testing in 2008 that four of these remedies showed significant success against worms, and one particularly successful plant, *Momordia charantia,* was found to not only be used for worms but also as an ingredient in remedies for "cancer, fever, eye and cutaneous infections, liver problems, anemia, and loss of appetite" (Wolpert et al. 2008, 1158). In other words, healers identified an effective medicine, and began to use it in other concoctions to understand the extent of its benefits. This certainly could be an effective way to create "holistic" medications, where the combination of remedies that have demonstrated effectiveness physiologically and psychologically could be accompanied by spiritual stimulation in prayer or possession.

The effectiveness of Vodou healing practices does not end at worms and indigestion, either. The use of *Cuscuta Americana* has been effective in stymying the symptoms of hepatitis (Fleurentin 1990), *Psidium guava* leaves have been successfully tested as strong anti-microbial medicine against diarrhea

(Cáceres et al. 1987, Weniger 1990), and *Crescentia cujete* pulp has demonstrated effectiveness both as an anti-inflammatory and as an antibiotic, though its use has always been careful as it contains low levels of arsenic (Weniger 1990). In addition, there are a number of spices common in many places in the world including Haïti that are considered good for you by Vodou healers, including ginger, cayenne pepper, cinnamon, and bay leaves. Healers frequently tested every part of these therapeutic plants, determining whether the roots, leaves, or stems were the most potent medicine, and carried on the knowledge to the rest of the community (Beauvoir 2007).

Beauvoir makes the very convincing argument that it should come as no surprise that some Vodou remedies are proving effective, especially in regards to herb-derived regimens. He notes that the World Health Organization has stated that 25 percent of all prescription drugs are still derived directly from trees, shrubs, and herbs, and that among "119 plant-derived pharmaceutical medicines that are on pharmacy shelves today in the United States, 74 percent correlate directly with their traditional uses" (Beauvoir 2007, 116). To add to this point, a number of East and South Asian medicines have similarly tested well, though it is worth noting that some of those remedies seem to be more readily accepted in the medical community than those suggested in Vodou.

Finally, there are the less-tangible benefits of the kind of community provided by Vodou. Support structures such as what Priester et al. (2009) refer to as "faith communities" are conducive to mental health outcomes. A number of studies across south and eastern Asia and east and southern Africa have suggested that traditional healers can provide substantial help in regards to mental health, and use practices that both the healers and Western psychologists alike would consider sound, helpful therapy (Prasadarao 2009). Furthermore, the common knowledge medicine and the concern for the community ensure that followers of Vodou comprise a holistic support structure, bringing the sick closer to the community and its ideals rather than ostracizing them. It is this level of support that lends to confidence in the medical practices and can help reduce negative feelings about sickness among those stricken.

Multicultural Approaches

The bonds between Western medicine and traditional medicine have frequently been tenuous; both approaches have historically been suspicious of the other, and rightly so. They are foreign solutions for either community, suggested by foreigners in such a way that usurps the other community's beliefs about the process of hurt or sickness and how to help it. As

Bellegarde-Smith observed, "Foreign structures that are superimposed do not easily take root nor thrive well in non-native soils" (2005, 65). That comment applies in both directions in regards to Western medicine and Vodou, though the West has always held a dominant position in regards to dictating health care practices.

In more recent years, though, attempts have been made to compromise between Vodou and Western medicine. Primarily, there is recognition that Western medicine cannot physically or spiritually penetrate some communities to a certain degree (Weniger 1991, Bellegarde-Smith and Michel 2007). Whether that is due to lack of resources, reception among Vodou followers, or a lack of sincerity on the part of Western medical practitioners, it has not been reasonable to expect that Western medicine should assume preeminence among the Haitian Diaspora. In fact, it has seemed to be more conducive to recognize areas where Western medicine can and should help and areas where manbos and houngans will be more effective.

It is in this spirit that above groups like TRAMIL have sought to understand Vodou medicine and determine which medicines have tangible physiological benefits over those which are far more therapeutic spiritually. The ultimate goal for both is to maintain Vodou in the face of Western medical and cultural bias, on the premise that there is neither deficiency nor anything inherently wrong in practicing Vodou and its remedies (Weniger 1991, Bellegarde-Smith 2005). The hope for Vodou scholars and healers is to be allowed to approach Western medicine from their own perspective, rather than being forced to engage a paradigm wherein Western medicine is the established, appreciable norm and Vodou essentially has to prove itself (Bellegarde-Smith 2005).

The cooperation between traditional healers and Western medical practitioners is not altogether unprecedented, even in terms of neo-African medicine. In Ghana, Asante herbalists were long noted for their extensive knowledge of herbal remedies and their active interest in sharing and using these remedies. Their tireless activity meant that they were effective much further into the countryside than Western medical practitioners, and thus had greater trust and better results with patients (Yeboah 2000). Interestingly, in 1978 the military Ghanaian government began to explore supporting "indigenous healer" organizations to improve the reach of quality health care, which culminated in an early joint-indigenous healing and Western medicine venture called Primary Health Training for Indigenous Healers in 1979. This organization encouraged small adjustments to some rituals by suggesting washing hands, talking about midwifery techniques, and conversely examining the effectiveness and creating a library of traditional medicine (Warren and Tregoning 1979). This initiated a long history of cooperation between Western medicine and traditional healers through-out Ghana with promising results; Ghana consistently has one of the high-est life expectancies in sub-Saharan Africa (World Bank 2012).

Since the 1980s, cases like Ghana's have increased greatly, to the point now where traditional remedies from many regions and cultural back-grounds are being touted and released in the marketplace—for better and for worse, in some cases (Waldram 2000). Regardless, the growing positive reception to traditional medicine suggests that, to some degree, health care systems such as Vodou will be able to maintain their integrity rather than be forced to constantly defend themselves.

Going Forward

Vodou's long, difficult history in forging a new identity in the Americas and creating a support structure for millions of disaffected Haitians has solidified it as an important presence in the lives of members of the Haitian Diaspora. A major reason for Vodou's survival is its flexible, incorporative nature, and adaptability to new challenges. Nowhere was this more appar-ent than in the Republic of Haïti itself, through the perils of enslavement, revolution, and the influence of European institutions. It is humanist, and rejects hierarchy among human beings; this equality goes into infinity—the ancestors and the unborn are all people that must be treated with full respect to their humanity, whenever that might be or might have been.

The flexibility and humanism must not be confused for weakness; Vodou carries a cogent set of ideals and structures that are shared and form the backbone of the theology. It has long maintained itself despite conscious attempts to eradicate it, and those who follow Vodou identify strongly with this resistance to cultures (particularly, European) that have sought to chal-lenge it.

At the same time, Vodou is inclusive of new ideas, and it intellectually engages new ideas with a mind towards seeing how it might fit a commu-nity formed around Vodou. It is for these reasons that organizations such as TRAMIL and KOSANBA exist, and why Western medical practitioners should not feel that their time is wasted on a patient that practices Vodou. On the contrary, if such a patient is consulting the help of Western medi-cine, they are demonstrating the syncretic nature of Vodou. A few impor-tant points regarding these patients:

- *Like any other healer, a Western medical practitioner must prove him or herself to a prospective patient.* Recall that it is not uncommon for followers of Vodou to determine on their own whether they agree with the diagnosis. A white-clad physician becomes part of a "priesthood."

- *Western medical practitioners must understand the legacy of resistance in Vodou.* Condescending European and American attitudes and distortions of Vodou are tired themes for followers.
- *Consult the help of KOSANBA to find local manbos and houngans.* Meeting with local healers is an even better way to understand the local Vodou community, and gain the confidence of the Vodou community's members that you are truly interested in cooperating. Remember that there are variances in practices from one place to another.
- *Learn about and understand Vodou.* But a Western medical practitioner should never presume that they know more than another about the theology. Vodou is about community and cooperation, not hierarchy.

A potential healer that follows these tips will very likely be in the ideal place to respect the patient's religion and perhaps create some plans for therapy that will avoid infringing upon it. Additionally, the medical care practitioner could discover new remedies and methods that they might use in their own practice, even for patients that do not follow Vodou.

Conclusion

In this chapter, we examined the long history of Vodou, tracing its origins back to the African continent and drawing attention to its belief and constructs. We have also discussed how personhood, health, and sickness are defined within these constructs, and how Vodou has provided its solutions for maintaining the balance identified with wellness. Vodou medicine and methods have provided tangible positive results, both physiologically and psychologically, and the practices of its adherents must be understood and respected.

The value of learning Vodou constructs stretches beyond helping the Haitian Diaspora and patients; as Bellegarde-Smith has demonstrated, Vodou's organization and beliefs are reflective of many characteristics of African and neo-African religions, particularly in West and Central Africa (2005). Communalism, the individual as inextricable from the community and the universe, the spiritual plane as inextricable from the physical plane, and the use of plants for therapy, are all common characteristics of this large body of religions. Vodou provides a window into understanding them all.

References

Aborampah, O-M. 2005. "Out of the Same Bowl: Religious Beliefs and Practices in Akan Communities in Ghana and Jamaica." In *Fragments of Bone: Neo-African Religions in a New World,* edited by Patrick Bellegarde-Smith, 124–142. Chicago: University of Illinois Press.

Beauvoir, M.-G. 2007. "Herbs and Energy: The Holistic Medical System of the Haitian People." In *Haitian Vodou: Spirit, Myth, and Reality*, edited by Patrick Bellegarde-Smith and Claudine Michel, 112–133. Bloomington, IN: Indiana University Press.

Beauvoir, M. G., B. J. Wolpert, R. A. DeFilipps, and J. Crepin. 2001. *Selected Medicinal Plants of Vodou.* Washington, D.C.: Smithsonian Institution.

Bellande-Robertson, F. 2007. "A Reading of the Marasa Concept in Lilas Desquiron's les Chemins de Loco-Miroir." In *Haitian Vodou: Spirit, Myth, and Reality*, edited by Patrick Bellegarde-Smith and Claudine Michel, 103–111. Bloomington, IN: Indiana University Press.

Bellegarde-Smith, P., ed. 2005. *Fragments of Bone: Neo-African Religions in a New World.* Chicago: University of Illinois Press.

Bellegarde-Smith, Patrick. 2005. "The Spirit of the Thing: Religious Thought and Social/Historical Memory." In *Fragments of Bone: Neo-African Religions in a New World*, edited by Patrick Bellegarde-Smith, 52–69. Chicago: University of Illinois Press.

Bellegarde-Smith, P., 2011. "The Man-Made Disaster: The Earthquake of January 12, 2010—A Haitian Perspective." *The Journal of Black Studies* 42: 264–275. doi: 10.1177/0021934710396709

Bellegarde-Smith, P., and C. Michel, eds. 2007. *Haitian Vodou: Spirit, Myth, and Reality.* Bloomington, IN: Indiana University Press.

Boddy, J. 1994. Spirit Possession Revisited: Beyond Instrumentality." *Annual Review of Anthropology* 23: 407–434. doi: 10.1146/annurev.an.23.100194.002203

Bootzin, R. R. and E. T. Bailey. 2005. "Understanding Placebo, Nocebo, and Iatrogenic Treatment Effects." *Journal of Clinical Psychology* 61: 871–880. doi:10.1002/jclp.20131

Cáceres, A., L. M. Girón, S. R. Alvarado, and M. F. Torres. 1987. "Screening of Antimicrobial Activity of Plants Popularly Used in Guatemala for the Treatment of Dermatomucosal Diseases." *Journal of Ethnopharmacology* 20: 223–237. doi: 10.1016/0378-8741(87)90050-X

Christophe, M. A. 2007. "Rainbow over Water: Art, Vodou Aestheticism, and Philosophy" In *Haitian Vodou: Spirit, Myth, and Reality*, edited by Patrick Bellegarde-Smith and Claudine Michel, 84–102. Bloomington, IN: Indiana University Press.

Colon, S. H. 1976. *The Traditional Use of Medicinal Plants and Herbs in the Province of Pedernales, Santo Domingo.* New York: Hunter College.

Crosley, R. 2007. "Shadow-matter Universes in Haitian and Dagara Ontologies: A Comparative Study." In *Haitian Vodou: Spirit, myth, & reality*, edited by Patrick Bellegarde-Smith and Claudine Michel. Bloomington, IN: Indiana University Press.

Daniels, K. M. 2007. "Appendix: Table of Haitian Lwa." In *Haitian Vodou: Spirit, Myth, and Reality*, edited by Patrick Bellegarde-Smith and Claudine Michel. Bloomington, IN: Indiana University Press.

Desch-Obi, T. J. 2005. "Deadly Dances: The Spiritual Dimensions of Kongo-Angolan Martial Art Traditions in the New World." In *Fragments of Bone: Neo-African Religions in a New World,* edited by Patrick Bellegarde-Smith, 70–89. Chicago: University of Illinois Press.

Fandrich, I. J. 2005. "Defiant African Sisterhoods: The Voodoo Arrests of the 1850s and 1860s in New Orleans." In *Fragments of Bone: Neo-African Religions in a New World,* edited by Patrick Bellegarde-Smith, 187–207. Chicago: University of Illinois Press.

Fennell, C. 2007. "BaKongo Identity and Symbolic Expression in the Americas." In *Archaeology of Atlantic Africa and the African Diaspora,* edited by Akinwumi Ogundiran and Toyin Falola, 210–250. Bloomington, IN: Indiana University Press.

Fleurentin, J. 1990. *Recensement du savoir traditionnel: Recherche et valorisation des plantes médicinales de la Caraïbe.* 1st Conference on Ethnopharmacology, Martinique, 16–19 April 1989. Martinique: Journal of Ethnopharmacology.

James, C. L. R. 1963. *The Black Jacobins: Toussaint L'Ouverture and the San Domingo Revolution.* New York: Random House.

Jordan, W. C. 1975. "Voodoo Medicine." In *Textbook of Black Related Diseases,* edited by Richard Allen Williams, 715–738. New York: McGraw Hill.

Kail, T. M. 2008. *Magico-Religious Groups and Ritualistic Activities: A Guide for First Responders.* Florence, KY: CRC Press.

Kloss, J. 1987. *Back to Eden.* Revised Edition. Loma Linda, CA: Back to Eden Books.

Laguerre, M. 1987. *Afro-Caribbean Folk Medicine.* Hadley, MA: Bergin and Garvey.

Michel, Claudine. 1996. "Of Worlds Seen and Unseen: The Educational Character of Vodou." *Comparative Education Review 40*: 280–294. doi:10.1086/447386

Michel, Claudine. 2007. "Of Worlds Seen and Unseen: The Educational Character of Haitian Vodou." In *Haitian Vodou: Spirit, Myth, and Reality,* edited by Patrick Bellegarde-Smith and Claudine Michel, 32–45. Bloomington, IN: Indiana University Press.

Mitchell, P. 2005. *African Connections: Archaeological Perspectives on Africa and the Wider World.* Walnut Creek, CA: AltaMira Press.

Montilus, G. 2007. "Vodun and Social Transformation in the African Diasporic Experience: The Concept of Personhood in Haitian Vodun Religion." In *Haitian Vodou: Spirit, Myth, and Reality,* edited by Patrick Bellegarde-Smith and Claudine Michel, 1–6. Bloomington, IN: Indiana University Press.

Neptune-Rozier, M. 1997. *Plantes Médicinales d'Haiti: Description, Usages, Propriétés.* Port-au-Prince: Editions Regain.

Ogundiran, A. and T. Falola, eds. 2007. *Archaeology of Atlantic Africa and the African Diaspora.* Bloomington, IN: Indiana University Press.

Prasadarao, P. S. D. V. 2009. "International Perspectives on Culture and Mental Health." In *Culture and Mental Health: Sociocultural Influences, Theory, and Practice,* edited by Sussie Eshun and Regan A. R. Gurung, 149–178. Oxford: Riley-Blackwell.

Price-Mars, J. 1928. *Ainsi parla l'oncle.* Compiègne, France: Compiègne Printing.

Price-Mars, Jean. 1953. *La République d'Haïti et la République Dominicaine.* Port-au-Prince: Collection du Tricinquantenaire de l'Indépendance d'Haïti.

Priester, P. E., S. Khalili, and J. E. Luvathingal. 2009. "Placing the Soul Back into Psychology: Religion in the Psychotherapy Process. In *Culture and Mental Health: Sociocultural Influences, Theory, and Practice,* edited by Sussie Eshun and Regan A. R. Gurung, 91–114. Oxford: Wiley-Blackwell.

Sager, R. 2012. "Transcendence through Aesthetic Experience: Divining a Common Wellspring under Conflicting Caribbean and African American Religious Value Systems." *Black Music Research Journal 32:* 27–67. doi: 10.5406/blacmusiresej.32.1.0027

Santillo, H. 1987. *Natural Healing with Herbs.* Prescott Valley, AZ: Hohm Press.

Solomon, S. 2002. "A Review of Mechanisms in Response to Pain Therapy: Why Voodoo Works." *Headache: The Journal of Head and Face Pain 42:* 656–662. doi:10.1046/j.1526-4610.2002.02155.x

Statistics Canada. 2007. "The Haitian Community in Canada." <http://www.statcan.gc.ca/pub/89-621-x/89-621-x2007011-eng.htm>

U.S. Census Bureau. 2010. "Selected Social Characteristics in the United States. 2006–2010 American Community Survey Selected Population Tables: Haitian (336–359)." http://factfinder2.census.gov/bkmk/table/1.0/en/ACS/10_SF4/DP02//popgroup~581

Waldram, J. 2000. "The Efficacy of Traditional Medicine: Current Theoretical and Methodological Issues." *Medical Anthropology Quarterly 14*(4): 603–625. doi: 10.1525/maq.2000.14.4.603

Warren, D. M. and M. A. Tregoning. 1979. "Indigenous Healers and Primary Health Care in Ghana." *Medical Anthropology Newsletter 11*(2): 11–13. doi:10.1525/maq.1979.11.1.02a00110

Weniger, B. 1990. *Elements for a Caribbean Pharmacopoeia: TRAMIL 3 Workshop, Havana, Cuba, November 1988.* Enda-Caribe, Cuba: Ministerio de Salud Publica.

Weniger, Bernard. 1991. "Interest and Limitation of a Global Ethnopharmacological Survey. *Journal of Ethnopharmacology 32:* 37–41. doi:10.1016/0378-8741(91)90101-I

Wolpert, B. J., M.-G. Beauvoir, E. F. Wells, and J. M. Hawdon. 2008. "Plant Vermicides of Vodou Show in Vitro Activity against Larval Hookworm." *The Journal of Parasitology 94:* 1155–1160. doi:10.1645/GE-1446.1

World Bank. 2012. "Life Expectancy at Birth, Total (Years)." http://data.worldbank.org/indicator/SP.DYN.LE00.IN/countries/ZF-SN?display=default

Yeboah, T. 2000. "Improving the Provision of Traditional Health Knowledge for Rural Communities in Ghana." *Health Libraries Review 17:* 203–208. doi:10.1046/j.1365-2532.2000.00297.x

CHAPTER FOURTEEN

Santería as a Culturally Responsive Healing Practice

Rafael Martinez, Matthew J. Taylor, Wilma J. Calvert, Jami L. Hirsch, and Cheryl K. Webster

> *. . . it's the healing [outcome] that matters, not the techniques or explanation.*
> (*The Dancing Healers*, Carl Hammerschlag 1988, 141)

Within Western culture, physical and mental illnesses are largely defined as biologically-rooted phenomena, with secondary consideration given to other contributory elements. As such, the most widely sanctioned mechanisms of treatment for physical and mental health sequelae are often viewed using a similar lens. Medication-driven, scientifically validated treatments are explicitly understood to be the gold standard as practitioners steer their patients toward successful health outcomes framed as the absence of disease. However, the clinical setting and interplay between clinician and patient are framed within a culturally constructed cognitive reality. Both participants have culturally born expectations about the therapeutic experience and employ learned worldviews that impact everything from an understanding of illness causality to the perceived efficacy of treatment modalities. A disease-centered, medicalized model of illness conceptualization and treatment has come to dominate the health landscape and other healing traditions have come to be viewed with less legitimacy. This serves to devalue and downplay the sociocultural and humanistic aspects of patient care. It is imperative that the treatment of illness not merely entail a unilateral, clinician-generated plan that simply "cures" symptoms in a re-ductionistic clinical sense, but rather is constructed as a joint venture that affords patients the opportunity to actively participate in their healing. A critical element of this, which is often deferred to in lieu of "efficacious Western medicine," is the creation of a complementary space for other heal-ing traditions. At its core, healing is the liberation from discomfort, anxiety, and fear. It would make sense that an undertaking towards this goal would involve collaboration with non-traditional, culturally-based healing tradi-tions both familiar to and perceived as efficacious to patients.

The goal of this chapter is to elucidate the relationship between culture, health beliefs, and the outcomes of these beliefs, and in doing so, educate healthcare professionals, (defined to include any culturally validated indi-viduals with healing acumen), about the importance of recognizing, ac-cepting, and incorporating culturally diverse interpretations and remedies. The chapter will briefly discuss the role of culture on health and then focus on the unique worldview conceptualizations of the Creole religion, Santería. We elucidate how the cultural meaning systems of Santería chal-lenge mainstream health practitioners' traditional Western paradigms of "normal" vs. "abnormal" patterns of behavior, thoughts and feelings. Fi-nally, the chapter will discuss how these beliefs and rituals can (and should be) utilized as complementary elements to Western-based therapeutic practices when appropriately aligned with client/patient belief systems.

Culture and Worldview Conceptualizations: Implications for Views of Health

Culture is "the sum total of knowledge passed on from generation to gen-eration within any given society (Castillo 1997, 20; Purnell and Pontious). It is through culture and its resultant worldview that humans protectively attempt to categorize and bring meaning to the world. D'Andrade (1984) refers to the specific paradigmatic entities that drive this process as cultural meaning systems and adds that by means of their four functions, they are the tools used by a society to structure cognitive reality.

The *representational* function refers to how a cultural group comes to represent the world symbolically. Meaningful symbolic systems are arbitrary and, at times, open to misinterpretation by those outside of the group. Where one person sees a swastika as representations of Nazi Germany, an-other sees a decorative Hindu form. This has implications for the realm of health in that both clients and practitioners view symptoms through a spe-cific representational lens of meaning, whereby symptoms are ultimately "symbolic" of specific sequelae.

The *constructive* function refers to the manner in which a society constructs or builds various cultural elements. For example, a couple is considered "married" after following a set of constructed rules designed specifically with this as the end result. Moreover, what even constitutes a marriage has been constructed (and altered) over time across the globe. The DSM classification system is a health-related example of the constructive function of cultural meaning systems. Specific symptoms noted over a specified time period are "bundled" together and subsequently given cultural meaning as they are viewed as a specific disorder. Castillo (1997) notes that prior to 1800, there were few descriptions of schizophrenia as we know it today, as society had not yet "constructed" it as an illness.

The *directive* function refers to the role of cultural meaning systems in guiding human behavior. In some societies, it is taboo or very frowned upon for members of different groups (e.g., castes, racial, tribal/village of origin) to associate with each other. In terms of health, the directive function influences perception of what constitutes inappropriate and maladaptive behavior and how practitioners come to view a "sick" person. Moreover, how a disorder is viewed in terms of causality will impact the course of treatment taken, specifically, where the ill person will go for treatment, be it a clinician practicing Western medicine or a traditional folk healer, as well as the degree of adherence to a specific treatment. For example, if a patient believes that their epilepsy is caused by sprit possession (Fadiman 1997), an exclusively medication-oriented treatment may be contraindicated as their attitudes, values, and treatment behavior may be culturally directed toward another option.

The final function of cultural meaning systems is the *evocative* function. It refers to the cultural rules about emotions, by which emotions are linked to specific events, in what constitutes an appropriate emotional display. An example of this is behavior at funerals; some are quite somber reserved affairs, others involve prolonged and demonstrative open displays of grief, and still others are more upbeat and festive, and almost suggest a party atmosphere. The emotional meaning linked to health is quite diverse. An individual with an external locus of control and a highly fatalistic life orientation may not appear as emotionally devastated by a cancer diagnosis as someone else. Emotional displays of an individual from an emotionally reserved culture may appear muted to their psychotherapist and thus open to misinterpretation (i.e., s/he doesn't care about the topic at hand because the clinician is not seeing the "expected" emotion).

Culture, and its associated worldview and cultural meaning systems, play a role in how health is viewed within a given society and by individuals. Culture gives shape to the Gestalt of health for both those who are unwell and their treatment providers. A number of authors have noted the meaningful distinction between disease and illness; where disease is a pathological biological state (with an associated diagnosis) and illness is a patient's subjective experience of being sick (Castillo 1997, Green, Carrillo, and Betancourt 2002, Kleinman 1988). Both are socially recognized states in that their conceptualization is the result of cultural communication codes, meanings, and context offered by the client and subsequently understood through a similar set of cultural interpretations by a clinician.

It is the interplay between patient and practitioner, and their use of personal and professional experiences, definitions of health and causality, and other meaning making schemas, which ultimately form the clinical reality of the therapeutic endeavor. It is from these perceptual lenses that the ill and their healers view what is happening, why, and how to remedy it (Castillo 1997, Kleinman 1980). When client and clinician bring different cultural schemas to their understanding of illness, the risk of a failed therapeutic endeavor is increased. To this end, clinicians should be aware of four ways that culture impacts health and health-related behaviors (Castillo 1997).

The first is in the subjective experience of illness. This describes the way in which both patient and clinician come to understand the experience of the patient's illness. How a patient experiences her illness will certainly impart some influence on where she seeks treatment, yet variations in the treatment seeking approach can occur (Fadiman 1997, Gany et al. 2006). A patient who believes that their illness is caused by a spiritual force may seek treatment in a hospital emergency room in lieu of or in addition to more culturally-based options, which may not be available. Moreover, from the clinician's viewpoint, it should not be assumed that just because an unwell person walks through the doors of the (Western) clinic that they will immediately buy into all elements of the brand of healing being offered. While the subjective experience of the patient is easily understood, the clinician also "experiences" the illness, largely through the cultural lens of his/her training and experience (both professional and personal). A psychiatrist may think about illness in biological terms, whereas a shaman may consider causality rooted in supernatural or spiritual forces and apply this causal model to the diagnosis and treatment.

Castillo (1997) speaks of idioms of distress, and this is a second way that the thread of culture impacts the therapeutic endeavor. These are the ways in which the client behaviorally or verbally expresses that he/she is ill. Symptoms have meaning as symptoms due to culturally-rooted communiqués. Within one culture, dreams of the dead may be viewed as meaningless, whereas in others, such dreams signify serious illness (Putsch 1988).

Guilt is a common symptom of depression among individuals from Western cultures, whereas somatization, which could be thought to be more readily associated with another class of disorders, is common among depressives elsewhere (Castillo 1997). These culture-specific messages about illness can be dismissed, overlooked, or misunderstood if practitioners are not attuned to their possibility.

Aside from the nature and cause of illness, the third way in which culture impacts health is in the diagnosis of the problem. Note culture's potentially consistent and self-fulfilling influence on the pathway from the patient's subjective experience of illness to the objective diagnosis offered by healers. Recall that diseases and diagnoses are socially agreed upon constructions of reality, and it is presumed that in any given patient-practitioner dyad both parties actually agree. From the diagnosis comes the culturally-proscribed treatment, defined by the clinical reality of the care-provider, but also the patient, who ultimately has to buy in and adhere to it. If clients do not have the cultural framework to understand a diagnosis, or clinicians offer a diagnosis foreign to a client's cultural meaning systems, adherence to treatment is unlikely. Fadiman (1997) presents a powerful case where physicians and patient's family utilized different cultural constructions of disease and causality which resulted in dire consequences where a relatively nondescript yet efficacious treatment failed.

The final way that culture affects health is in what is viewed as or deemed an acceptable outcome of illness. Depending on the illness and culture, complete alleviation of symptoms is generally seen as a successful and acceptable outcome (e.g., remission of cancer). This outcome is especially sought within Western medicine, as health is often defined as the absence of disease; however, other frameworks are not as rigid in their conceptualization of healthy or normal functioning. An acceptable culture-based outcome elsewhere may be more related to the reestablishment and maintenance of life balance. This approach may conclude that a treatment was a success even when it did not yield complete and lasting symptom alleviation, but rather a (potentially) temporary state whereby symptoms abate, yet can reappear if this balance within life is not maintained (e.g., dhat syndrome; see Castillo 1997).

Santería: A Brief History and Overview

The African Diaspora in the Americas resulted in a number of syncretized religions that combined elements of Christianity, particularly Roman Catholicism, and the African religious traditions brought by the slaves to the New World (Brandon 1993, Sandoval 2006, Schmidt 2006). Additionally, some of these religions also absorbed native indigenous elements, as in the case of the Maria Lionza cult in Venezuela and Haitian Voudou (Courlander 1976, Metraux 1959; see chapter 13 this volume). Afro-American religions such as Santería, Candomble, Obeah, and Voudou, to name a few, are grounded and structured in African myths and rituals. However, these religious practices have incorporated symbols, rituals and myths borrowed mostly from Roman Catholicism. These religions have spread over the years to include not only individuals of African descent, but many other nationalities and ethnic groups. Currently, it is estimated that over one million individuals (mostly Cuban-Americans) practice Afro-Cuban Santería in the United States (Gonzalez-Wippler 1973/2007, 1989a). According to the 2010 U.S. Census, individuals of Cuban-American descent are concentrated in South Florida, New Jersey, and New York. Santería is also popular with other Hispanic groups, such as Puerto Ricans, who are found in large concentrations in the states of New York and Florida (U.S. Census Bureau 2011).

The Afro-Cuban religions' (i.e., Santería, Palo, and Abakua) inheritance can be linked to selected African cultures such as the Ibo, Efik, Yoruba, and Mahi from West Africa, and the Bantu-speaking tribes from Central Africa (Cabrera 1954, Courlander 1976, Martinez 1979, Palmie 2002). The word *Santería* derives from the Spanish word *santo* and can be traced to the Spanish colonists' derogatory characterization of the West African slaves' religious practices, which included a heavy emphasis on worshipping the saints or *santos* of the Roman Catholic faith. The saints were worshipped by the slaves as representations of the Yoruba divinities known as *orishas*. Over time this term has been used by the general population, and current practitioners self-describe as *santeros,* and their practice as *Santería*. Additionally, statues and lithographs of the Roman Catholic iconography are found in Santería altars, however, these are frequently referred to by their African orisha names. Other terms used to identify this Afro-Cuban Diaspora religion are *Lukumi* and *Ocha* religion. The ethnographer William Bascom tells us that "the African elements of Santería are predominantly Yoruba, or Lucumi, as the Yoruba of Nigeria are called in Cuba" (1950, 64).

Present Day Manifestations of Santería

The worship of the supernatural in the Santería religion centers on the *Orishas,* or divinities, that control the universe and everything connected with human existence. This religion recognizes a supreme creator variously known as *Olodumare* (The Supreme Judge), *Olorun* (The Lord of Heaven), *Oba-Ogo* (The King of Glory), etc. (Ortiz 1908). Practitioners of Santería describe this supreme deity as an abstract character who created the universe and is detached from human affairs. *Olodumare* designated a number of orishas to rule over different aspect of life and nature, thus establishing distance from direct worship by humans.

In the Santería cosmology, each person is believed to be born under the protection of a specific orisha that must be worshipped throughout life. This orisha or *santo* (saint), as they are also popularly called, play a central role in all the ceremonies and healing rituals performed by practitioners. Followers of Santería will participate in a number of divinatory or consultation rituals where an initiated priest of the religion will use either a necklace known as the *opele* chain (used by *babalawos* or *Ifa* priests) or the *di-loggun*, consisting of 16 cowrie shells (used by *obas* or *italeros*) to determine who is the guardian orisha that rules over the follower's head.

Selected orishas of the Santería religion are recognized as possessing different manifestations or "avatars" where they are described with unique personality characteristics, likes and dislikes, and other idiosyncratic traits. For example, the orisha Eleggua is recognized in as many as 101 avatars or *caminos,* variously known as *Echu AgbóBará,* described as a trickster that listens to everything humans say; *Echu Agbálonké,* a strong and mature Eleggua that punishes with fire and guides the souls of the departed; *Echu Achi kuelú,* an elder Eleggua that lives underground and owns all minerals and metals such as gold, etc. (Bolivar-Arostegui 1990, Cabrera 1954). Other Eleggua avatars are recognized by practitioners and described as astute and tricky, a thief who only accepts offerings that have been stolen, a liar who loves to create confusion and misunderstandings, etc. (Bolivar-Arostegui 1990). Table 14.1 describes the attributes, powers and other elements associated with selected orishas of the Afro-Cuban Santería pantheon.

Rites and Rituals

Religious participation in the Santería religion is broadly observed in two contexts: (1) rituals conducted by a follower alone or performed by an initiated *santeros* or *santeras* (Santería priest or priestess) on a follower, or (2) organized rituals presided by a santero with the participation of other santeros and followers known as *aleyos*. These rituals follow a continuum of symbolic gestures, drumming and dancing, the ritual sacrifice of selected animals, trance states, uses of herbs, roots and plants, and other

Table 14.1 Characteristics of Selected Afro-Cuban Santería–Orishas

ORISHA/SANTO	ATTRIBUTES/POWERS	COLOR(S)/OFFERINGS/ SYMBOLS
Olofi; Olodumare; Olorun	Creator and source of all power	Invoked in selected prayers
Eleggua (the Christ Child; St. Anthony)	Owner of destiny and the cross-roads; trickster; warrior deity	Red and Black; roasted corn, smoked possum; blood of young roosters
Oggun (St. Peter)	God of iron and warrior deity. Owner of metals	Green and Black; offerings placed in the railroad tracks; knives, railroad spikes, horseshoes; blood of roosters, pigeons, etc.
Ochosi (St. Norberto)	God of justice and warrior deity	Gold and Blue; the crossbow, deer antlers, handcuffs; blood of pigeons, etc.
Obatala (Our Lady of Mercy; Resurrected Christ)	Son of Olofi - father of the orishas; god of peace and wisdom	White; silver bell called "agogo," white pigeons and other four-legged white animals (e.g., goats)
Yemaya (Our Lady of Regla)	Goddess of the Oceans; primordial mother of the santos	Blue; Seashells and anything from the ocean; Watermelons, sugar cane syrup, pork rinds; blood of ducks
Oshun (Our Lady of Charity)	Goddess of the rivers, sensuality, love and money	Yellow and Gold; mirrors, gold, copper; blood of hens and female goats
Chango (St. Barbara)	An impulsive and warrior-like god; promiscuous and womanizer	Red and White; apples, bananas, the double-edge ax; blood of rams, lambs, goats and roosters
Babalu Aye (St. Lazarus)	God of illnesses and skin diseases	Black, Purple and Yellow; crutches, cigars, pennies
Oya (Our Lady of La Candelaria)	Goddess of the cemetery and death; impulsive and mighty	Nine colors; eggplants; offerings placed in cemeteries

magico-religious performances (Brandon 1991, Martinez 1979, Martinez and Wetli 1982).

Consultation with the Oracle

In the Santería religion there are three primary divinatory systems used to identify the source of troubles, confirm the orishas' acceptance of offerings, and establish a course of religious action. The divination systems are: the "Obi" or coconut divination (referred in Spanish as *tirar los cocos* ("throwing of the coconuts"); the *Dilogun* or seashell divination (referred in Spanish as *leer los caracoles* or *registro* ("to read the shells" or "to search"); and the *Opele* chain, a system used only by a class of Santería priests known as *Babalawos* (McNeill et al. 2008).

The simplest and most frequently used form of divination is the *Obi*. It consists of four pieces carved from inside a coconut and shaped into round pieces measuring two to three inches. Beginning with prayers invoking the ancestors and the powers of the orishas, the santero throws the pieces of coconut on the floor with the chances of falling with the white side up. There are five positions in which these 4 pieces can fall. *Obi* divination is a yes or no system for questions posed by the santero priest. For example, four white rinds showing up is called *Alafia* and it is interpreted as an absolute yes to the question posed; it is interpreted as a message of happiness and harmony. The other four positions are called *Itague* or *etawa* (three white rinds up); *Ellife* or *ejife* (two white rinds up); *Okana* (one white rind up); and *Oyekun* (four black or woody rinds up). This last sign is negative and announces misfortune and unfavorable outcomes (Martinez 1979, Lele 2001).

Seashell divination or *Diloggun* is a crucial system based on interpreting the positions of 16 cowrie shells (Gonzalez-Wippler 1989b). In fact, without the seashells, the santero cannot perform any of the major rituals of the Santería religion. The cowries are combined with five divination aids called *igbo*, which include a black stone called *ota*, a long seashell called *aye*, the head of a tiny doll called *eriaworan*, a small ball of compacted powdered eggshell called *efun*, and a tiny animal vertebra called *eggun*. *Diloggun* divination is complex and it begins with a series of prayers and invocations to the spirits of the dead and the orishas. These prayers are known as *moyugbar*. The seashells are thrown on a straw mat used for the reading. There are sixteen patterns or *odus*, with each having a name, a refrain, and several legends. It is the role of the priest to interpret for the consultant each of the *oddus*. The divination aids or *igbos* are selectively used by the santero priest to confirm the messages contained in certain seashell patterns.

Opele divination is conducted only by the Babalawo priest and consists of a metal chain that connects eight oval shaped pieces of coconut rinds or tortoiseshell. The Babalawo priest throws down the opele and interprets any of the 16 possible patterns or *oddus*. The combination of the 16 patterns can form 256 new designs, each containing verses, legends and proverbs that are applied to the consultant's situation. The *oddus* are accompanied by invocations called *suyeres*. Babalawos believe that the *Opele* oracle includes all the knowledge and understandings of mankind (Martinez 1979).

The Necklaces Ceremony

Receiving the necklaces is considered the baptism or entrance into the Santería religion. It is a ceremony where an individual receives five necklaces connected to these orishas: Eleggua, Obatala, Oshun, Yemaya, and Chango. It is a celebratory ritual where the initiate is welcomed into the religion and is structured around the three phases of rites of passage proposed by Arnold van Gennep (1909/1960): separation, transition and re-incorporation. A feature of all Santería rituals is the presence of a *padrino* or *madrina* (godfather or godmother) to lead the rituals performed on followers. This person is chosen by the devotee based on trust, familiarity, and/or good religious reputation in the Santería community. In the process of consulting the seashells for whatever reason, the Santería follower is told that she/he is to receive the *collares* (necklaces) as read in the messages of the seashells *registro*. If the *santero* conducting the divination is the *padrino/madrina* of the devotee, they will agree on a date and time for the ceremony. Additionally, a second officiant called a *yugbona* will become an assistant in the ceremony and will establish a religious relationship to the person going through this initiation, thus becoming sort of a second godfather/godmother (Martinez 1979, Gonzalez-Wippler 1989a).

The initiate that is to receive the necklaces is asked to come to the *yugbona's* house the night before the ceremony so that a *rogacion de cabeza* ("prayer of the head") ritual is performed. This involves a series of prayers performed by the *yugbona* and culminates with the initiate being anointed with a paste prepared with coconut, *cascarilla* (ground egg shell), palm oil, guinea pepper, and other ingredients. The paste is placed on the initiate's head and held in place with a white cap. Other cleansing rituals are performed in order to prepare the person for the necklaces ritual the following day.

This *rogacion* ritual officially begins the *separation* stage in this rite of passage. The initiate is to wear white clothing for the ritual, abstain from sexual activity, avoid partying, drinking alcohol or engaging in other mundane activities. The person is severed from common activities. The receiving of the necklaces ritual will then be conducted the following day by the padrino, yugbona, and other santeros invited to participate in the ceremony. Most often, this ritual is conducted in the *padrino/madrina's* home. The rites of passage *transition* stage can be identified as the day of the ceremony, when the initiate is asked to wear old clothing, preferably white or light colored. She/he is also asked to bring a set of brand new white clothing, including underwear, socks, shoes, hat or cap, etc. After the usual prayers and invocations to the ancestors and the orishas, conducted in a ritual room, the *padrino/madrina* will proceed to symbolically tear away the old clothing from the initiate, thus symbolizing the destruction of the old person.

Immediately after this, the initiate is led to a bathroom where a tub has been prepared with a liquid known as *omiero*, which contains a variety of leaves, roots, flowers and other ritual ingredients. The initiate is then asked to kneel, and every santero/santera participating in the ceremony, starting with the padrino/madrina and the yugbona, will come in and place a little of the omiero on the person's head. Afterwards, the person is left alone and asked to bathe using a special white odorless soap known as *jabon de castilla* (castille soap). The initiate is asked to dress up with the new white clothing brought for this occasion and asked to rejoin the santeros in the ritual room for the imposing of the five necklaces (Martinez 1979, Fernandez-Cano 2008).

The imposition of the necklaces ritual is led by the padrino/madrina, however, all santeros in the room participate in the placement of the necklaces on the initiate. Upon completion of the ceremony, the person receiving the necklaces is asked to wear them for the rest of the day while wearing the all-white attire. The ceremony concludes with a dinner or brunch. The rites of passage *re-incorporation* stage occurs when all the restrictions (such as dressing in white, wearing the necklaces, abstaining from sexual activities, etc.) are lifted the day after the necklaces are received.

The necklaces ceremony serves as a way to establish social bonds in a fictive religious family. The bond of godfather/godmother is established in this ceremony as well as with other initiates in the Santería community. The cleansing rituals, receiving the necklaces with the power of orishas, and similar rituals empower the individual to take control of whatever situation she/he was facing before the initiation.

Receiving the Warriors

The initiation of receiving warriors (*Eleggua, Esun, Oggun, and Ochosi*) represents another major step in joining the Santería religion. The warriors are powerful and mighty entities that protect the initiate and help them to fight and overcome any and all obstacles. They also provide the devotee a sense of control and mastery when confronted with difficult situations. There is a significant degree of personalization with the warriors as they are aligned with each devotee's needs and prepared and tailored to each initiate. Each is specially prepared or *cargados* (charged) by the padrino/ madrina; for example when molding Eleggua's effigy in the shape of a head with cement and cowrie shells, the padrino/madrina will ask the person who will be receiving it to provide a stone, a jewel, or some other personal item that will be included in the effigy.

Because Eleggua is the guardian of the gates and destiny, the warriors are symbolically kept close to the home entrance or else in the ritual room. The most personalized warrior is Esun. It is depicted as a metal pedestal holding a cup-like compartment fringed with tiny bells and a rooster standing on top of it. The cup-like compartment contains cotton, roasted corn, coconut, and other roots and herbs (Brandon 1991). Some santeros include the name of the initiate inside the cup. Esun is recognized as one's self or personal essence. Oggun and Ochosi are both depicted in the mythology stories or *patakis* as fearless warriors. Ochosi is the orisha of justice and rules over courts, jailhouses, police stations, etc. Oggun is the god of metals represented by railroad spikes, knives, and all things metal. The symbolism surrounding the warriors guides the Santería practitioner in the daily struggles that all humans deal with in different contexts. The warriors empower the devotee to confront obstacles head-on with the conviction that victory is assured (Martinez 1979, Fernandez-Cano 2008).

The Priesthood Initiation

Becoming a priest or priestess in the Santería religion is a one-year process that includes multiple rituals, observance of taboos, dress code, and numerous rules governing daily activities. Not every Santería practitioner moves on to this initiation level, however, it is a crucial step for those persons confronting serious health issues and other major obstacles in their lives. The first step in the priesthood initiation process is to identify the orisha that rules over the devotee's head. All of the rituals, including the preparation before the actual initiation, are going to be dictated by the orisha that is to be *coronado* (crowned). This initiation is called *hacer santo* (to make saint) or the *asiento* (settlement), the latter referring to the settling of the orisha on the initiate's head.

Each Orisha has specific preliminary rituals before the actual inititation. For example, sons/daughters of Oya, the goddess of death and the cemetery, will participate in rituals nine days before the actual initiation (nine is Oya's number). Each day, ceremonies are conducted at the railroad tracks, the cemetery (at midnight), at the foot of the Royal Poinciana tree, at a Catholic church, etc. The day before the initiation, the novice is taken to the river by the *yugbona,* or the godfather/godmother, to be ritually cleansed and bathed in the river. It is also customary to perform a *misa de entrada* (entrance mass) to identify the spirits of the dead that must be worshipped or propitiated before the initiation. This ritual is actually based on *espiritismo* (spiritualism) beliefs that have been incorporated in this Diaspora religion. Various other rituals are performed to prepare the person for the initiation (Sandoval 2006).

The day of the initiation numerous santeros will gather for an all-day event that includes preparing the herbs and plants sacred to each orisha into a liquid called *omiero,* the sacrifice of animals specific to each orisha, numerous prayers, songs and invocations performed on the novice, etc (Brandon 1991). The focus of the ritual is on the initiate's head, which is shaven and painted with various designs and concentric circles representing the orishas and particularly the one that is being 'crowned'. The initiate will wear white during this ceremony as well as a couple of other special dresses made for the occasion.

The initiation ceremony will continue for seven days with each day having unique activities. Some of these include an open house celebration immediately following the day of the initiation called *dia del medio* (day in the middle) to welcome family and friends and present the new initiate to the Santería community, and the *Ita* which is conducted the day after the open house. This is a divination ritual conducted by an *oba* or a *babalawo* and results in a blueprint of religious activities, do's and don'ts, and other observances. Each orisha received during the initiation is consulted (Gonzalez-Wippler 1989a).

The initiate will remain in the house where the initiation was conducted for seven days, meditating and learning about the religion. She/he is treated like a newborn. For example, they are the first ones to be served food, are walked to the restroom when needed, and are referred to as *Yawo,* a name used for all neophytes in the Santería religion. The complete initiation into the Santería priesthood lasts a year. It is a period marked by strict taboos and observances. Neophytes are forbidden from drinking any alcohol or attending parties. Females are not allowed to put on make-up and both males and females must cover their heads with a white hat, cap or shawl as well as dress in white. It is a period marked by frequent interaction with the godfather/godmother while learning from the santeros associated with the particular family called *ile* or *casa de santo* (House of Saint) into which they were initiated. All restrictions are lifted at the end of the one year period, and the person is now recognized as a full-fledged priest or priestess (santero or santera) in the religion. The individual is re-incorporated (van Gennep 1909/1960) into the community while recognized in his/her new role (Fernandez-Cano 2008, Garcia-Cortez 2000, Martinez, 1979).

Santería Themes as Healing Practice

The history of 21st century Western medicine has rarely considered indigenous healing practices, such as, herbal remedies, magic, witchcraft, and religious practices as legitimate forms of healing (Airhihenbuwa 1995). As the Western medical perspective gains prominence, it has insisted that the field and its practices be exclusively scientific in nature, objectively measureable, and consistently replicable. The increased emphasis on scientific medicine has left little space for traditional approaches and has unnecessarily constructed a rigid reality that overlooks the fact that there is more to healthcare than medical (biological) care. This is a critical oversight as these "local" tools and explanations of sequelae have not been universally replaced by scientific explanations. Furthermore, these traditional frameworks are rooted in cultural knowledge, and not only serve as a lens through which to view a group's system of culture and its potential influences on perception, judgment, communication and behaviors, but, in a practical sense, address a number of psychosocial dimensions which will impact healing (Mphande and James-Meyers 1993, Thomas, 2001). The power of the practitioner (and treatment) comes in part from the client's belief in the ability of the healer, as inferred from their analysis of the practitioner's training, educational degree, experience, or community status (Moodley and Sutherland 2010). So in spite of the fact that traditional healing and Western approaches to medicine are often viewed in binary opposition to one another, especially from the perspective of medical professionals, the reality is that the two are often cultural bedfellows which can be compatible, used simultaneously, and ultimately may result in a more efficacious treatment undertaking (Baez and Hernandez, 2001; Del Castillo, in press; Moodley and Sutherland 2009).

The previous discussion of Santería's history and its basic tenets offers insight into how followers view themselves, the world, and the events therein. Not only does this constructed reality have implications for how self is viewed, along with linkages to others, but equally as important, self-in-relation to the material and spiritual world (Holliday, 2008). Rites and rituals serve a number of roles in the development of (individual) self and are also individual behavioral expressions of cultural identity. Not only are rites and rituals an expressions of shared commonality among individuals, they are often done in the presence of others. Thus, they also serve to promote group solidarity and reaffirm an individual's connection with the group.

Santería can function as a supportive system of culturally meaningful symbols and healing processes, both of which can serve to bring about enhanced treatment (Martinez and Welti 1982). The initial step in all major Santería rituals is to consult the oracle (i.e., the *Obi*, the *Dilogun* or the *Opele*) to identify the source of trouble or diagnose the consultant, determine a course of ritual steps, and establish a follow up strategy. The divination rituals always begin with a series of invocations to the ancestors and the orishas (*moyugbar*). These prayers tie the consultant to a spiritual realm of ancestral spirits and divinities, and provide psychological connectedness to other Santería followers protected by the same supernatural entities. The divination ritual provides a mechanism to structure the situation of the consultant and provide a sense of control, which is a common psychotherapeutic theme. An individual arrives at the divination session (*consulta*) full of questions and uncertainties and walks away with a blueprint for action, including specific religious rituals believed to bring back normalcy in everyday living (Lefley 1981).

On matters related to health, it must be noted that Santería followers sometimes seek western medical diagnoses and the corresponding treatments (Ness and Wintrob 1981; Suarez, Raffaelli, and O'Leary 1996). Religious rituals are performed to ensure the success of the medical intervention. Still, the etiology or ultimate cause of the problem can be traced to supernatural causation such as punishment by the orishas due to their neglect by the follower, sorcery or *brujeria* performed by an enemy wishing harm on the person/victim, and on occasion, disruptions may be caused by spirits of dead ancestors who have been neglected in rituals. Common or minor rituals are called *addimus* and include offerings of flowers, fruits, incense, glasses or rum or aguardiente, etc. to please the spirits of the dead (*los muertos* or *egun*) and/or the orishas. Major offerings known as *ebbos* will include the sacrifice of birds and four-legged animals (e.g., roosters, pigeons, goats). In more serious health crises or situations, the follower may be told that he/she needs to receive the necklaces, the warriors, selected orishas (e.g., *Yemaya-Olokun*, *Babalu Aye*), or even proceed with initiation into the Santería priesthood.

In these ritual performances, the Santería follower is actively involved in seeking his/her cure or solution to the problem. There is intense and frequent interaction with the *padrino/madrina* who conducts or prescribes rituals aimed at symbolically sending away any negative forces or hexes through religious cleansings known as *limpiezas, despojos* or *rogaciones*. These rituals strive to attract good karma (known as *ashe*) as well as the blessings of the ancestors and/or the orishas. These ceremonies help transition the consultant from a passive agent to an active participant in the healing process (Santi, Jr. 1997).

Martinez and Wetli (1982, 35) offer that Santería rites and rituals are "cathartic techniques in which anxieties and intrapsychic conflicts are objectified," and thus laid bare for treatment. For example, the Santería priest/priestess may identify the source of trouble to be a particular person who may be working evil sorcery against the consultant. It is possible that the recommended course of action be to magically retaliate by preparing a doll resembling the enemy (e.g., a male or female figurine) and include a personal item once touched by the target of the magic (e.g., clothing, hair, saliva, etc.). This doll once prepared will be placed upside down in a glass of water that is placed in a refrigerator freezer. By performing this magic, the enemy is symbolically frozen or immobilized from further evil action against the victim and all of her/his life activities will turn upside down with negative consequences (i.e., the inverted doll in the glass). Other similar rituals may involve writing the name of a person on a piece of paper and placing the paper inside a small honey jar in order to "sweeten" their disposition towards another person or situation. A number of similar symbolic rituals allow the person to objectify his/her fears and conflicts without using direct confrontation or violence against the enemy.

Rites and rituals, as part of the socialization process, aid in epistemological development (i.e., knowledge of the world), which in turn, forms the foundation of interpretations of the world. In terms of health related processes, cultural knowledge and interpretation link directly with perceived causality of illness and this, in concert with an individual's disposition, has implications for treatment (Sandoval 1979). In reviewing the diverse characterizations of each orisha and their corresponding avatars, we observe a comprehensive list of human traits, behaviors and dispositions. The fact that each follower of Santería is believed to be a "son" or "daughter" of a specific orisha points to an affinity between the personality of the follower and the avatar of a specific orisha. For example, sons and daughters of Eleggua tend to be playful, tricky, and sometimes prone to creating misunderstanding while others are helpful and facilitate or prevent situations from happening; followers of Chango are impulsive and combative; the children of Yemaya are wise and moody; and so on (Sandoval 2006).

Each orisha is also believed to be responsible for specific afflictions, illnesses and disruptions should the follower fail to properly worship the deity. For example, Obatala punishes with paralysis and birth deformities; Oshun is connected with abdominal distress, domestic strife, etc. Yemaya inflicts respiratory distress; Oya is associated with marital separation, etc. (Sandoval 2006). The Santería practitioner is careful to always follow and align with the behaviors and lifestyles expected of a son or daughter of specific orishas. In fact, those who get initiated as *santeros/a* will have a divination ritual known as *ita* performed on the third day of the initiation. At this time, a lifetime blueprint of do's and don'ts and other prescribed behaviors and taboos are established for the initiate. Any deviation or misalignment with one's Orisha will result in punishment by the supernatural (Pasquali 1994).

Many traditional worldviews consider all elements of the world to be connected and view health as equivalent to harmony (Mphande and James-Meyers 1993). Maintaining a harmonious connection to the ancestors or familial spirits of the dead is also important in the Santería religion. As mentioned, all major rituals begin with invocations calling for the ancestors' blessings. Failure to remember the departed or acting in ways that dishonor their memory, may trigger their anger and punishment, resulting in disruptions such as chronic illnesses, general misfortune, accidents, etc. Santería practitioners will find out through divination the cause of their problem(s) to be the neglect of the ancestors. They will be advised as to what ritual offerings and/or ceremonies must be conducted in order to bring back harmony and avoid the ongoing ancestral wrath. In this sense, Santería rituals serve to connect the living and the dead, thus establishing a continuity of tradition, values, family and community ties (Lefley 1981).

Another situation involving spirits of the dead is when the suffering presented by the consultant is related to the presence of an evil or dark spirit (*muerto oscuro*) that was sent by an enemy santero/a. In such situations, rituals involving cleansing and purification rituals will be prescribed to exorcise and "send away" such malevolent entitites. At times, rituals are performed where the evil intruder is removed by the officiating santero/a. These rituals are considered dangerous and performed only by the seasoned priests or priestesses who at times go into trance states, convulsing and displaying the symptoms of an intruding evil spirit just removed from a victim. The santero/a will eventually get rid of the evil spirit, thus liberating the consultant from further suffering (Suarez et al. 1996). These rituals are frequently performed during spiritist masses (*misas espiritistas*), which are a religious syncretism of *Espiritismo* and Santería practices.

Conclusion

Many health service delivery systems and treatment modalities are dominated by Western-based approaches and conceptualizations. Culturally responsive practice does not mean the supplanting of evidence-based practices, rather that clinicians remain open to the complementary use and incorporation of other belief systems that unwell people bring to the therapeutic encounter. Ill people ultimately want answers about life and alleviation from their symptoms and a variety of treatment approaches can offer these. As culture and its belief systems impact and determine an individual's worldview and interpretive lens, clinicians must be acutely aware of this and the potential boon and bane of alternative worldviews. Understanding the variety of folk beliefs that patients hold will increase the likelihood of a successful treatment endeavor and the betterment of patient outcomes, which at the most basic level is the true role of *all* healers.

References

Airhihenbuwa, C. O. 1995. *Health and Culture: Beyond the Western Paradigm.* Thousand Oaks, CA: Sage.

Baez, A. and Hernandez, D. 2001. "Complementary Spiritual Beliefs in the Latino Community: The Interface with Psychotherapy." *American Journal of Orthopsychiatry* 71: 408–415.

Bascom, W. 1950. "The Focus of Cuban Santería." *Southwestern Journal of Anthropology* 6: 64–68.

Bolivar-Arostegui, N. 1990. *Los Orishas en Cuba.* Havana: Ediciones Union.

Brandon, G. 1991. "The Uses of Plants in Healing in an Afro-Cuban Religion, Santería." *Journal of Black Studies* 22: 55–76.

Brandon, G. 1993. *Santería from Africa to the New World.* Indianapolis: Indiana University Press.

Cabrera, L. 1954. *El Monte.* Miami: Mnemosyne Publishing Co.

Castillo, R. J. 1997. *Culture and Mental Illness: A Client Centered Approach.* Pacific Grove, CA: Brooks/Cole.

Courlander, H. 1976. *A Treasury of Afro-American Folklore.* New York: Crown Publishers.

D'Andrade, R. G. 1984. "Cultural Meaning Systems." In *Cultural Theory: Essays on Mind, Self, and Emotion,* edited by R. A. Shweder and R. A. LeVine, 89–119. Cambridge: Cambridge University Press.

Del Castillo, R. In press. "Institutionalizing *Curanderismo* into a Mainstream Healing System: Boundary Spanners and Innovation in Action." In *Hispanics in the Southwest: Issues of Immigration, Education, Health, and Public Policy,* edited by A. H. Benavides, E. Midobuche, and P. H. Carlson, 116–134. Tempe, AZ: Bilingual Review Press.

Fadiman, A. 1997. *The Spirit Catches You and You Fall Down.* New York: Farrar, Straus and Giroux.

Fernandez-Cano, J. 2008. "Ocha, Santería, Lucumi o Yoruba: Los Retos de Una Religion Afro-Cubana en el Sur de Florida." [Ocha, Santería, Lucumi or Yoruba: The Challenges of an Afro-Cuban Religion in South Florida]. (Doctoral dissertation Universidad de Granada, Spain.)

Gany, F. M., A. P. Herrera, M. Avallone, and J. Changrani. 2006. "Attitudes, Knowledge, and Health-Seeking Behaviors of Five Immigrant Minority Communities in the Prevention and Screening of Cancer: A Focus Group Approach." *Ethnicity and Health 11*: 19–39.

Garcia-Cortez, J. 2000. *The Osha: Secrets of the Yoruba-lucumi Santería Religion in the United States and the Americas.* New York: Athelia Henrietta Press.

Gonzalez-Wippler, M. 1973/2007. *Santería: African Magic in Latin America.* New York: Anchor Books.

Gonzalez-Wippler, M. 1989a. *Santería: The Religion.* New York: Harmony Books.

Gonzalez-Wippler, M. 1989b. *Introduction to Seashell Divination.* New York: Original Publications.

Green, A. R., J. E. Carrillo, and J. R. Betancourt. 2002. "Why the Disease-Based Model of Medicine Fails Our Patients." *Western Journal of Medicine 176*: 141–143.

Hammerschlag, C. A. 1988. *The Dancing Healers: A Doctor's Journey of Healing with Native Americans.* New York: Harper One.

Holliday, K. V. 2008. "Religious Healing and Biomedicine in Comparative Context." In *Latina/o Healing Practices: Mestizo and Indigenous Perspectives,* edited by B. W. McNeill and J. M. Cervantes, 249–270. New York: Routledge.

Kleinman, A. 1980. *Patients and Healers in the Context of Culture: An Exploration of the Borderland Between Anthropology, Medicine, and Psychiatry.* Berkeley: University of California Press.

Kleinman, A. 1988. *The Illness Narratives: Suffering, Healing, and the Human Condition.* New York: Basic Books.

Lefley, H. P. 1981. "Psychotherapy and Cultural Adaptation in the Caribbean." *International Journal of Group Tension 11*: 3–16.

Lele, O.N. 2001. *Obi: Oracle of Cuban Santería.* Rochester: Destiny Books.

Martinez, R. 1979. "Afro-Cuban Santería among Cuban-Americans in Dade County, Florida: A Psycho-Cultural Approach." Master Thesis. Department of Anthropology, University of Florida, Gainesville.

Martinez, R. and C. V. Wetli. 1982. "Santería: A Magico-Religious System of Afro-Cuban Origin." *The American Journal of Social Psychiatry 2* (3): 32–38.

McNeill, B. W., E. Esquivel, A. Carrasco, and R. Mendoza. 2008. "Santería and the Healing Process in Cuba and the United States." In *Latina/o Healing Practices: Mestizo and Indigenous Perspectives,* edited by B. W. McNeill and J. M. Cervantes, 63–79. New York: Routledge.

Metraux, A. 1959. *Voodoo in Haiti.* New York: Schocken Books.

Moodley, R. and P. Sutherland. 2009. "Traditional and Cultural Healers and Healing: Dual Interventions in Counseling and Psychotherapy." *Counseling and Spirituality 28*: 11–31.

Moodley, R. and P. Sutherland. 2010. "Psychic Retreats in Other Places: Clients Who Seek Healing with Traditional Healers and Psychotherapists." *Counselling Psychology Quarterly* 23: 267–282.

Mphande, L. and L. James-Meyers. 1993. "Traditional African Medicine and the Optimal Theory: Universal Insights for Health and Healing." *Journal of Black Psychology* 19: 25–47.

Ness, R. C. and R. M. Wintrob. 1981. "Folk Healing: A Description and Synthesis." *American Journal of Psychiatry* 138: 1477–1481.

Ortiz, F. 1908. *Los Negros Brujos*. Miami: New House.

Palmie, S. 2002. *Wizards and Scientists: Exploration in Afro-Cuban Modernity and Traditions*. Durham: Duke University Press.

Pasquali, E. A. 1994. "Santería." *Journal of Holistic Nursing* 12: 380–390.

Putsch, R. W. 1988. "Ghost Illness: A Cross-Cultural Experience with the Expression of a Non-Western Tradition in Clinical Practice." *American Indian and Alaska Native Mental Health Research* 2: 6–26.

Sandoval, M. C. 1979. "Santería as a Mental Health Care System: An Historical Overview." *Social Science and Medicine* 12: 137–151.

Sandoval, M. C. 2006. *Worldview, the Orichas, and Santería*. Gainesville: University Press of Florida.

Santi, A., Jr. 1997. "Santería Compared to Psychology as a Mental Health Care System." *Dissertation Abstracts International: Section B: The Sciences and Engineering* 58(3-B): 1545.

Schmidt, B. 2006. "The Creation of Afro-Caribbean Religions and Their Incorporation of Christian Elements: A Critique against Syncretism." *Transformation* 23: 236–243.

Suarez, M., M. Raffaelli, and A. O'Leary. 1996. "Use of Folk Healing Practices by HIV-Infected Hispanics Living in the United States." *AIDS Care* 8: 683–690.

Thomas, R. M. 2001. *Folk Psychologies across Cultures*. Thousand Oaks, CA: Sage.

U.S. Census Bureau. 2011. *The Hispanic Population: 2010*. http://www.census .gov/prod/cen2010/briefs/c2010br-04.pdf.

Van Gennep, A. 1960. *The Rites of Passage*. (M. V. Visedom and G. L. Caffee, Trans.) Chicago: University of Chicago Press. (Original work published 1909).

About the Editor and Contributors

EDITOR

Regan A. R. Gurung is Ben J. and Joyce Rosenberg Professor of Human Development and Psychology at the University of Wisconsin, Green Bay. Born and raised in Bombay, India, Dr. Gurung received a B.A. in psychology at Carleton College (MN), and a Masters and Ph.D. in social and personality psychology at the University of Washington (WA). He then spent three years at UCLA as a National Institute of Mental Health (NIMH) Research fellow.

He has received numerous local, state, and national grants for his health psychological and social psychological research on cultural differences in stress, social support, smoking cessation, body image and impression formation. He has published articles in a variety of scholarly journals including Psychological Review and Personality and Social Psychology Bulletin, and Teaching of Psychology. He has a textbook, *Health Psychology: A Cultural Approach*, relating culture, development, and health published with Cengage (now in its third edition) and is also the co-author/co-editor of ten other books. He has made over 100 presentations and given workshops nationally and internationally (e.g. Australia, India, Saudi Arabia, New Zealand).

Dr. Gurung is also a dedicated teacher and has strong interests in enhancing faculty development and student understanding. He was Co-Director of the University of Wisconsin System Teaching Scholars Program, has been a UWGB Teaching Fellow, a UW System Teaching Scholar, and is winner of the CASE Wisconsin Professor of the Year, the UW System Regents Teaching Award, and the UW-Green Bay Founder's Award for Excellence in Teaching, as well as the Founder's Award for Scholarship, UW Teaching-at-its-Best, Creative Teaching, and Featured Faculty Awards.

He has strong interests in teaching and pedagogy and has organized statewide and national teaching conferences, is a Fellow of the American Psychological Association, the Association for Psychological Science and the Midwestern Psychological Association, and has served on the Div. 2 (Teaching of Psychology) Taskforce for Diversity, as Chair of the Div. 38 (Health Psychology) Education and Training Council, and as President of the Society for the Teaching of Psychology.

CONTRIBUTORS

Leticia Arellano-Morales, Ph.D, is a counseling psychologist. She is currently an Associate Professor within the Department of Psychology at the University of La Verne. Her research interests include Latina/o health and mental health, multicultural counseling competencies, multiracial feminism, and ethnic minority college students.

Kavita Avula, PhD, is a licensed clinical psychologist who is an associate with the KonTerra Group and practitioner for Greenleaf Integrative Strategies, firms that provide organizational and individual support to humanitarian aid organizations and their employees, who work in conflict-affected areas around the globe. In addition, she is a consultant for The World Bank Group Personal & Work Stress Counseling Unit and has a private practice in Washington, DC where she provides individual and group psychotherapy. Dr. Avula specializes in cross-cultural and international psychology, trauma and resilience, group dynamics and critical incident response.

Patrick Bellegarde-Smith, Professor Emeritus of Africology, received his PhD in international politics, history and comparative politics from The American University in 1977. He has taught in the fields of international development, Caribbean cultures, gender, religions, and national identity, and currently publishes in the areas of African metaphysics and cosmology, and Haitian religious thought. He is the recipient of the Lifetime Achievement Award for scholarship from the Haitian Studies Association, and is an oungan asogwe, a priest in the Vodou religion.

Amina Benkhoukha, B.S., is a doctoral student in the clinical psychology (health emphasis) PhD program at Ferkauf Graduate School of Psychology, Yeshiva University. Ms. Benkhoukha's research interests involve culturally specific stressors associated with acculturation, discrimination and acculturation.

Lauren Brinkley-Rubinstein is a PhD student in the community research and action program at Vanderbilt University and has conducted public health-relevant research for seven years. Her primary research interests include investigating the social context of health, the impact of incarceration and drug laws on health, health equity, and health policy. She has an educational background in sociology/criminology and social policy and practical research experience and specific training in public health research methodology with a focus on health disparities and the social determinants of health

Wilma J. Calvert is an assistant professor in the College of Nursing at the University of Missouri-St. Louis. Her research interests focus on the effects of alcohol, tobacco, and other drugs on vulnerable populations in urban and rural communities. Her most recent research projects focused on health promotion in low-income fathers of color residing in urban communities, and prevention efforts aimed at school-aged children living in communities with a high prevalence of methamphetamine use and production. She has also examined how protective factors, including religion and spirituality, may reduce participation in various health compromising behaviors, including the use of alcohol, tobacco, and other drugs in various populations.

Ayşe Çiftçi is an Associate Professor in counseling psychology at Purdue University. Her research interests focus broadly on cross-cultural psychology and diversity issues specifically related to immigrants and international students. Dr. Çiftçi serves as the editorial member of several journals and is actively engaged in the American Psychological Association.

Sabrina Crawford earned her doctorate in Psychology from The George Washington University in Washington, DC and her bachelor of arts in Psychology from Rider University in Lawrenceville, NJ. Dr. Crawford has a private practice providing individual therapy, as well as psychological assessments to culturally diverse clients. She also serves as a consultant to COPE Inc., where she conducts therapy and provides psychoeducation to managers, employees, and spouses of international organizations in the Washington D.C. area. Her research interests include cultural competency, acculturation, trauma, and abuse.

Miriam Frankel, M.A. is a PhD candidate in psychology (health emphasis) at the Ferkauf Graduate School of Psychology of Yeshiva University. She has special interests in the effects of socioeconomic status and chronic disease on health, and incorporating multicultural sensitivity into clinical practice.

Yvette Fruchter, M.A., is currently in her fourth year at Ferkauf School of Psychology in their Clinical Psychology (Health Emphasis) Program. Yvette's research interests focus on understanding the psychosocial components of chronic illness. She is currently completing her dissertation on the impact of anxiety and depression on kidney disease patients' quality of life and treatment adherence.

Pilar E. Gauthier (Menominee Nation) is a graduate of Western Washington University with an M.S. in Mental Health Counseling. Her areas of interest include trauma-informed care, systemic oppression, retraditionalizing Native American family systems, and evaluating culturally appropriate and responsive case conceptualization, assessment, and treatment in mental health. As a Native American, she strives to further the development of Indigenous methodology and meaningful community-based research.

Julii M. Green is African American & Eastern Band Cherokee. She is an Assistant Professor at Alliant International University/CSPP in San Diego, CA. Her research interests are intimate partner violence and the impact on ethnically diverse families; Native American/Alaska Native/& Indigenous mental health and wellness; ethnicity and underage substance use; trauma and attachment; mixed methods research. Dr. Green was the 2012 recipient of the University of North Dakota's Allery Award for Native Research.

Lauren Hagemann is a PhD candidate in the clinical psychology program with health emphasis at Yeshiva University's Ferkauf Graduate School of Psychology in Bronx, New York. Her research interests include investigating how the structure and quality of social relationships impacts stress and health and associated health behaviors.

Jami L. Hirsch holds a Bachelor of Liberal Studies degree from the University of Missouri-St. Louis, where she focused her studies on combining the complementary fields of Psychology and English. She currently works as an Intake Specialist for Community Psychological Service, a nonprofit agency in the St. Louis area dedicated to bringing services to under-served populations. Her developing research interests include minority group access to, and experience of, mental health treatment in the United States.

Kimberly L. Howell is a doctoral candidate in depth psychology at Pacifica Graduate Institute. Her dissertation is entitled, *"Peek-A-Boo! I See You: Capturing The Stories and Images of Invisible Beauty in Los Angeles"* which addresses issues of body image and the effects of place on psyche and soma. Kimberly is an international speaker on issues related to feminism and somatic aesthetics and is a facilitator of therapeutic workshops geared toward helping build healthy levels of bodily self-acceptance.

Chun Nok Lam, MPH, is a research project manager at the University of Southern California in the Department of Emergency Medicine. He is involved in various research projects focusing on HIV, diabetes, healthcare utilization, Latino and Asian health and innovative mobile health technology. He has a special interest in Traditional Chinese Medicine and has conducted a study assessing the utilization of TCM among Chinese-Americans during his academic training.

Soh-Leong Lim, PhD (MFT), is an Associate Professor at San Diego State University in the Marriage and Family Therapy Program. Her research focuses on cross cultural issues in mental health. She is a Licensed Marriage and Family Therapist and an Approved Supervisor with the American Association for Marriage and Family Therapy (AAMFT).

Abbey Mann, M.S., is a PhD Student in community research and action with a certificate in women's and gender studies at Vanderbilt University. Her current research focus is on sexual minority wellbeing, and her interests include health disparities, stigma, social support, and access to health care. She completed her thesis on stigma towards children with emotional behaviors in August 2012.

Carlos Marquez is a third year doctoral student at Ferkauf Graduate School of Psychology. He has a masters in forensic psychology and is currently doing a concentration in neuropsychology and is an extern at Montefiore Hospital Neurology Department. His current research includes looking at cognitive and motor abilities in the geriatric population.

Rafael Martinez holds a Master of Arts degree in Cultural Anthropology and Master of Science and Doctor of Education degrees. Dr. Martinez is the Director of Education Programs and Undergraduate Psychology Program at Carlos Albizu University, Miami Campus. His professional interests include cultural studies, Afro-Caribbean syncretic religious systems, and higher education. He is a nationally recognized law enforcement training consultant in matters of ritualistic crimes and cult movements.

Gen Nakao, MSEd., is a second year doctoral student in clinical psychology at Yeshiva University's Ferkauf Graduate School of Psychology. His research interests include self-construal as the basis of cross-cultural psychology, qualitative study on multicultural counseling competence, and the interpersonal theory of psychotherapy. He is an international student scholar of Japan Student Services Organization (JASSO).

Wendy M. K. Peters is a Clinical Assistant Professor, faculty fellow, and member of the Native Health Research Team in the Center for Rural Health at the University of North Dakota School of Medicine & Health Sciences. Dr. Peters is Native Hawaiian and specializes in human and cultural development and multicultural adaptation. She is an inaugural fellow for the Council of National American Psychological Associations for the Advancement of Ethnic Minority Interests (CNAPAAEMI).

Sherry Pontious, PhD, RN, CRNA (Honorary), retired associate dean/ HSA chair and professor at College of Nursing and Health Sciences Florida International University.

Larry Purnell, PhD, RN, FAAN is Professor Emeritus at the University of Delaware. Dr. Purnell is the creator of the Purnell Model for Cultural Competence, which has been translated in multiple languages.

Natasha P. Ramanayake, M.A., is a doctoral student in the clinical psychology (health emphasis) program at Yeshiva University. She completed her master's work at Teachers College, Columbia University. Her current research involves understanding the role of ethnic identity in culturally homogenous societies, and understanding psychosocial risk factors for cardiovascular disease.

Laura Reid-Marks is a doctoral student in counseling psychology at Purdue University. She is originally from Kingston, Jamaica. Her research interests are broadly in the area of health disparities. More specifically, she is interested in the psychosocial factors that lead to mental and sexual health disparities.

Rocio Rosales Meza earned her PhD in Counseling Psychology from the University of Missouri-Columbia. She is currently an Assistant Professor at the University of La Verne in the Psychology Department. Her research focuses on Latina/o mental health and Latina/os in higher education. Dr. Rosales Meza is Mexican, bilingual in Spanish and English, and is the first generation in her family to be born in the United States.

Anthony F. Santoro, M.A., is a second year doctoral student in clinical psychology at Yeshiva University's Ferkauf Graduate School of Psychology. His interests include religiosity, spirituality, cultural differences, and the ways in which these variables interact with physical and mental health. He is a Leadership Education in Neurodevelopmental Disorders (LEND) Fellow at Albert Einstein College of Medicine.

Lamise Shawahin is a counseling psychology doctoral student at Purdue University. Her research interests focus primarily on multiculturalism and diversity issues, with an emphasis on the experiences of Muslim-Americans.

Sonia Suchday, Ph.D., Professor and Chair, Psychology Department, Pace University. Dr. Suchday is a Health Psychologist with research interests in globalization, immigration, acculturation,and stress and stress-related disorders.

Matthew J. Taylor is an associate professor of psychology at the University of Missouri-St. Louis. Holding a doctorate in clinical psychology, his research interests fall under the broad category of minority mental health and multicultural psychology. At the core of his work is describing how sociocultural themes impact the lives and mental health of minority individuals. During the last 15 years, he has written extensively and developed local, regional, national, and international projects focused on racial identity, substance use, and culturally competent therapeutic practices with minority populations.

Mario Tovar holds a PhD in Clinical Psychology from Walden University. He is an Associate Faculty of Anthropology at Ashford University, Adjunct Faculty of Psychology at The University of the Rockies, Adjunct Faculty at Everest University Online, and the Director of Psychological Services at the Rio Grande State Center in Harlingen, Texas. His research interests are folk medical practices, mind body interactions, the relationship between martial arts and physical and mental health, group dynamics in sports, and Mexican-American psychology.

Jesse N. Valdez PhD, Associate Professor and Professional Psychologist, Counseling Psychology Program, University of Denver. Licensed psychologist in Colorado PSY 1224 and California PSY 13824. Registrant #50600 National Register of Health Service Providers in Psychology. Clinical and research interests include bicultural/bilingual (English/Spanish) behavioral health psychology, mental health, and psychotherapy. Author of: Valdez, J. N. (2000). "Psychotherapy with Bicultural Hispanic Clients." *Psychotherapy: Theory, Research, Practice, Training,* 37, 240–246 and Valdez, J. N. (2006). "Stress." In J. Jackson (Ed.) *Encyclopedia of Multicultural Psychology* (pp. 445–450). Thousand Oaks, CA: Sage Publications.

Cheryl K. Webster is an alumna of Howard University, where she studied Classical Civilization and Biology; she also holds a Certificate of Specialization in Bio-Technology from St. Louis Community College through the Danforth Research Center (St. Louis, MO). Ms. Webster is currently an Applied Behavior Analysis (ABA) Child Behavior Therapist with the Missouri Special School District and is pursuing a PhD in clinical psychology. Her research interests are in the diagnoses and treatment of mental health issues in minority populations.

Benjamin Wendorf is a doctoral candidate and lecturer in the Department of Africology at the University of Wisconsin-Milwaukee. His primary research interests include societal and infrastructural constructs of the African Diaspora, Ghanaian post-independence history, and the history of infrastructure and trade routes. He is a recipient of the George W. and Winston A. Van Horne Prize for graduate students.

Index

acculturation, 5, 29, 31, 60, 62, 63, 75–76, 77, 80, 99, 118, 128, 157, 173, 180, 268; of African immigrants, 100–101; bilinear model of, 104–105; definition of, 103; as a factor in health disparities among immigrants, 54–56; and group dynamics, 108–109; and health risk behaviors among immigrants, 111–112; impact of on the family, 109–111; impact of on traditional versus modern mental health practices, 109–110, 116–117; models for the measurement of, 104–106, 249–250; specific identity measures of, 106; two dimensions of, 54–55; two-by-two acculturation matrix, 105. *See also* acculturative stress; Concordance Model for Acculturation (CMA)

acculturative stress, 53, 56, 57, 99, 106, 107, 111; in recent immigrants, 107

acupuncture, 152, 154, 197, 202, 203, 208, 213, 214, 215, 234; demand for in the United States, 209–210; the FDA's view of, 206–207; practice of in the United States, 207; use of by Asian Americans, 207–208

Africa, 55, 99, 228, 321; Central Africa, 101, 309, 311, 318, 324, 334; migration from, 100–101, 110, 112; and the origins of Vodou, 312–313;

sub-Saharan Africa, 323; West Africa, 100, 101, 334

African Americans, 22, 76, 100, 112, 127, 129, 141, 233, 310

African Diaspora, 333–334

African immigrants, 112, 115; number of African immigrants living in the United States, 101; overview of, 100–101; prevalence of mental health issues among, 115–116

Afro-Cuban Diaspora, 334

Agency for Healthcare Research and Quality, 19

Aguirre-Molina, H., 233

Ahmad, I., 57

Ahn, A. C., 208, 209

Alaska Natives (ANs). *See* Native Americans

alcohol consumption/abuse, 12, 19, 38, 62, 75, 115, 126, 205; among Asians, 112; among Native Americans, 174–175, 176, 177

Alegria, D., 235, 253

allopathic medicine, 152, 154, 157, 158, 164, 165, 206

altered states of consciousness (ASC), 132, 281, 288, 298; and shamanism, 282–283, 286–287, 290

alternative medicine, definition of, 283

American Indians (AIs). *See* Native Americans

Amish, the, 5–6